BRAINSTORMING

BRAINSTORMING

VIEWS AND INTERVIEWS ON THE MIND

Shaun Gallagher

ia

imprint-academic.com

Published in the UK by Imprint Academic
PO Box 200, Exeter EX5 5YX, UK

Published in the USA by Imprint Academic
Philosophy Documentation Center
PO Box 7147, Charlottesville, VA 22906-7147, USA

ISBN 9 781845 400231 (pbk)
ISBN 9 781845 401474 (hbk)

A CIP catalogue record for this book is available from the
British Library and US Library of Congress

Contents

In memory of

Jacques Paillard and Francisco Varela

Chapter One

Introduction

I did not write this book, I constructed it. And in regard to its content, let me admit at the beginning that in this book I beg, borrow, and steal (well maybe not steal, since I have observed copyrights) as much wisdom as I can from some of the best minds of our time. These are people who think about brains and minds professionally. Although this is a book about the philosophy of mind, it is also interdisciplinary, so I have made use not only of philosophers, but also of psychologists, neuropsychologists and neuroscientists, people who have gained their understanding of how brain and behavior and mental experience go together through experimentation. I've borrowed from people in person — in a series of interviews, many of which have been published in the *Journal of Consciousness Studies*. I've borrowed by means of e-mail exchanges that I've had with numerous people over the past several years. And of course, I've borrowed from books.

This book includes interviews, but is not strictly a collection of interviews. I have mixed in explanations and descriptions that are meant to clarify and explicate the issues under discussion. More specifically, this book is intended to be an unorthodox but very accessible introduction to certain themes that cut across the philosophy of mind and psychology. This might rightfully seem a contradiction. An introduction to a certain subject matter is supposed to be orthodox, if nothing else. That is, if one intends to introduce someone to a subject matter, one normally intends to review the established and received views that define the field. So in what sense can this be at the same time an introduction and unorthodox? Well first, the genre of this book is not standard for introductory textbooks since it consists in large parts of interviews rather than straight explanatory discourses. In addition, I can honestly say that there was no preconceived plan to the book, although this does not mean that a plan did not emerge in its construction. The topics and themes that we cover have emerged from the interviews themselves. But this is also why this can be considered an introductory text. The interview style, I believe, makes the various topics and themes very accessible, in the way that conversation tends to be more accessible than formal lecture. And as in a conversation, topics tend to emerge on their own and can be deeply engaging. Furthermore, the fact that these are the topics that emerged in conversations with some of the most important researchers in the field means that we will be exploring views that are close to the cutting edge of contemporary philosophy and science. So what we find expressed here are not so much the received and established views but a set of ongoing questions and discussions that define the field. If these are the issues that the leading researchers are concerned about and find exciting, it seems appropriate to think that these are the most appropriate issues to begin with, and that these are the issues that beginning students, or even experts who are approaching these topics from different fields, might find the most interesting.

As I begin to construct this book I'm sitting at a very large desk in my office. On the desk is my computer, and in my computer I have stored in electronic form hundreds of relevant papers, interviews, e-mails, and some of my own thoughts as I have recorded them. I also have lined up on my desktop (the actual one rather than the virtual one) a large number of books. Books that I consider some of the best written on the topic of the mind. When I say that they are the best, I don't mean that all of the ideas they contain are true or that all of the theories they propound are correct. In fact, amongst all of these papers and books, on my estimate, there are thousands of contradictions — so they couldn't all be right. Some of these works are scientifically outdated. Actually that is a rather easy claim to make since the practice in science seems to be to exclude references published more than five years ago. Philosophers have a different practice, going perhaps to the other extreme. In any case, as a philosopher I have no problem keeping Aristotle's *De Anima* (350 BCE) on my desk next to Marc Jeannerod's *The Cognitive Neuroscience of Action* (1997). Gilbert Ryle's *The Concept of Mind* (1949) is uncomfortably sandwiched between Descartes' *Meditations* (1641) and Daniel Dennett's *Consciousness Explained* (1991). Patricia Churchland's *Neurophilosophy* (1986) is lying there orthogonal to Edmund Husserl's *Lectures on Internal Time Consciousness* (1928), which is piled on top of Davidson's *Essays on Actions and Events* (2001). And Gerald Edelman's *Bright Air, Brilliant Fire* (1993) is leaning lightly against Merleau-Ponty's *Phenomenology of Perception* (1945).

Someone familiar with the contents of these various works might complain that I keep a very messy desk — perhaps both physically and metaphysically. They might question the mind that puts one or two materialist Churchlands (Patricia and Paul) next to a transcendental Husserl, for example, or that keeps Descartes so close to Dennett, and mixes empirical science with pure philosophy. But all of these thinkers (and I haven't mentioned the ones on the bookcases that surround me, or the ones on my list of books still to read) have something important, or at least something interesting, to say about the mind.

I've given myself license in this introduction (to be quickly revoked for the rest of the book) to be polemic – for just a minute. I want to point out that there have been many false barriers erected, many silly lines drawn across the last century of philosophy. For example, the so-called analytic-continental divide, which often prevents philosophers who cite Davidson, Dennett or the Churchlands from citing Husserl or Merleau-Ponty. There may be reasoned and productive disagreements between these groups of thinkers, but to discover them and to move beyond them, if that is possible, one must at least consider them together. The discipline called philosophy of mind has traditionally been associated with analytic philosophy in the 20th century. In this book I will not hesitate to redefine the philosophy of mind to include some of the continental phenomenologists – Husserl, Merleau-Ponty, and even more contemporary thinkers in this tradition – when it makes sense to do so.

I think there is another, slightly older divide that needs to be closed if we are to move forward in our understanding of the mind. This is the overly simplified division between philosophy and empirical science. Prior to the 20th century, philosophy by its very nature was trans-disciplinary. It was practiced as such by people like Descartes, Newton, and Locke in the 17th century. They were thinkers who were philosophers and scientists at the same time. Even through the 18th and the late 19th centuries the lines were not clearly drawn between philosophy and psychology, philosophy and economics, philosophy and physics. Indeed, scientific experimentation was still called 'natural philosophy'. Things started to come apart when universities started to make their curricula more cohesively specialized, when the natural and then social-behavioral sciences started to divide into their own departments. The divide that separates philosophy from these sciences is reflected in the 19th century positivist movement, but it has certainly characterized most of the 20th century. There were always some philosophers, however, who stayed close to the psychological sciences. William James was a good example at the end of 19th century; Maurice Merleau-Ponty stayed the course around the mid-20th century; and in regard to cognitive science, and the more recent neurosciences, Daniel Dennett and Patricia Churchland provide good examples of a growing number of philosophers who carry on that more original 17th-century conception of philosophy. In this book I suggest that we think of philosophy in that very wide and comprehensive sense, going back, even to ancient times, to its original meaning as an all-encompassing term for the pursuit of knowledge.

For those philosophers who are paying attention to the empirical sciences of psychology and cognitive neuroscience, and to the ongoing work on artificial intelligence and robotics, it becomes easier to span the two aforementioned divides with one bridge. Researchers in both the European tradition of phenomenological philosophy and the analytic philosophy of mind are today working together with scientists, and are considering the implications of empirical studies for addressing philosophical issues. In doing so they naturally meet up at the frontier of empirical science. This convergence of science, phenomenology, and philosophy of mind turns out to be a fruitful and refreshing approach that exemplifies in a specific way what Owen Flanagan and others call a method of 'triangulation' (e.g., Flanagan 1992). The idea is that to understand something as complicated as the nature of the mind *or* the brain (where the 'or' is still in question), one needs to exploit many different disciplines and to find a coherent way to integrate the results of these different kinds of studies. This is the approach we want to pursue here.

The interviews

A further introductory word about the title, *Brainstorming*. There is an intended echo of Daniel Dennett's book entitled *Brainstorms*, and I intend it as a bit of homage to him. Although I disagree with him in multiple ways, I think Dennett has done more than anyone to move philosophy of mind in the empirical direction. His thinking is both challenging and accessible — an excellent model for everyone who aspires to this particular genre of philosophy. I should note, however, that the original inspiration for *Brainstorming* was a series of interviews I did with neuroscientists and neuropsychologists, which naturally focused on how our understanding of the brain can contribute to solving philosophical problems about the mind. In those interviews I was brainstorming in every sense of the word. It seems appropriate, therefore, to introduce my fellow brainstormers, the scientists I interviewed and who contribute to this book with those interviews.

Michael Arbib was born in England, grew up in Australia, and studied at MIT where he received his Ph.D. in Mathematics in 1963. He helped found the Department of Computer and Information Science and the Center for Systems Neuroscience, the Cognitive Science Program, and the Laboratory for Perceptual Robotics at the University of Massachusetts at Amherst. Today he is Fletcher Jones Professor of Computer Science, a Professor of Neuroscience and the Director of the University of Southern California Brain Project at the University of Southern California. The title of his first book, *Brains, Machines and Mathematics* (1964, 1987 second edition), gives a good indication of his scientific interests. For all his extensive research in these areas, however, Arbib has not ignored philosophical, social, and even theological topics (Arbib 1985a; Arbib and Hesse 1986). He was one of the original founders of the Society for Neuroscience where his membership number is 007. This, he says, gives him a license to think.

Jonathan Cole is, amongst other things, a clinical neurophysiologist practicing at Poole Hospital in Bournemouth, England, an author of extraordinarily interesting books, and an experimental neuroscientist who conducts his experiments in many of the major laboratories in Europe and North America, and at least once while floating weightless in mid-air some 40,000 feet above earth. In all of these endeavors, Cole is an explorer of human experience in its many variations, and most often at the frontiers or extremes of such experiences. In his first book, *Pride and the Daily Marathon* (1995) Cole presented the neurology and the phenomenology of an extreme and unusual condition of deafferentation in his patient and friend, Ian Waterman. Cole's other books, *About Face* (1998) and *Still Lives* (2004), explore, respectively, the personal and social difficulties faced by people who live with facial pathologies and those who suffer from spinal cord injury. These encounters with extraordinary people have put Cole in a unique position to glimpse the significance of those things that form part of our everyday and ordinary lives, but that we take for granted and hardly ever notice.

Christopher Frith is emeritus research professor at the Functional Imaging Laboratory of the Wellcome Department of Imaging Neuroscience at University College, London, and now Research Professor at Aarhus University in Denmark. He explores, experimentally, using the techniques of functional brain imaging, the relationship between human consciousness and the brain. His research focuses on questions pertaining to perception, attention, control of action, free will, and awareness of our own mental states and those of others. Frith investigates brain systems involved in the choice of one action over another and in the understanding of other people. Some of his investigations are aimed at understanding the brain basis of schizophrenia. In his widely cited study, *The Cognitive Neuropsychology of Schizophrenia* (1992), Frith argues that many of the positive symptoms of schizophrenia, such as delusions of control, auditory hallucinations, and thought insertion, involve problems of self-monitoring. Patients, in effect, lose track of their own intentions and mistakenly attribute agency for their own actions to someone else. His most recent book is *Making Up the Mind: How the Brain Creates our Mental World* (2007)

Michael Gazzaniga is a professor of psychology at the University of California, Santa Barbara, and head of the SAGE Center for the Study of the Mind. As a graduate student he worked with Roger Sperry on human split-brain research, and he continued work on brain lateralization. Gazzaniga is the author of *The Social Brain* (1995), and most recently *The Ethical Brain* (2005). He has also edited multiple editions of the comprehensive reference work, *The Cognitive Neurosciences*. He recently participated in the public television special *The Brain and The Mind*, to make our growing knowledge about the brain more generally accessible to the public. He is Editor-in-Chief of the *Journal of Cognitive Neuroscience*, and a member of the US President's Council on Bioethics.

Marc Jeannerod is former director of the Institut des Sciences Cognitives in Lyon. His work in neuropsychology focuses on motor action. Experimental studies conducted by Jeannerod and his colleagues at Lyon have explored the details of brain activity, not only as we are actively moving, but as we plan to move, as we imagine moving, and as we observe others move. His work also captures important distinctions between pathological and non-pathological experience. In *The Cognitive Neuroscience of Action* (1997) Jeannerod focused on object-oriented actions. At the very end of that book he raises questions that seem quite different. How is it possible to understand the intentions of others? Precisely what mechanisms allow us to imitate other people's actions? In more recent years much of Jeannerod's work has been in pursuit of these questions about interaction with others, and he has helped to show that there are intimate connections between moving ourselves and understanding others. His most recent book is *Ways of Seeing: The Scope and Limits of Visual Cognition* (2003) with the philosopher Pierre Jacobs.

Anthony Marcel is a psychologist who has worked most of his professional life at the Medical Research Council's Cognition and Brain Sciences Unit in Cambridge. He currently conducts his research at Cambridge University's Experimental Psychology Department, and teaches at the University of Hertfordshire, just north of London. In the 1980s, he conducted several famous experiments on subliminal priming which contributed to developing a theory of nonconscious perception. Much of his work focuses on the study of brain damage and such conditions as Blindsight, Neglect, and Agnosognosia. Most recently, with John Lambie he has been working on a theory of emotion. Tony also is an actor who spends his summers doing Shakespeare and such in and around England.

Jacques Paillard (1920–2006), was a well-known scientist who studied the psychophysiology of the motor system. His focus on the motor system prompted Marc Jeannerod to all him a 'man of action' at a memorial in honor of his work in 2007 in Paris. He was Professor Emeritus at the University of Aix-Marseille, and headed the neurobiology laboratory at the National Center for Scientific Research (CNRS). Paillard also did research at the Université de Laval in Quebec where he worked with GL, a woman who, like Jonathan Cole's patient Ian Waterman, lacks a sense of body position (having no proprioception or sense of touch from the chin down). Paillard's work lives on through his webpage at http://jacquespaillard. apinc.org/, where you can find his papers.

Jaak Panksepp is the Distinguished Research Professor Emeritus of Psychobiology at Bowling Green State University in Kentucky. His Ph.D. from the University of Massachusetts in Amherst is in physiological psychology, and he did postdocs in at the University of Sussex and the Worcester Foundation in Massachusetts. He is the author of over 200 scientific articles and the book *Affective Neuroscience: The Foundations of Human and Animal Emotions* (1998). He earned the NIMH Research Scientist Development Award for his work in hypothalamic mechanisms of energy balance. In his current research he investigates social bonding and emotion, play and pleasure mechanisms of the brain. He also works as a psychiatrist at the Medical College of Ohio, Toledo and focuses on childhood disorders. He edits a book series, *Advances in Biological Psychiatry*, and he is a director of the Memorial Foundation for Lost Children, founded to help parents and children with neuropsychiatric disorders.

Francisco Varela (1946–2001) was a neurobiologist and philosopher who was born in Chile and studied with Humberto Maturana, with whom he developed the concept of autopoiesis, an important biological principle. He completed his Ph.D. at Harvard and went, eventually, to live and work in Paris. His research in biology and in the cognitive neurosciences has been extremely influential for a number of disciplines. In addition he was good friends with the Dalai Lama, with whom he helped to found the *Mind and Life* Institute. Francisco recognized the importance of first-person methods for studying consciousness, including approaches based on Buddhist meditation and European phenomenology (see especially his book with Evan Thompson and Eleanor Rosch, *The Embodied Mind*, 1991). Although I did not conduct a formal interview with Francisco, I enjoyed numerous conversations with him over several years. Based on my recollections from those conversations and a variety of published interviews, the segments of 'interview' with Francisco presented here are constructions which I believe to be faithful to his own views.

I've met and discussed related issues with a number of other people on my travels and with whom I had wanted to do formal interviews. But due to limitations imposed by space, time and physical bodies, I was unable to arrange the meetings. These include Alain Berthoz, Jean-Pierre Changeaux, Edmund Rolls, and Sandra Witelson. If their interviews are absent from this book, their views do not go unrepresented. Furthermore, I've drawn on a number of interviews that others have conducted as a way to round out some of the ideas presented here. Finally, Chapter 3 contains what one might call two quasi-interviews. In effect, I've constructed interviews out of some written texts that are in some ways like interviews —a Platonic dialogue, and some philosophical correspondence between Descartes and a number of thinkers. These quasi-interviews set the broad stage on which contemporary questions about the mind and the brain continue to be asked.

How to Study the Mind

The philosophy of mind, as a distinct sub-discipline of philosophy, had its start in the 1940s in the writings of the Oxford philosopher Gilbert Ryle. In a wider sense, signaled by Ryle himself, the philosophy of mind goes back to the 17th century, and especially to the writings of Descartes. If, for Descartes, the mind was beyond doubt, there are plenty of doubts about the mind to be found in 20th-century philosophy of mind, including doubts about whether there is such a thing as 'the mind'. In Ryle's book, entitled *The Concept of Mind*, we find the challenging thought that what Descartes called the mind, the mental substance, may not exist in any real sense. The referent of the concept of mind may be something quite different — perhaps a kind of mental behavior or a set of activities against which any story about mental substance amounts to a fiction.

On the other side of the English Channel, in Paris, around the same time that Ryle was writing his book, phenomenologists were digging into the deep structures of consciousness. They seemed to have no doubt that the mind was something that could be investigated philosophically. In 1960, when analytic philosophy of mind was characterized by methods that involved conceptual and linguistic analysis, and computational modeling, phenomenology continued to employ methods that depended on close description of experience. Although both approaches focused on questions about the mind, consciousness, the self, and the various features of mental life, there seemed to be little connection between phenomenological schools on the European continent and the philosophers of mind in Oxford or their cousins at the Cambridges (England and Massachusetts).

In 1960, however, there was a gathering of philosophers at Royaumont, an abbey outside of Paris, with the expressed intention of discussing just these issues. Present were Gilbert Ryle and another philosopher from Oxford, A. J. Ayer. W. V. O. Quine from Harvard rounded out the team of analytic philosophers of mind. The phenomenologists were represented by Maurice Merleau-Ponty, a French phenomenologist also trained in psychology, and H. L. Van Breda who was a scholar of Husserl's philosophy (and founder of the Husserl Archives in Leuven). Following a talk by Ryle, Ayer suggested that there was some justification for the kind of phenomenological project that Husserl and his followers engaged in. And this was followed up by Merleau-Ponty.[1]

> **Ayer:** [I]t seems to me … that one can legitimately pose some question about the whole ensemble of processes, of manners of being, of actions, of sensations, or of impressions that one cannot consider as objects — let us say — memory; in what does memory consist? Is it essential to reserve this notion to designate only those experiences that are our own? … And it is not impossible that this is the genre of research that certain disciples of Husserl recommend, in which case their curiosity seems to me perfectly legitimate.

> **Merleau-Ponty:** I have also had the impression, while listening to Mr. Ryle, that what he was saying was not so strange to us [phenomenologists], and that the distance, if there is a distance, is one that he puts between us rather than one I find there.

The phenomenological approach involves the development of a reflective description of one's own experience in order to discover how conscious processes relate to the world — a relation that Husserl, following Brentano, called 'intentionality'. Phenomenology begins with a description of one's own experience, but it also goes on to develop a conceptual analysis of what it finds in experience. It was this kind of analysis that Merleau-Ponty found familiar in Ryle's work, even if Ryle's method was more keyed to the analysis of how we talk about the mind.

Ryle, however, resisted the idea that his analysis was anything close to phenomenology. He also resisted suggestions made by Quine who proposed a naturalized epistemology, that is, an approach where most of the philosophical work would be done by sciences like psychology. Ryle seemingly rejected any contribution from science, which he calls the 'research of fact', and which he characterizes, and perhaps caricatures by the example of chemists working with test tubes.

> **Ryle:** See here what comes to my mind when speaking of research of fact. Nothing very mysterious, as you see. But what matters is that the questions of fact of this order are not the province of philosophy. One will never say that so and so is a better philosopher than so and so because so and so knows facts of which the other is ignorant.

This short conversation captures the methodological state of affairs that dominated 20th-century thought about the mind. The question we want to ask here is: How have things changed? The answer, I propose, is that there has been significant change in regard to how methodologies relate to one another.

---

1   The following brief exchange is found in Merleau-Ponty 1996, 59–72.

Neurophilosophy, heterophenomenology, neurophenomenology

First, in the eyes of most philosophers of mind, Quine has won the debate, at least in the sense that most philosophers of mind today are seeking to naturalize consciousness and mental processes, that is, to show how the mind is caused by, or emerges from or is identical to brain processes that are best explained by science, and sometimes a science dominated by computational models. Patricia Churchland, for example, has developed a 'neurophilosophy', which follows the path of eliminative materialism, the idea that explanations of mental processes are reducible to explanations of brain processes. So, for her, 'philosophy at its best and properly conceived is continuous with the empirical sciences' (1986, 2). Daniel Dennett, who studied with both Quine and Ryle, pursues a similar route and champions the importance of empirical science for understanding the mind. For Dennett, computational science still holds great promise for understanding mental processes.

> **Dennett:** If you go back 200 or 300 years, you'll see that there was one family of phenomena that people just had no clue about how it could possibly be, and those are mental phenomena. It's the very idea of thinking, and perception, and dreaming and sensing—and we didn't have any model for how that was done physically at all. Descartes and Leibniz, great scientists in their own right, simply drew a blank when it came to figuring these things out. And it's only really with the computational ideas that we now have some clear and manageable ideas about what could possibly be going on. We don't have the right story yet, but we have some good ideas. At least one can now see how the job can be done. And I think this is a breakthrough, one of the great breakthroughs in the area of human understanding. And that is, coming to understand our own understanding, to see what kind of parts it can be made of. If you compare it just with life itself, or reproduction and growth, those were deeply mysterious processes a hundred years ago, and forever before then. Now we have a really a pretty clear idea about how it's possible for things to reproduce, how it's possible for them to grow, to repair themselves, to fuel themselves, to have a metabolism—all of these otherwise stunningly mysterious phenomena are falling into place, and when you look at them you see that at the very fundamental level they are basically computational. ... What governs those effects is the software level, the algorithmic level. If you want to understand how ... orderly cognition takes place, you need to have this high-level understanding of how these billions or trillions of pieces [neuronal cells] interact with each other. ... There is nothing magical about a

computer. ... It's good old push-pull traditional material causation. (Brockman 2001).

Dennett, however, as well as Churchland and many other analytic philosophers of mind, keep their distance from phenomenology. Dennett, for example, provides a short history of his relation to phenomenology.

> **Dennett:** I studied Husserl and the other Phenomenologists with Dag Føllesdal at Harvard as an undergraduate, and learned a lot. My career-long concentration on intentionality had its beginnings as much to do with Husserl as with Quine. But part of what I thought I learned from those early encounters is that reading the self-styled Husserlians was largely a waste of time; they were deeply into obscurantism for its own sake. I may have picked this attitude up from my graduate advisor, Gilbert Ryle, who was himself a masterful scholar of Husserl and Phenomenology. In any case, when we discussed my own work on intentionality he certainly didn't encourage me to follow him in attempting to plumb the depths of the Continental Husserlians. (Dennett 1994).

Dennett goes on to tell of the poor reception he received in Paris and Nice where he was invited to give some lectures.

> **Dennett:** The French Husserlians either were aghast or found me beneath notice, in spite of my attempt to convey my sense of my Husserlian heritage.

In some sense, despite what seems to be Dennett's wholesale rejection of phenomenology, he does take it seriously (see Roy 2007). And he says so, mentioning the work of a contemporary Husserlian phenomenologist, Eduard Marbach.

> **Dennett:** I take very seriously Eduard Marbach's recent and forthcoming attempts to build a bridge between my heterophenomenology and (his refreshingly clear version of) Husserl's autophenomenology (Dennett 1994).

Dennett's 'heterophenomenology' is not phenomenology understood in the Husserlian tradition (which Dennett calls autophenomenology), but an attempt to incorporate first-person reports about experience (reports generated especially in experimental settings) into scientific investigations. The heterophenomenologist integrates the subject's self-reports with other more objective evidence from empirical science. The goal is to use first-person data (that is, reports generated by the subject about her experience) to understand the subject's experience, but without taking those reports as veridical. There is much about our own experience that we don't understand, and, in contrast to claims made by Descartes, we can be wrong about our own mind. Since we are not authoritative about out own experience, a healthy skepticism about first-person reports is necessary.

> **Dennett:** The total set of details of heterophenomenology, plus all the data we can gather about concurrent events in the brains of subjects and in the surrounding environment, comprise the total data set for a theory of human consciousness. It leaves out no objective phenomena and no subjective phenomena of consciousness. (2003, 11).

On the other side, phenomenologists, or those inspired by the work of phenomenologists like Merleau-Ponty, have also been turning their attention to the sciences and have been working with some of those empirical scientists who on their part are open to the ideas of philosophers (see Gallagher and Zahavi 2008 for an introductory account). Francisco Varela is a good example of a scientist who found phenomenology essential for an understanding of the mind. In an interview with Claus Otto Scharmer in 1996 Varela expressed this view.

> **Varela:** I maintain that there is an irreducible core to the quality of experience that needs to be explored with a method. In other words, the problem is not that we don't know enough about the brain or about biology, the problem is that we don't know enough about experience. ... We have had a blind spot in the West for that kind of methodical approach, which I would now describe as a more straightforward phenomenological method. ... Everybody thinks they know about experience, I claim we don't. (Scharmer 2000).

The method Varela has in mind is phenomenology, but not phenomenology alone. In my own conversations with him, he expressed this very clearly.[2]

> **SG:** You want to integrate phenomenology with science, and specifically, cognitive neuroscience, but in a different way from Dennett's heterophenomenology.

> **Varela:** You know about Husserl and Merleau-Ponty's work on perception and action. It goes back to Husserl's lectures on *Thing and Space* where he shows that perception always involves motor kinaesthesia. Well this, which is a real precision in phenomenological description, is clearly confirmed by contemporary neuroscience. One can't reach this kind of correlation by a pure external, third-person analysis, as you find in someone like Dennett, and more generally in

---

2   Over the four or five years that I knew and worked with Francisco we had many conversations about neurophenomenological approaches to consciousness. The following (and similar interchanges in later chapters) is a reconstruction based on my recollections of conversations with him, and a compilation of conversations and interviews that others had with Francisco. They include bits and pieces of my conversations with Francisco and interviews/conversations by Benvenuto (2001); Brockman 1995; Davis (1994); Haywood and Varela (1992); Mulder 2000; Scharmer (2000); and Walker (2000).

analytic philosophy. Phenomenologists take a methodological first-person approach in their search for the structures of consciousness, and such structures are open to confirmation by third-person cognitive neuroscience. Both first-person and third-person are necessary and need to be integrated.

This combination is what Varela (1996) called 'neurophenomenology', and it differs from Dennett's heterophenomenology in that it takes a different attitude toward first-person reports. If Dennett starts with first-person reports, he remains skeptical about their validity, and very quickly attempts to transform them into neutralized data — texts to be interpreted in the light of third-person measurements. Moreover, the original first-person reports are not guided by phenomenological method; they are the product of naïve introspection, informed at best by folk psychology. Varela, in his interview with Scharmer (2000), indicates the problem with this sort of data.

> **Varela:** It is totally mainstream in psychology or in cognitive science to have experiments where you ask people, Did you see this? Did you see that? Were you aware of this? This is the classical technical verbal report, which is used widely. … However … it doesn't do justice to the richness and complexity of what is experienced. The verbal report requires somebody there who says, 'Yeah, I saw it,' so there is some kind of access to experience. But it remains extremely impressionistic. [It] needs to be developed further. … One key thing: disciplined regular training. Without really specific regular training, like everything else in human affairs, you stay a beginner.

Phenomenological practice consists of a methodically, intersubjectively guided reflection on how the world appears to the conscious subject. This kind of approach becomes a full-fledged neurophenomenology when the phenomenological method is integrated into experiments that involve correlating mental experience with brain processes (see Lutz et al. 2002). The fact that phenomenology is not a method that is confined to first-person subjectivity is important. Varela notes that this method is intersubjective, and involves the second person.

> **Varela:** So this is a very important antidote to the myth or the belief or the dogma that anything that has to do with introspection or meditation or phenomenological work is something that people do in their little corners. That really is a mistaken angle on the whole thing. Although there are some reasons that it is a very common mistake. This is perhaps the greatest difficulty within science. The first reaction people have is that [first-person experience is] just a personal thing. That it's private. But the notion that the first person is private is a disaster. The first-person access is as public as the third person,

okay? When you have a third-person point of view, clearly you need a first person who does the measurement and does the writing, etc., but [provides] a social network to which it is going to be addressed. So a key point is that it's really not very meaningful to speak about consciousness or experiences being private. There is a quality to experience where you need a mode of access that you might want to call the first-person access. That doesn't make it private. It's just as social as everything else. And that's something it took me a long time to discover. I had a blind spot on that like everybody else.

The distance between Varela and Dennett is even clearer concerning the status of computational models. Varela's phenomenological turn was at the same time a turn away from computationalism, and a turn toward embodied cognitive science. He explains this in his interview with C. Walker (2000, 2).

Walker: will you describe how cognitive science evolved from its view of the mind as an information processing system to its view of the mind as a system of embodiment?

Varela: The discipline of the study of the human mind—cognitive science—was born after WW II. At that time, the dominant tradition in the West held that the human mind and its processes had to do with logic, with being, as Descartes would say, 'clear and distinct'. This tradition, from Descartes through the entire rationalist tradition—which is very strong in the Anglo-Saxon world—led early cognitive scientists to ask: How can we understand clear ideas chaining into one another to produce very coherent principles? At roughly the same time, the computer was invented. The principle of a computer's logical 'symbol manipulation' was just perfect—it seemed the perfect way of couching what the human mind was all about. Such was the origin of cognitive science, and it became known as the cognitive tradition. People picked it all up very intuitively. Remember how people used to say the mind was a computer? That the mind was software and the body was hardware? Ridiculous. The problem is that such a view was in fact intuitive within the context of its moment in the history of the West. … As people looked into cognitive neuroscience, they found that neither perception nor movement nor memory nor emotion could be addressed on a basis of logic. People were attempting to corner the human mind with basic principles of reasoning and categorization, which are, of course, rather poor. So people began to re-evaluate what had been done and began to tilt the balance more and more toward 'embodied cognitive science', as it is now called.

Embodied cognitive science has been called the third wave in cognitive science, following the early emphasis on computationalism, and then a second wave motivated by the exciting work in neuroscience especially in the 1990s. Varela, who was trained as a biologist and who together with Humberto Maturana explicated the important biological principle of autopoiesis, suggested that the implications of a situated embodied understanding even reaches to our understanding of life itself, in strict counterpoint to Dennett's claim that life is computational.

> **Varela:** In fact, with genetic engineering we can see the exact same conceptual tension that we saw with early cognitivism. Cognitive science saw the mind as a collection of programs and symbol manipulations, just as genetic engineers see life as a collection of genes ready for programming and arranging. All life has come to be seen as programs that can be adjusted and conditioned to whatever we imagine we need. Now we're beginning to learn — in parallel, as it so happens with the embodied mind — that life is wholly embodied. The principle of life is not in its genetic components and building blocks but the entire situatedness of an organism. (Walker 2000, 2).

Triangulation and a plurality of methods

What emerges then in these various concerns about how one goes about studying the mind is the present situation where philosophers of mind, empirical scientists, and phenomenologists are all talking with each other and starting to see value in a process that has been called 'triangulation'.[3] The realization is that the complexity of the mind-brain is so great that no one discipline can capture it all. One has to pool a diverse set of methods in order to capture all aspects of mental experience. (see Figure 2.1)

We find confirmation of this strategy of reaching out to different disciplines in the work of two leading cognitive scientists, Michael Arbib, originally a mathematician who then took his mathematical talents into the areas of cognitive computational neuroscience, and Jaak Panksepp, a leading proponent of affective neuroscience. In an interview with Michael Arbib I asked him how he approaches the relations between empirical science and the more philosophical, less empirical approaches to the mind.

---

3   Owen Flanagan uses this term to describe what he calls the 'natural method'. 'I propose that we try the most natural strategy, what I call the natural method, to see if it can be made to work. Tactically, what I have in mind is this. Start by treating three different lines of analysis with equal respect. Give phenomenology its due. Listen carefully to what individuals have to say about how things seem. Also, let the psychologists and cognitive scientists have their say. Listen carefully to their descriptions about how mental life works and what jobs consciousness has, if any, in its overall economy. Finally, listen carefully to what the neuroscientists say about how conscious mental events of different sorts are realized, and examine the fit between their stories and the phenomenological and psychological stories.' (Flanagan 1992, 11)

Philosophical
Conceptual
Analysis   Experimental
                                            Science

Phenomenological
Description and Clarification

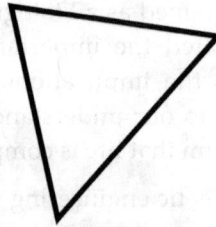

Figure 2.1 Triangulation

Is this a two-way street — should philosophical concerns also guide empirical research? He framed his answer by describing his own work and how he came to an appreciation of philosophy.

Arbib: Detailed study of animal brains is now augmented by the use of brain imaging to look at what big chunks of brain are doing in ways that can be linked to human experience. To aid the building of these new bridges between cognitive phenomena and the detailed study of neural networks I've worked on something called Synthetic PET, which is basically using models inspired by, for example, the detailed circuitry of the monkey to predict what might be seen in imaging of a human brain (Arbib, Fagg and Grafton 2003). I am particularly concerned to use such studies to begin to fill in the gaps in the evolutionary theory of brain mechanisms of language.

But this is a linkage between psychology and neuroscience rather than philosophy. ... I think the turning point for me philosophically was when I was teaching at Stanford in the late 1960s. David Armstrong, a great Australian philosopher of mind (see, e.g., Armstrong 1968), came for a sabbatical and I decided to sit in on his course, which was based on Ryle's *Concept of Mind*. But we only got through two chapters of the book during the whole quarter! David's style was to encourage reflection rather than deliver facts, and I ended up writing far more of what I was thinking as he was speaking than of what he actually said. This helped me begin to become somewhat more articulate about philosophy of mind. I had a joke about 'brainless philosophers of mind' who somehow imagined that you could talk about the mind without knowing about the brain. Today, 35 or so years later, there is a real dialogue between brain and mind researchers but that was not the case back then as I tried to get myself into a position where I could learn from the conceptual issues raised by the philosophers while making my own brain-based contribution to philosophy of mind.

A few years later, I was invited to be a discussant for an American Philosophical Association workshop to discuss what I think was Dan Dennett's first book, *Content and Consciousness*. This provided an occasion to get into an interesting discussion with a philosopher who was very sympathetic to the need to understand the brain and to try and see what the issues were (Arbib 1972, Dennett 1971). In this way, I was actively engaged in the transition from philosophy of mind as a purely abstract exercise to a philosophy of mind integrated with cognitive science and cognitive neuroscience. The effort to understand the network of interactions between what seems to us the reality of the person on the one hand and the reality of the lab bench on the other remains very much a driving force.

Jaak Panksepp captures the possibilities and the limitations introduced when theorists attempt to combine various philosophical and scientific approaches. He draws a middle course between those represented by Dennett and Varela, since he thinks both a computational approach to cortical-cognitive systems, and a dynamic systems approach to sub-cortical-affective systems are necessary. I asked him about recent experiments that he was excited about, and about how one might apply the kind of basic research he was doing.

Panksepp: Well, the experiments that really excite me are connecting some of the basic neuroscience, which can only be done in animal models, to human psychiatric issues. We are interested in the neurochemistries that mediate human anger, sadness, joy, and various desires. We now know some of the underlying neuropeptide circuits that seem to mediate specific affective states. ... The role of many emotion-modifying neuropeptides discovered in animals now desperately needs to be characterized affectively as well as cognitively in humans. Many are already relatively low-hanging fruit for the development of mediations for specific psychiatric symptoms albeit not conceptual syndromes. A symptom-based psychiatry, based one emotional endophenotypes, is one goal of my vision for affective neuroscience (Panksepp 2006).

Also, we need to go in the opposite direction, probing the molecular changes that arise from emotional experiences. Might we one day be able to monitor emotional changes by following changing neurochemical patterns? When animals go into primal emotional states, many changes are transpiring in the brain. Another critically important thing to decipher at the organic chemical level is the gene expression patterns that are modified by experience. As animals play joyously, might we be able to identify new play instigating molecules ('luderons') and neural pathways for happiness?

SG: And such progress can only come through research and experimentation?

Panksepp: Yes, but sometimes it can come out of serendipity. The medications of the first generation of biological psychiatry were all discovered by chance. Our current work is mainly research with a therapeutic eye; it's basic science with, hopefully, a practical end-point. For a while my bias had been to select research questions that I envision to have some kind of a useful endpoint. Unfortunately, most research in this area has little consequence for clinical practice. I spent a good part of my research career doing electrical recordings from the brain. None of that connected up with clinical practice. So now I am more committed to neurochemical approaches. I think basic emotional systems are organized much more in terms of distinct neurochemical profiles than easily demonstrable neurophysiological profiles.

SG: If one methodology, like the use of EEG, or brain imaging is not adequate, is the solution to use a number of different disciplines or perspectives to put together the complete picture?

Panksepp: Surely. I would say understanding in this area must use a triangulation strategy; a combination of (i) *brain* measures and manipulations, careful (ii) *behavioral* and (iii) *psychological-mental* analyses. In my estimation, neurochemical analyses will be the most likely to yield the most practically useful knowledge — especially if we concurrently pay attention to cultural/ecological issues. But we must remember that science only clarifies functional *parts* of a complex phenomenon. Other disciplines, from art to philosophy, are needed to reconstruct an image of the whole. ...

SG: So then is it possible to be led astray if we focus too narrowly on one methodology or one model? For example, have we misunderstood cognition by staying too close to the computational model? I think I know how you would respond to this. You suggest its not computations or representations all the way down but that at some point we need to talk about embodied, nonlinear dynamics, and still you do want to leave some place for the computational model. Is it the difference between the cortical (as computational) and the subcortical (as more nonlinear) or is it more complicated than that?

Panksepp: Yes, comparatively narrow information-processing approaches have been much oversold in the mind sciences. Endogenous global state-control system of the brain cannot be clarified in those ways. Likewise, in neuroscience narrower and narrower approaches give you ever better knowledge of smaller and smaller parts. One big question is how to move creatively toward synthetic wholes. Certainly one coarse way to parse useful sensory-percep-tual, *channel-control* information-processing and global attentional and affective state-control approaches is at cortical vs. subcortical levels of brain function. Information processing models are espe-cially useful for studying cognitions, where mental functions are strongly linked to external stimuli impinging on the senses that then get transformed into perceptions in the neocortex. Affective analog, state-control functions are more embodied, with large-scale net-works having intrinsic patterns that control large numbers of bodily processes. Also, the one thing that all scholars should agree upon at this point is that mind as truly manifested in the world is fundamen-tally organic, with information-processing being just one aspect of a more complex whole.

Information-processing as a comprehensive model of mind, has not only been oversold, but it is imbued with more than a residue of dualism. The idea that mind can be simply computed on any type of sufficiently complex computational platform seems to leave the real body and brain behind. One wonders what the computationalists do with the simple reality that minds, as they currently exist on the face of the earth, are most surely organic processes and are in some deep and perhaps essential way grounded in non-mental organic pro-cesses.

Computationalism became an attractive intellectual enterprise because of the ease of computation with the onset of the computer revolution. We're a lazy species but also one attracted by new glitz, and if we have a great new tool we will use it for everything that we can possibly think of. So we've now had this metaphor of a computa-tional mind for almost four decades, and I think it is a highly mis-leading metaphor for the emotional mind. Many in robotics are now heading toward embodied architectures, and making more progress. The allure of the modern computer has prevented too many brilliant people from pursuing more useful approaches such as organic, neuroscientific ones.

[...] One way to look at it is that too much of cognitivism is stuck with the belief-based view that external information-processing is the foundation of what organisms do, rather than the embodied emo-tional and motivational states that depend on large non-linear attrac-tor landscapes, arising from below, that control bodily actions and associated feelings. In fact, there is probably an organismic center, a core self process, for most things animals do. Information-processing revolves around an affectively self-centered, 'What's in it for me?' type of process. If we gave those ancient systems primacy, I think we would have a dramatically different view of learning—namely how informational schemes become embedded within the finer neurodynamics of those ancient, lumbering, emotional 'beasts of the mind' (large 'attractor landscapes'?) that are gradually educated to put on some cognitive clothes.

SG: So it appears to be extremely difficult, even with an arsenal of methods, to undress the mind, so to speak, to explain the mind-brain system.

Panksepp: I tend to accept that there is a level of complexity in the system that is not capable of being observed directly, just like in particle physics, and that the only way to penetrate the internal organizations of such processes is by theory. That's where I differ from quite a few of my colleagues. I do not believe in ruthless reductionism, and the dangerous, value-free, and culture diminishing view that the need for mental concepts disappears when all the neural firings have been tabulated. A key function of the brain is to generate global network states that are the raw foundational stuff of mentality, and much of the underlying organization currently has to be inferred rather than directly observed.

Anyone who says that behaviorism was killed by the cognitive revolution has not been paying attention. The behaviorists made a transformation. They became neuroscientists. The behaviorist biases are with us to this day but they are among the neuroscientists who still refuse to make inferences. For instance, in the realm of emotion they will say an emotion cannot be seen, ever. I tend to agree with them that yes a neurodynamic process can only be seen indirectly. Just as in particle physics the internal structure of matter at some point can only be seen by theoretical inference. In physics the inference is based completely on mathematics. Mathematics will not work on the brain. But an understanding of neuro-systems, neuro-chemistries, where you can translate from animal experiments to potential studies of human experience can generate predictions. As soon as you have a coherent logical prediction you're doing science.

The arts and sciences of cognition

How far afield from mainstream science can we travel to find insights into the mind? Varela and his colleagues have looked to Buddhist meditation for a methodological access to first-person experience (Varela, Thompson, and Rosch 1991). One could also think, not unlike mainstream analytic philosophers, that there is something in language that might throw some light on the organization of the mind. But does the language have to be propositional in nature? Could we discover something about the mind in poetry? Could we use both the arts and the sciences to study the mind? I'm drawn to what John Searle once said in a television interview: that we should use anything at our disposal to understand the mind.

There is an old poem by Robert Browning called 'How They Brought the Good News from Ghent to Aix' (1895). It's about the speed of moving information around different centers of commerce in Medieval times. Slower than e-mail, and certainly slower than synaptic connections in the brain, they depended on horses to deliver the mail. But that was speed in those days. Someone (I forget who, but it may have been Galen Strawson) recommended this poem to me because I had mentioned that I was going to be traveling from Aix-in-Provence in France to the modern city of Ghent in Belgium, from one academic conference to another one (this was in 2001). I took trains rather than a horse. But one piece of news that had traveled very fast and that was mentioned to me both in Aix at a conference on gestures, and in Ghent, at a conference on embodiment, was a new journal entitled *Neuro-Psychoanalysis*. I asked Jaak Panksepp, who is on its editorial board, about the concept behind the journal.[4]

> **SG:** I was in Ghent recently at an academic conference. The philosophers there are extremely enthusiastic about something relatively new, which you yourself mentioned in one of your articles: neuropsychoanalysis, which is also the name of a new journal.

> **Panksepp:** Well, I think neuropsychoanalysis is the attempt to bring depth psychology into traditional science. We know that psychoanalysis did not develop in a scientific tradition, for various reasons. Now psychoanalysis has two aspects, one is the theory of depth psychology that Freud and his followers and other people generated. This is a phenomenological theory. And then there is the treatment of psychiatric disorders with psychoanalysis. The treatment aspect had been very thoroughly evaluated and found wanting in regard to many disorders. Psychoanalysis is not anymore useful than any other talk therapy for schizophrenia, or autism. It's not effective. Now a lot of people say that means the theory of depth psychology was disproved, which is not the case; it was never tested. There is not a large experimental literature. And Freud himself was enough of a biologist that he stated over and over that many of the structures that he built would eventually be grounded on biology. For instance, he says we will find many, many chemicals in the brain controlling

---

4   This is part of the interview that was not published in the *Journal of Consciousness Studies*.

many specific psychological processes. On his deathbed, in a 1940 paper (he died in 1939), he says that we will eventually be able to harness these chemistries and therefore change the mind. Now those were statements of future possibilities that could never have emerged without a solid neuroscience. Now we have a solid neuroscience, but we have no respect for psychology. As a matter of fact most neuroscientists don't know anything about psychology at all and don't care to know about psychology. They are not ready to move between disciplines if they think that the other discipline is of no relevance to their activity. But, of course, for philosophers the most interesting issue is how do you link mind issues with brain issues. I think we will have a variety of strategies for docking mind/brain and my own endeavor in the study of emotions has been one example. I accept the phenomenology as being foundational and essential. There are feelings, emotions. Description of these is every important but does not suffice for science. But when you begin to try to dock them to brain issues then you have very traditional science. So neuropsychoanalysis is another endeavor to promote docking. I think it emerges from psychoanalysts who are also neuropsychologists working with brain-damaged individuals.

For instance, it's well known that if you have right parietal damage you can show contra-lateral neglect, that is, you no longer notice anything in the left visual field. Such patients neglect their body on the left side. They may even say this is not a part of my body. They just deny the existence of their own physical body. When Mark Solms, and his wife Karen Capland Solms, analyze these individuals in a psychoanalytical free association setting then periods of recognition of their deficits can emerge. Islands of psychological activity. They describe how bad they feel that they are paralyzed. So there is a level of mental organization that is suppressed, repressed, although it is not obvious in neurological examination. So neuropsychoanalysts would certainly promote that kind of research. And they are interested in brain emotional processes and an affective neuroscience approach to understanding emotions. The bottom line is they are psychoanalysts that are interested in promoting an empirically connected intellectual discipline. And that's great!

Psychoanalysis may be both a science and an art. Medicine is too. In both one can find opportunities to explore the human and experiential side of the embodied cognitive system. This is something that Jonathan Cole insists upon. One of his friends, Ian Waterman, is also one of his patients and his experimental subject. Ian has an unusual condition of deafferentation (loss of proprioception [body position sense] and sense of touch) involving the whole body from the neck down. As a result he has profound problems with motor control.

SG: Jonathan, you are an experimental scientist, but you are also a physician who treats patients. Is it important to do both kinds of work?

Cole: I get paid as a clinical doctor, and I grew up with an academic, neurophysiological background. And as you say, I am an empirical scientist. Much of my writing is — well, you could describe it as about narrative, about biography.

SG: It concerns, in the broad sense, how people live with neurological problems.

Cole: Yes, I am trying to look at both sides. I've studied Ian as a scientist, but I have also written his biography, informed by science, but also by my crude readings of philosophy. When you approach what it is like to be someone else, you can do that scientifically in a lab, to find out how someone can create a motor program or how someone can time action, but you also need to go out of the lab to ask how they live. And I know that Ian always says that he would not have done the amount of scientific work, over more than a dozen years, if I hadn't also been as interested in what it is like to be him, with his condition. I would say that this phenomenological approach to the subjective experience, the lived experience of illness, is just as important and informative as the lab science.

SG: Yes, well you know that I agree with that. Your work is a good example of how this combination can lead to very productive outcomes in regard to our understanding of illness. One very practical result is that because of your genuine interest in Ian as a person, he was willing to do more science with you. I'm also reminded of one of my favorite pieces by John Dewey (1928). He once gave a lecture to a college of physicians in which he chastised them for focusing in a very mechanical way only on the physical condition, the body of the patient, and ignoring the environment in which the patient lived. To understand illness one needs to know about the body, but also about the person's way of life. To cure the body and then to send the patient back into a noxious environment is to ignore an important aspect of the illness.

Cole: Yes, and the same goes for empirical science. Science is defined as knowledge — certainly it is in my OED. And it has come to be known as empirical science, which is a wonderful tool, and I am not in any way criticizing that. It produces results and data which allow the verification or refutation of hypotheses, which has been such a powerful technique. Most people are not aware of how power-ful it has been. We know infinitely more about the natural world and about how we all work because of empirical science. But we should also not forget the wider, more personal, more subjective experience. To leave that to novelists—and I have nothing against novelists— neglects something in between, an informed interest. I quote Merleau-Ponty (1964) at the beginning of *Still Lives* (Cole 2004): 'Science manipulates things and gives up living in them'.

It's not clear that we have to give up anything if we are willing to take a multi-disciplinary approach to explaining the mind, and to include data that reflects not only brain and behavior, but embodied experience in a physical and social and culturally mediated environment.

Chapter Three

Preliminaries, Prerequisites and Precedents

The questions that we have to deal with have been posed and debated for over 2500 years. But do we really have to pay attention to precedent in this regard? Do any of the old answers, often framed in terms of 'the soul', still make sense? Let's consider two possible answers to this question. The first one is 'Yes'. Since there has been a long-standing discussion about things like the mind, the soul, the self, consciousness, and more generally, cognition, there may be a good deal of wisdom to be found in these discussions. So it may certainly be worth a look at what some of the traditional philosophers have to say. The second possible answer is 'No'. Assuming that we've taken a look, it seems that the traditions are so conflicted, so full of contradictions, so lacking in consensus, that it is best to start over and begin the investigation from scratch.

The first answer is the ancient one, clearly discernable in the originators of western philosophy, the Greeks like Plato and Aristotle. They begin their investigations in dialog with those thinkers who had pursued the same questions before them. They are not naïve about this, however. That is, they do not expect simply to find the answers to these questions in the wisdom of the ages. Rather, they tend to approach previous thinkers in a skeptical way. Indeed, they find all of the contradictions of previous thought to constitute an inspiring way to set out the problems, or what the Greeks called the *aporiai* [perplexities]. The second answer reflects a modern way of thinking, and is represented most clearly by Descartes. Descartes sought to start from scratch, from a presuppositionless zero-point; and to do this he advised us to throw away all of our philosophy books. Before we do that, however, let's take a look at the very first systematic philosophical discussion that addressed many of the issues that we will be concerned with.

Think of this chapter as setting the stage for the later ones. If the contemporary philosopher Jerry Fodor is right, if 'in intellectual history, everything happens twice, first as philosophy and then as cognitive science'

(1981, 298), and if Alfred North Whitehead is right, that all of philosophy is but a series of footnotes to Plato, then the problems that cognitive scientists wrestle with today have their roots in Plato. Furthermore, in almost every case, when philosophers of mind, and cognitive scientists seek to lay the blame for most of the problems they confront, they almost always point at Descartes. So it seems practical, if not essential, to familiarize ourselves with some of the thinking of these two philosophers.

A conversation with Socrates

Let's reach back to an early discussion of how souls and bodies and minds are related. One of the most influential of the Platonic dialogues is called the *Phaedo*, and it features Socrates in prison, in conversation with his friends, discussing what he feels to be his physical and metaphysical imprisonment in his body, and the possible liberation that he may experience when he drinks his hemlock and dies. Not the most pleasant starting point, but it seems to be *the* starting point for much that comes after it, shaping the mysticism of Plotinus, the early Christian thought of the Gnostics, St. Augustine, and the Neoplatonism of medieval schools—the very influential tradition that Descartes consciously dismissed, and unconsciously repeated.

The *Phaedo* is a conversation amongst friends, some of whom are quite worried about the impending death of Socrates, and about their own future and the future of a certain way of questioning and challenging common sense and the status quo. The importance of the conversation for us is that it sets out a number of theories about the relationship between the body and the soul. Back then the majority of people in the world believed that there is such a thing as the soul. Actually, this is still the case. The majority of people in the world still believe that individuals have or are souls—and they do so religiously. In academic and scientific circles the existence of the soul is hardly open to question—that is, science has decided that there is no such thing (especially if we think of it as a *thing*). Yet all of the ancient questions about the soul have been translated into modern questions about the mind, consciousness, and self. Even contemporary thinkers who don't even want to think about the soul, do not shy away from considering the question of the immortality of the self, albeit conceived of in terms of mental existence prolonged by technological means.[1] But we'll set that question aside, since we have not even asked what the soul or the mind is yet.

---

1   For example, Dan Dennett, in an interview conducted by Wim Kayzer, suggests that if the self is reducible to information (see Chapter 11), then by means of information storage the self could be sustained indefinitely (Kayzer 1993).

Plato's dialogue addresses all of these questions — including questions about immortality, the nature of the soul, how the mind experiences the world, and so on — and it sets out a number of positions that are still in play today. The most basic question, however, is this: what is the relationship between the soul and the body. A position that is not far from a certain contemporary view is set out by Simmias, one of Socrates' friends who is participating in the prison conversation.

Here is the setting. Socrates, condemned by the city of Athens, is in prison, getting ready to drink his sentence, a cup of hemlock, and die. His friends are hanging around quite worried about this development, and whether they might face the same fate. They want to know what Socrates thinks about death and the possibility of an afterlife. They want to know how to think about the soul and body. Socrates has been going on about the idea that the soul needs to be in a kind of harmony in order to survive death. In this context, Simmias, one of his followers, puts forward a proposal. As you'll see, this simply increases the worry. As we listen in on the Platonic conversation, let's not pretend that we are flies on the wall, sitting back in an observer's role. Plato always encourages his reader to engage in the conversation, so let's do that. With all apologies to Plato, I'm going to take some liberties with the text and allow myself (SG) to interrupt their conversation when I need some clarifications.[2]

> **Simmias:** I dare say that you, Socrates, feel, as I do, how very hard or almost impossible the attainment of any certainty about these questions is in the present life, I mean this life before we die. So please, let me make a proposal. First, let me say that anyone who doesn't ask these ultimate questions is a coward, or someone who is too busy going about their everyday life to bother considering the most important issues about that life. We should be courageous and pursue these questions until we have attained one of two things: either we will discover or learn the truth about them; or, if this is impossible, we should take the best and most irrefutable ideas, and let this be the raft upon which we sail through life. Not without risk, as I admit, especially if one does not have religious faith. So, as you bid me, I will make a proposal, since I should not like to reproach myself later about not having said what I think. For when I consider the matter either alone or with our friend Cebes here, your arguments about harmony and the immortality of the soul do not appear to me to be sufficient, Socrates.

> **Socrates:** I dare say, my friend, that you may be right, but I should like to know in what respect they are not sufficient.

---

2   The following extracts from the Phaedo (360 BCE) are based on the translation by Benjamin Jowett (1871).

Simmias: In this respect. Might not a person use the same argument about harmony and thinking about a musical instrument, like the lyre, might he not say that harmony is something invisible, incorporeal, fair, and divine (as music often is). This harmony lives in the lyre when it is in tune, but, let's face it, the lyre and the strings are composed of matter—physical material, which is composite and earthy. Moreover, this material doesn't last forever. Now, according to your argument, if or when someone breaks the lyre, or cuts and rends the strings, the harmony nonetheless survives and does not perished. You cannot imagine, as we would say, that the lyre without the strings, or the broken strings themselves, remain, and yet that the harmony, which is of divine and immortal nature has perished. The harmony, you would say, certainly exists somewhere, even if the wood and strings decay.

SG: Yes, I see where you are going. Socrates may think that a harmony, like the mathematical ratios that define it, exists Platonically, if you know what I mean. The harmony exists independently of whether anyone plays it, or regardless of whether anyone discovers it. But you don't think so. For a harmony to exist, you think, a composer has to compose it, or a musician has to perform it.

Simmias: Plato is sitting over there in the corner, and he can speak for himself. But I mean something different. Please, pay attention. I think that for Socrates, and for most of us, the theory of the soul which we are all inclined to entertain, suggests that the body is strung up, and held together, by physical elements—hot and cold, wet and dry, and the like—and that the soul is the harmony or the appropriate proportional admixture of these physical elements. And, if this is true, the inference clearly is that when the strings of the body are unduly loosened or overstrained through illness or injury, then the soul, like a musical harmony, perishes at once, even if the material remains of the body may last for a considerable time, although they eventually decay or burn. So, if someone maintains that the soul, being the harmony of the elements of the body, perishes when the body dies, how shall we answer him?

Socrates: (at this point looking round at his friends and smiling, the way he always did—as if he already knew how to answer this challenge) Simmias proposes a very reasonable theory; can any of you answer him?

SG: I agree, Simmias has a good point here. Perhaps what we call the soul, or the mind, or consciousness, is totally dependent on the body, or more specifically, on the proper functioning of the brain. If something goes wrong with these physical aspects, it often seems to be the case that something goes wrong with the mind; and if the physical body dies, is seems quite reasonable to think that the soul dies and consciousness ceases to exist.

Socrates: Actually, I meant my question to be rhetorical — I'm quite ready to provide an answer.

Actually, before Socrates offered his answer to Simmias, he digressed to important considerations about method. Questions about method are important, because one needs to know what will count as a good answer to the kind of question that we are considering here. Really, what sort of approach should we take to answering questions that seem almost unanswerable? Indeed, in this conversation we might start to think that there are two questions that are being confused. One has to do with the immortality of the soul — Simmias suggesting that it is not immortal. The other is about how the soul relates to the body. There seems to be some agreement that the answer to the first question depends on the answer to the second. If the soul is a harmony of physical processes, as Simmias suggests, then it is not clear that it can survive the destruction of such physical processes. But how do we determine the proper way to think about the soul and the body? Some people contend that natural science can tell us everything there is to know about these matters. Others suggest that these are metaphysical questions that are irreducible to science.

Socrates: When I was young, I had a prodigious desire to pursue knowledge about the natural processes of the world. This enterprise appeared to me to have lofty aims because science has to do with the causes of things, and it teaches why a thing is, and how it is generated and destroyed. I was always getting excited by these kinds of questions: Is the growth of animals the result of some decay which the hot and cold principle contracts, as some have said? Is it the blood, or the air, or the fire, the element with which we think, or perhaps nothing of the sort. Perhaps the brain may be the originating power of the perceptions of hearing and sight and smell, and memory and opinion may come from them, and science itself may be based on just the kind of information accumulated in memory and opinion.

SG: Okay, I'm not sure about the air or the fire, but it seems right that we should look at the brain in this regard. But I know you have more general things to say about method.

Socrates: (continuing as if he had not heard me) I went on to examine the decay of physical processes, and then to the study of astronomy, and at last I concluded that I was wholly incapable of these inquiries, as I will satisfactorily prove to you. For I was fascinated by them to such a degree that my eyes grew blind to things that I and others thought we knew quite well. I forgot what I had before thought to be self-evident, that people grow as a result of eating and drinking; for when by digestion flesh is added to flesh and bone to bone, and whenever there is an aggregation of congenial elements, the lesser bulk becomes larger and the small man greater. Was not that a reasonable notion?

Cebes: Yes, I think so.

SG: Actually, I'm not entirely sure I follow your meaning. You seem to prefer what we call common sense rather than scientific investigation.

Socrates: Well; but let me tell you something more. There was a time when I thought that I understood the meaning of greater and less pretty well; and when I saw a tall man standing by a small one I fancied that one was taller than the other by a head; or one horse would appear to be greater than another horse: and still more clearly did I seem to perceive that ten is two more than eight, and that two cubits are more than one, because two is twice one.

Cebes: Now I'm not sure I understand. Have you changed your mind about these things?

Socrates: The problem is that I was far enough from imagining that I knew the cause of any of them. Really, I cannot satisfy myself that when one is added to one, the one to which the addition is made becomes two, or that the two units added together make two by reason of the addition. For I cannot understand how, when separated from the other, each of them was one and not two, and now, when they are brought together, the mere juxtaposition of them can be the cause of their becoming two: or is it possibly that the division of one is the way to make two; for then a different cause would produce the same effect. … Nor am I any longer satisfied that I understand the reason why one or anything else either is generated or destroyed or is at all, but I have in my mind some confused notion of another method.

SG: Okay. I'm confused too. But at least I understand that you were confused about whether you actually had something like a causal explanation of how these things worked. So if this natural scientific approach wasn't working for you what did you do?

Socrates: Well, I ran into someone who had a book by Anaxagoras, and he quoted this. Anaxagoras proclaimed that mind [*nous*, the rational principle] was the disposer and cause of everything. In other words he was treating mind as a principle that could explain everything. I was quite delighted at this notion, and I said to myself: If mind is the disposer, and it works on a rational principle, then mind will dispose all for the best, and put each particular thing in the best place. In any case, I argued that if we desired to find out the cause of the generation or destruction or existence of anything, then we simply had to find out what state of being or suffering or doing was best for that thing. In other words, we only had to consider what was best for something — its best place or function in the big picture, the rational picture, and then we would understand it. So I rejoiced to think that I had found in Anaxagoras a teacher of the causes of existence such as I desired, and I imagined that he would tell me first whether the earth is flat or round; and then he would further explain the cause and the necessity of this, and would teach me the nature of the best and show this was best. So, if he said that the earth was in the centre, he would be able to explain that this position was the best, and I should be satisfied if this were demonstrated, and not want any other sort of causal explanation. And I thought that I would then ask him about the sun and moon and stars, and that he would explain to me their comparative movement, and their cycles and various states, and how their various properties, active and passive, were all for the best. For I could not imagine that when he spoke of mind as the disposer of them, he would give any other account of their being as they are, except that this was best; and I thought when he had explained to me in detail the cause of each and the cause of all, he would go on to explain to me what was best for each and what was best for all. I had hopes, which I would not have sold for a great deal of money, and I seized the books and read them as fast as I could in my eagerness to know the better and the worse.

SG: This sounds like quite an enlightened plan.

Socrates: What hopes I had formed, and how grievously was I disappointed! As I proceeded, I found my philosopher altogether forsaking mind or any other principle of order, but having recourse to air, and ether, and water, and other eccentricities. I might compare him to a person who began by maintaining generally that mind is the cause of the actions of Socrates, but who, when he endeavored to explain the causes of my various actions in detail, went on to show that I sit here because my body is made up of bones and muscles; and the bones, as he would say, are hard and have ligaments which divide them, and the muscles are elastic, and they cover the bones, which have also a covering of skin which contains them; and as the bones are lifted at their joints by the contraction or relaxation of the muscles, I am able to bend my limbs, and this is why I am sitting here in a curved posture. That is the sort of explanation he would give, and he would have a similar explanation of my talking to you, which he would attribute to sound, and air, and hearing, and he would assign ten thousand other causes of the same sort, forgetting to mention the true cause, which is that the Athenians have thought fit to condemn me, and accordingly I have thought it better and more right to remain here and undergo my sentence. Indeed, I am inclined to think that these muscles and bones of mine would have gone off to Megara or Boeotia — by the dog of Egypt they would — if they had been guided only by their own idea of what was best, and if I had not chosen as the better and nobler role, instead of playing truant and running away, to undergo any punishment which the State inflicts.

SG: So, if I understand you, the kind of explanations you were looking for were not the kind of physical explanations that can be given by natural or physiological science. You wanted an explanation according to reasons. Why am I still sitting here? Why did I reach for a drink? You would not accept the explanation that would be framed in terms of neurons firing and motor control mechanisms. You would rather say that 'I was thirsty, and that given my belief that water quenches thirst, I decided to reach for the drink.' Yet, if we ask *how* I was able to reach for a drink, rather than *why* I did, wouldn't the physiological explanation in terms of neurons and motor control be sufficient?

Socrates: There is surely a strange confusion of causes and conditions in all this. It may be said, indeed, that without bones and muscles and the other parts of the body I cannot execute my purposes. But to say that I do as I do because of them, and that this is the way in which mind acts, and not from the choice of the best, is a very careless and idle mode of speaking. I wonder if it would be useful to distinguish between the cause and the condition, which the many, feeling about in the dark, are always confusing and misnaming. ... Still, since I have failed either to discover myself or to learn from anyone else the nature of the best, I will exhibit to you, if you like, what I have found to be the second best mode of inquiring into the cause.

Cebes: I, for one, should very much like to hear that.

Socrates: I thought that as I had failed in the contemplation of true reasons, I ought to be careful that I did not lose the eye of my soul; as people may injure their bodily eye by observing and gazing on the sun during an eclipse, unless they take the precaution of only looking at the image reflected in the water, or in some similar medium. I thought of this and I was afraid that my soul might be blinded altogether if I looked at things with my eyes or tried by the help of the senses to apprehend them directly. And I thought that I had better have recourse to ideas, and seek in them the truth of existence. I dare say that the simile is not perfect, for I am very far from admitting that he who contemplates existence through the medium of ideas, sees them only 'through a glass darkly', any more than he who sees them in their empirical functions and effects. However, this was the method which I adopted: I first assumed some principle which I judged to be the strongest, and then I affirmed as true whatever seemed to agree with this, whether relating to the cause or to anything else; and that which disagreed I regarded as untrue.

Perhaps we could think of this as starting with a model and then testing it out using a principle of rational consistency. I'm not sure. But where does this get us in regard to the question about the body and soul? When Socrates comes back to this issue, he turns the tables on Simmias. Rather than worrying about the specific question of how the soul relates to the body, which is a metaphysical question, Socrates appeals to rational consistency between what must be the case in this regard, and what we believe in regard to the immortality of the soul. To answer Simmias, Socrates appeals to an epistemological concept he had outlined previously in the dialogue. This is the famous Platonic doctrine of recollection. According to this idea, we do not learn by experience so much as use experience as the occasion to remember things that we have learned in a previous life. If Simmias accepts this doctrine, which he does, then the soul can't be related to the body in the way that he proposes. That is, if the soul is reincarnated from a previous life to the present one, something which is implied by the theory of recollection, then the soul cannot depend on the physical processes of the body.

This response by Socrates seems a bit unfair, since Socrates himself likely never believed in the theory of recollection, and it is not even clear that Plato believed in it. But one question that is nicely raised by this move is whether we need to settle epistemological questions before we can settle metaphysical ones, or whether an understanding of how we come to know things will help us understand the nature of the mind. Do we need to understand cognitive functions before we can say precisely what the mind is and how it relates to the body? The discussion of method raises the same kind of question. Assuming that *how* we do things is not equivalent to *why* we do things, does a causal explanation in terms of physical processes (an answer to the 'how' question) give us a complete understanding of the mind, or do we need to appeal to something else — something that would answer the 'why' question?

As I said earlier, Plato doesn't set out to provide definitive answers to questions like these; he seems perfectly happy to raise the questions and to move us into a state of *aporia* or perplexity, a state in which we have to seek our own answers.

Cartesian communications

Perplexity is not something that Rene Descartes liked at all. He favored the
certainty of 'clear and distinct' answers. Today the only clear and distinct
certainty about Descartes is that in the contemporary consensus amongst
philosophers of mind and cognitive scientists, he, more than any other
philosopher, has the most to answer for. His *Meditations* set body and
mind in metaphysical and scientific opposition. Descartes and his
mind-body problem continue to haunt contemporary discussions, under
various titles such as 'the hard problem' of consciousness (Chalmers 1995),
or the 'explanatory gap' (Levine 1983). How can physical processes generate something like consciousness, which seems to be irreducible to physical processes, and certainly different from them. There are great efforts
taken by philosophers and scientists to debunk Descartes for conceiving
the mind as a 'Cartesian theater' (Dennett 1991), totally divorced from the
embodied emotions (Damasio 1994). Furthermore, his *Meditations* are the
very opposite of dialogue or conversation, unless one thinks of it as a conversation with himself. Descartes could conduct his meditations in a dark
closet if he wanted, or as he seemed to do, alone in his sitting room.
Wouldn't it be good to barge in on him and be able to ask for some clarifications, if not for some retractions.

Actually, Descartes did agree to answer some pointed questions about
all of this, in his various correspondences with princesses, physicians, and
philosophers. And, almost as if we have access to Descartes' e-mail, we
still have some of that correspondence in the form of letters.[3] We can look
at these missives where he defends and explains himself to others, as an
ongoing interview with Descartes through which we can get an inside or
inner view of his thoughts in his *Meditations*.

Let's start with his correspondence with Elisabeth of Bohemia [1618–80].
She was the granddaughter of James I of England and, a true bohemian,
had a healthy interest in philosophical questions. In May of 1643, Elisabeth
wrote to Descartes to ask him to explain how a soul can 'determine the
spirits of the body to produce voluntary actions.' She noted that movement requires some kind of contraction or extension of muscles, but she is
puzzled at how the mind might be able to effect this, since, as Descartes
had concluded in his *Meditations*, the mind and body are two different
kinds of substances and cannot interact. It is interesting to note that Descartes himself did some scientific experiments on just this issue. He
showed that muscles worked in pairs, one 'retracting' and the other 'relax-
ing' in each movement (Hauptli 2005). Furthermore, even in his *Meditations*, his views are more complicated than strict denial of interaction

---

3   Letter-writing was something that people did before they were able to communicate
     electronically.

between body and mind, since Descartes also thinks that in some mysterious way the mind and the body do interact. I've edited Descartes' reply to make him get to the point faster,[4] and I've interrupted where I thought it might help. Our princess is puzzling over the following issue: if one wants something to move, one can give it a push with one's hand; but if one wants one's hand to move, can we say that the mind pushes the hand? Here, in part, is Elisabeth's question.

> **Elisabeth:** It seems to me that the accomplishment of movement happens by a kind of pushing (*pulsion*, propulsion) of the thing that is moved, and as such is determined by the manner in which it is pushed, and by the nature and shape of the thing that pushes. Contact is needed for the push to happen, and extension is needed to qualify the shape of the surface of the thing that pushes. But you exclude extension from your concept of mind, and something like contact seems to be incompatible with an immaterial thing.

> **Descartes:** Look, everything we can know about the human mind or soul depends on two things. The first is that it thinks; the second is that, since it is united to the body, it can act and be acted upon. In the *Meditations* I didn't say much about the second thing; rather I devoted all my efforts to clarifying the first, with the intent to prove that there is a distinction between the soul and the body. Only the former was useful for making that distinction, and the second would be a distraction from it. But since your Highness has asked such an insightful question, I shall try to explain how I conceive the union of the soul and body, and how the soul has the power to move the body.

> First, I note that we have certain primitive notions; they are like originals that we use as patterns out of which we construct everything we know.

> **SG:** Perhaps you mean what psychologists today call cognitive 'schemas'.

> **Descartes:** There are only a very few such schemas, or, as I prefer, notions. The most general ones apply to whatever we can conceive — being, number, duration, and so forth. In addition, with respect to our knowledge of body by itself, we have only the notion of extension, from which there follow notions of shape and motion. With respect to the soul taken by itself, we have only the notion of thought (including perceptions of the understanding and inclinations of the will). Finally, with respect to the soul and the body taken as a com-

---

4   I've provided very free translations, after consulting the original French (see http://www.ac-nice.fr/philo/textes/Descartes-Elisabeth/Descartes-Elisabeth.htm) and a number of English translations, including Smith (1958), Kenny (1970) and George MacDonald Ross, 1975–1999 at http://www.philosophy.leeds.ac.uk/GMR/hmp/texts/modern/descartes/dcindex.html.

posite, we have only the notion of their union. The power that the soul has to move the body, and the power the body has to act on the soul, and to cause its sensations and passions, depends on this notion of union.

Now to get good scientific knowledge we need to keep these notions properly distinct, and we shouldn't attribute them to things they do not belong to. If we use the wrong notion to solve a problem we'll clearly go wrong. Likewise if we try to explain one of these notions by means of another. Keep in mind that these are primitive notions, and each of them can be understood only through itself. One problem that we have is that we rely so much on our senses that the notions of extension, shape, and motion seem much more familiar to us than the others. This leads us to make mistakes when we want to use these notions to explain things they do not apply to. So, for example, when we use our imagination, a faculty that depends on sensory representation, to understand the nature of the soul, we are misled. Or when we think of the way in which the soul moves the body in terms of the way in which one body moves another body, we are misled.

SG: Okay, so we have to be careful to avoid these kinds of category mistakes, and if we want to explain movement, we need to understand it in terms of the notion of union, or the composite mind-body. But what precisely do you mean by union? Her Highness wants to know. We all want to know, because you didn't say much about it in your *Meditations.*

Descartes: Right, I'm getting to that. Her Highness was kind enough to read the *Meditations.* There I was trying to work out the notions that belong to the soul alone, by distinguishing them from those that belong to the body alone. So we end up with a kind of Platonic dualism.

SG: Perhaps we could call this a Cartesian dualism, since you were much more concerned with the mind and cogitations than with something like the Platonic soul.

Descartes: Well, I'm honored. I think I am, anyway. But to move on, the thing I have to explain, as you say, is how to understand the notions that belong to the union of the soul with the body, without using notions which belong to the body alone or the soul alone. The problem is that we have been confusing the notion of the power by which the soul acts on the body with the notion of the power by which one body acts on another body. We have also attributed such powers to various properties of bodies, such as weight, heat, and so forth, and we have imagined these properties themselves to be thing-like, that is, as things distinct from bodies, sometimes even calling them substances, rather than qualities or properties. And again we have been confused, because we sometimes use notions that pertain to bodies, and sometimes those that pertain to the soul, depending on whether we have attributed to them something material or something immaterial. For example, we have supposed that weight or gravity is like a thing, and that it has the power to move the body it inhabits towards the centre of the earth. In doing this, however, we are not puzzled about how it moves the body, or how it is joined to it. And we do not really think that it operates by pushing or contacting one surface against the other. I believe that we are misusing the notion of material thing in applying it to weight, which is certainly not a real thing distinct from the body. Here's the point. I believe that we can use this notion of weight as a way to understand how the soul moves the body.

Elisabeth: I'm not quite sure I follow your explanation. Do you mean that something like weight is what allows the soul to move the body? It would be easier for me to understand the soul to be material and extended, than that something immaterial have the capacity for moving a body. For, if movement occurred through a kind of informing process of vapors, the vapors that perform the movement would have to be intelligent, which you accord to nothing corporeal. And although in your metaphysical meditations you suggest the possibility of the second, it's very difficult to comprehend that a soul, as you have described it, after having had the faculty and habit of reasoning well, can lose all of it on account of some vapors.

Descartes: You have rightly challenged the very poor explanation I gave you in my last letter. Thank you for giving me the chance to respond, and the opportunity to take into account the things I left out. Here's what I forgot to say. I did distinguish between three kinds of primitive notions, each known in its own special way, and not by comparison with one another — namely the notions of the soul, of the body, and of the union between the soul and the body. I should have then explained the differences between these three notions, and between the operations of the soul by which we know them. Then I should have said why I used the analogy with weight. I should have explained that, although we might be tempted to think of the soul as material (which is strictly what it means to conceive it as united with the body), this does not prevent us from subsequently knowing that it is separable from it.

So here goes. First, there is a great difference between these three kinds of notions. The soul conceives itself only through pure understanding. Body (and those properties that define bodies, extension, shape, and motion) can also be known through the understanding alone, but is much better known through the understanding helped by the imagination especially the mathematical imagination. Finally, things that belong to the union of the soul and the body can be understood only obscurely through the understanding alone, or even through the understanding helped by the imagination. On the other hand, they are known very clearly through the senses.

SG: That seems a very strange thing for you to say, since you usually don't give much credence to the senses.

Descartes: Well consider people who never bother with philosophical theory, and who use only their senses and a practical way of thinking. They have no doubt that the soul moves the body, and that the body acts on the soul. By considering them as a union, they consider them as a single thing. In contrast metaphysical theory, which exercises the pure understanding, gives insight into the notion of the soul. Then the study of mathematics (where we use our imagination in regard to shapes and motions) promotes the habit of thinking of body in a variety of ways. So what I am suggesting, and what is certainly lacking in my *Meditations*, is that by immersing ourselves in real life and everyday social interaction, and not by metaphysical meditation or studying things which exercise the imagination, we learn to understand the union of the soul and the body.

SG: So, let me get this straight. Are you suggesting that we learn about the possibility of moving by moving, or through practice? And this is a different kind of knowledge than the theoretical stuff you were concerned about in the *Meditations*.

Descartes: I'm afraid that you might think that I'm not serious about what I have just suggested. But I am. Indeed, I recommend the following study rule: never spend more than a few hours a day on thoughts which exercise the imagination; never spend more than a very few hours per year on thoughts which exercise the understanding alone; and devote the remaining time to indulging in sensory experience, and giving one's spirit a rest. This is why I have retired to the country.

SG: Now I really am wondering whether you're serious.

Descartes: My point is this, that if you pay too much attention to metaphysical meditations, rather than to thoughts requiring less concentration, you will be able to discover some obscurity in the notion of the union between the soul and the body. But you will be demanding more than human understanding is capable of. I think that the human spirit is incapable of conceiving, at one and the same time, the distinction between the soul and the body, and their union. That would mean simultaneously conceiving them as one thing and as two — a contradiction. So if you are still occupied with the reasoning which proves the distinction between the soul and the body, that may in fact interfere with your ability to understand the notion of union. We all experience for ourselves this union as long as we are not philosophizing. An individual just is a single person, which is a combination of body and thinking, and is of a nature that this thinking can move the body, and can sense the contingencies involved. That's why I used the analogy of weight, something usually imagined to be united with a body in the same way as our thinking is united with our bodies. An imperfect analogy, I know, because such qualities are precisely not things, as we may imagine them.

Your Highness suggests that it is easier to attribute material and extension to the soul, than to attribute to the soul the capacity to move a body and to be moved by it since it is immaterial. But you are welcome to attribute such matter and extension to the soul; this is nothing more than to conceive it as united to the body. Once you have fixed this concept, and consulted your own experience, it should be easy to consider that the matter attributed to thinking is not the thinking itself, and that the physical extension is different from the extension of this thinking, in that the first is tied to a particular place from which it excludes all other physical extension, whereas this is not true of the second. One can thus return to the distinction between the soul and the body, despite the fact that you have verified the conception of their union.

Elisabeth: I agree that the senses demonstrate that the soul moves the body; but they fail to teach me (any more than the understanding and the imagination) the manner in which it does so. In regard to that, I think there may be unknown properties in the soul that might motivate a reversal of what your metaphysical meditations, with such good reasons, persuaded me: that the mind lacks extension. Although extension is not necessary to thought, it does not seem to be contradictory to it, and it could easily belong to some other, less essential function of the soul.

It is clear from this correspondence that once we buy into the metaphysical distinction between two substances, body and mind, it shapes the way we think of the mind to such an extent that it is difficult to imagine *how* it can do what it does, even if we know from practical experience that it does it. In his book, *The Passions of the Soul* [1649], which Descartes dedicated to Elisabeth, he attempts a different explanation, this time trying to say *how* the mind interacts with the body, and he locates that interaction in the brain.

[...] although the soul is joined to the whole body, there is yet in that a certain part in which it exercises its functions more particularly than in all the others; and it is usually believed that this part is the brain, or possibly the heart: the brain, because it is apparently in it that we experience the passions. But, in examining the matter with care, it seems as though I had clearly ascertained that the part of the body in which the soul exercises its functions immediately is in nowise the heart, nor the whole of the brain, but merely the most inward of all its parts, to wit, a certain very small gland which is situated in the middle of its substance and so suspended above the duct whereby the animal spirits in its anterior cavities have communication with those in the posterior, that the slightest movements which take place in it may alter very greatly the course of these spirits; and reciprocally that the smallest changes which occur in the course of the spirits may do much to change the movements of this gland.

Let us then conceive here that the soul has its principal seat in the little gland which exists in the middle of the brain, from whence it radiates forth through all the remainder of the body by means of the animal spirits, nerves, and even the blood, which, participating in the impressions of the spirits, can carry them by the arteries into all the members. And reconciling what has been said above about the machine of our body, i.e. that the little filaments of our nerves are so distributed in all its parts, that on the occasion of the diverse movements which are there excited by sensible objects, they open in diverse ways the pores of the brain, which causes the animal spirits contained in these cavities to enter in diverse ways into the muscles, by which means they can move the members in all the different ways in which they are capable of being moved ... let us here add that the small gland which is the main seat of the soul is so suspended between the cavities which contain the spirits that it can be moved by them in as many different ways as there are sensible diversities in the object, but that it may also be moved in diverse ways by the soul, whose nature is such that it receives in itself as many diverse impressions. (Descartes 1969, 347–48).

Actually, Descartes expressed this idea several years earlier than his exchange with Princess Elizabeth, specifically in his correspondence with Lazare Meyssonnier (1602–72) a physician at Lyon, and he continued to make clarifications for a number of years (1640–41), in correspondence with other friends, like Antoine Arnauld (1612–94) and Marin Mersenne (1588–1648). In order to work out a more complete response to Elisabeth's questions, I'll call these other interlocutors into the conversation. In response to Meyssonnier, Descartes attempts to resolve one of the problems introduced by his dualism by appealing to a kind of monistic structure in the brain.

Descartes: In my opinion, the pineal gland, which we call the conarium is the principal seat of the soul; it is the place where our thoughts occur. I think this is right because I can find in the brain no other part which is not doubled. Consider that we see something only once although we use two eyes, and we hear a sound only once although by two ears. Since we never have more than one thought at one time, then the species which enter the mind through the eyes or ears, etc., must come to be unified in some one part, and there be contemplated by the soul; now in the entire head the pineal gland is the only such non-doubled part to be found. In addition, it is most appropriately situated for this, since it is at the center and it is sustained and surrounded by the carotid arteries, which bring the animal spirits into the brain.

SG: Is this something like a theater then? A center where all thoughts are played out and inspected, or introspected by the soul? Or do you mean something more like a very short memory that we put to work, or a workspace in the mind? What are these things you call species, and are they processed in some way, or do they stand there for inspection?

Descartes: When I talk of corporeal forms or species, I mean those things that we must have in the brain in order to imagine anything. These are not thoughts themselves. Thought is the operation of the mind which imagines, i.e. which directs itself towards these species. These species may be preserved in memory, for example. Concerning such memories, I imagine that they are like the folds conserved in this piece of paper once it has been folded. It may be better to think of them as received principally in the whole substance of the brain. They may also in some way come into this gland, but if they did so, they would get in the way of what needs to be quickly dealt with. If memories were preserved here, or if things were kept around for showing, our spirits would be dulled; for I believe that people with the best and subtlest spirits must have the gland completely free of memories and perfectly mobile. Thus we see, in contrast with the other parts of the brain, the gland is smaller in humans than it is in animals.

Mersenne: Am I to understand that the mind interacts with the animal spirits in this part of the brain and gives direction to the body in a way that might satisfy the idea that the soul might be considered extended.

Descartes: Indeed, the soul also uses animal spirits (also known as physical vapors) that do not reside in this gland; for it is not the case that the soul is contained in the gland in a way that prevents it from extending its activity to other parts. I don't mean that the soul is identical to these vapors, since it is one thing to use, and a very different thing to be immediately joined or united. Again, my reasoning is that since our soul is not a set of distributed processes, but itself one and indivisible, then the part of the body to which it is most immediately united must also be one and not divided, and that is this gland, which is the only thing that meets this requirement in the whole brain.

We know through our own perceptual experience that the seat of the common sense, where different sense modalities must coalesce, the part of the brain in which the soul exercises all its principal functions, must be mobile or dynamic. There is also a dynamic interaction of the mind with the animal spirits. Now it makes sense that the conarium should be a gland, because a gland has its principle function to take in the most subtle parts of the blood from the vessels surrounding them, so the the conarium's function is accordingly to receive the animal spirits. Since it is the only uniquely solid part of the brain, then it necessarily must be the location of the common sense, of thought, and therefore of the soul. If this is not so, then we would be led to the conclusion that the soul is not immediately united to any solid part of the body, but only to the animal spirits which continually come and go, like water that runs in a river — but this would be absurd.

Mersenne: From what I know of the brain, however, I note that no nerve goes to the conarium. Furthermore, if the processing in the conarium is so dynamic, then how can it be the seat of the common sense?

Descartes: But these two facts support my view. Since every nerve leads to some sense-organ or moving part (the eyes, the ears, or the arms, and so forth), if only one led to the conarium, it could not be the seat of the common sense, all of them would have to lead to it in the same way; if it is impossible for all of them to lead there, it is possible for them to communicate by the agency of the spirits, and this is what happens in regard to the conarium. Certainly the seat of the common sense must be extremely dynamic in order to register all the impressions which arrive from the senses; it seems necessary that it is moved by the spirits which transmit these impressions; and only the conarium functions in this way.

Arnauld: But does this mean that the mind is aware of these animal spirits, or how else could it conduct its business with them?

Descartes: No, we are not aware of the way that our mind communicates the animal spirits from nerve to nerve. It doesn't depend on the mind alone, but involves the mind's union with the body. Still, we don't understand the action by which the mind moves the nerves, as such action exists in the mind, and it appears that it is just the inclination of the will to move the limbs. This inclination of the will is facilitated by the flow of the animal spirits into the nerves, and this happens because of the disposition of the body, of which we are unconscious. But if the mind is unconscious of the disposition of the body, at the same time it is not unconscious of its union with the body, for if it were not aware of this it could never will to move the limbs. So again I say that although we are not in a position to understand, by reason or by imaginative comparison of this with other things, how the mind, which is not a physical thing, can move the body, which is a physical thing, we cannot doubt that it does so, since experience certainly and self-evidenly makes us immediately aware of this. This is one of the things that we know immediately, in and by itself.

It is a common practice today among philosophers and scientists to circulate their ideas by sending around their latest papers to colleagues, or posting them on their webpages for people to read. It was more difficult in Descartes's day to accomplish a wide circulation, through the mails that depended on less than modern transportation systems. Yet Descartes, keen on getting feedback from significant thinkers, was able to get the manuscript of his *Meditations* around to a number of critical commentators, including the British philosopher Thomas Hobbes. The result was that seven sets of comments from various thinkers, and his replies, were published along with the *Meditations* (1641). The exchange with Hobbes, in Latin, happened while Descartes was in exile in Holland, and Hobbes was in exile in Paris. Mersenne facilitated the circulation of ideas. Hobbes's first point amounts to nothing; he simply accuses Descartes of rehashing some things that Plato said, e.g., about not trusting the senses. Descartes responds that he was not trying to take credit for these ideas, but he was trying to do something different with them. Hobbes's second point is more substantial. He defends a materialist position against Descartes's dualism. I'll frame it in the second person, as comments made to Descartes, and I'll slightly alter the translation and abbreviate the discussion to make sure we get to the main points as efficiently as possible.[5]

Hobbes: As you, Descartes, propose, from the fact that I am thinking it follows that 'I am', because what thinks is not nothing. But when

---

5   For the full text, see George MacDonald Ross's translation at www.philosophy.leeds.ac.uk/GMR/hmp/texts/modern/hobbes/objections/objects.html

you go on to say, 'That is, [what I am is] mind, soul, understanding, reason', there is room for doubt. It does not seem valid to argue from 'I am thinking' to 'I am thought', or from 'I am walking' to 'I am a walk'. You assume that an intelligent thing is the same as intellection, which is the action of an intelligent thing; or at least that an intelligent thing is the same as the intellect, which is the capacity possessed by an intelligent thing. You know that philosophers distinguish the underlying subject from its capacities and actions. ... Consequently, a thinking thing is the subject that underlies mind, reason, or understanding, and it must be something corporeal.

A thinking thing is corporeal because subjects of actions are incomprehensible unless they are conceived as corporeal or material. ... If knowledge of the proposition 'I exist' depends on knowledge of the proposition 'I think'; and knowledge of the latter depends on the fact that we cannot separate thought from thinking matter, then we must conclude that the thinking thing is material rather than immaterial.

Descartes: Well I admit that I did use words which were as abstract as I could find to refer to the thing or substance, with the intention of divesting it of everything that did not belong to it. In contrast, you, Mr. Hobbes, use words that are as concrete as possible (such as 'subject', 'matter', or 'body') to signify the thinking thing, just so it cannot be separated from body.

But enough of verbal quibbles: let us get down to the substantial issue. You rightly refer to our inability to conceive of action independently of its subject, e.g. to think of thought without a thinking thing; that which thinks is not nothing, as you say. But you go on to claim, contrary to all linguistic usage and logic, that a thinking thing is something corporeal because subjects of actions are comprehensible only if they are conceived as ... — what shall we say? 'Substantial', I would accept, or even 'material' if you want, provided this is understood in the sense of metaphysical matter. But it does not follow that they must be corporeal.

Now we call some characteristics physical — for example, size, shape, motion, and anything else that we cannot think about independently of their having extension in space. The substance these inhere in we call 'body'. It's not that one substance is the subject of shape, and a different substance the subject of motion, and so on, but all these characteristics are united by a single, common principle: they are all essentially spatial. Other characteristics we call mental, for example, understanding, willing, imagining, sensing, and so on. These all share the essential principle of thought, or perception, or consciousness. The substance underlying them is a thinking thing or mind. This is not to be confused with corporeal substance; acts of thought share nothing in common with bodily acts; thought, belongs to a completely different category of being from extension, which is the essential principle shared by the rest. If we form two distinct concepts of these two distinct substances, it becomes easy to judge whether they are one and the same or distinct.

Hobbes: You suggest that the idea of my own self is innate. Now if the self is my body, I get it from looking at my body; and if the self is the soul, we have no idea of the soul at all. Rather, by using reason, rather than our senses, we have to deduce that there is something internal to the human body, something which gives it the animal motion by which it senses and moves. That's what we call the 'soul', but we don't have an idea or percept of it. ... There is a great difference between imagining or perceiving, and conceiving with the mind, which involves reasoning to conclude that something is the case, or that a certain thing exists. But you give no explanation of how they are different. ... But what if we say that reasoning is nothing other than using the word 'is' to join names together, linking them into sequences? In that case reasoning can tell us nothing about things in the real world, but only about names. This is so even if names are agreed upon by convention. Accordingly, reasoning will depend on names; names will depend on images; and images I believe will depend on the motion of the bodily organs. Therefore, mind is nothing other than motions in various parts of an organic body.

Descartes: Well I disagree. Reasoning is not just the joining of names, but the joining of things signified by the names; and I am amazed you could think differently. For example, would you not say that a Frenchman and a German can reason about precisely the same things, even though they have completely different words in their minds? Furthermore, if you are justified in concluding that mind is motion, then you may as well conclude that earth is sky, or anything else you want to dream up.

On the question of whether mind is motion or how the mind is related to movement, however, Descartes does not have the last word. Today when we want to ask how the brain is mobile, or what it's dynamics are, we turn to neuroscientists. As philosophers who want to explain cognition, we need to ask about the details. What kind of movement, in the brain, or of the body, generates our cognitive experiences? To get some answers, then, we need to turn to the most recent research and the people who have been studying brain dynamics and the way that our bodies move as we move into action.

Chapter Four

Movement

Having provided some historical background, it's time to get down to business. Let's turn to the things that philosophy of mind and the cognitive sciences actually try to explain. Now it might seem strange to some that I want to start a broad discussion of cognition by talking about movement, and not just movement or processing in the brain, but bodily movement — the way we move around the environment, and the movement that allows us to do things, and therefore perform actions. But movement is a very good place to start because it is like starting from the bottom and working our way up. And at the bottom it is difficult to see where to draw a line between certain non-cognitive aspects of movement, and other aspects that seem to count as cognitive. Some movement seems to be highly informed by cognitive elements; other movement seems completely empty of such elements. All animals move or are moved; but just as some animals may not be conscious or capable of rational thought, not all animals (and maybe no animals at all) are in full control of their movement.

In the philosophical tradition there is an ancient link between movement and mind. Aristotle talked about our awareness of time as being linked to a certain kind of movement that occurs in the mind (*Physics* 218b21–24 and 219a5). But whatever concept of movement he would specify here (something he doesn't do), any concept of movement that we have is derivative from bodily movement. Indeed, as George Lakoff and Mark Johnson (1980) might suggest, the concept of mental movement in this case is likely a metaphor. Remember also that Descartes and Elisabeth were wrestling with questions about the relation between the mind and movement. Elisabeth noted that bodily movement clearly requires some kind of contraction or extension of muscles, but she is puzzled at how the mind might be able to effect this, since, as Descartes had suggested in his *Meditations,* the mind and body are two different kinds of substances and cannot interact. Descartes proposed that there was some kind of reciprocal interactive movement between animal spirits and pineal gland — so that 'that the slightest movements which take place in it [the pineal gland] may alter very greatly the course of these spirits; and reciprocally that the smallest changes which occur in the course of the spirits may do much to change the movements of this gland' (*The Passions of the Soul* [1649]). Today, of course, talk of animal spirits just won't do it.

Deafferentation and conscious movement

So how is this idea of the mind-movement relation explained today? Let's turn to some experts on movement and see what they say. First, let's go to Chicago where I've been participating in some ongoing experiments with Jonathan Cole in David McNeill's gesture lab at the University of Chicago. The experiments involved Ian Waterman (sometimes referred to as IW in the experimental literature). As we mentioned in Chapter 2, IW is a person who has lost proprioception (sense of posture and limb position) and touch from the neck down. This extremely rare condition is referred to as deafferentation (Cole 1995). Taking a close look at this case may help us to understand something about how consciousness and movement interrelate.

Ian's condition is the result of an illness he had at age nineteen. The result of the illness was damage to the large peripheral nerves that carry information about touch and proprioception to the brain. Ian is still capable of movement and he experiences hot, cold, pain, and muscle fatigue, but he has no proprioceptive sense of posture or limb location. Despite the initial loss of motor control that came with this, Ian regained controlled posture and movement but in an entirely different way from normal, specifically by consciously monitoring his body. Prior to the deafferentation he had normal posture and was capable of normal movement. When he lost proprioception, however, he was unable to sit up or move his limbs in any controllable way. For the first three months, even with a visual perception of the location of his limbs, he could not control his movement. In the course of the following two years, while in a rehabilitation hospital, he gained sufficient motor control to feed himself, write, and walk. He went on to master everyday motor tasks of personal care, housekeeping, and those movements required to work in an office setting.

To maintain his posture and to control his movement Ian must not only keep parts of his body in his visual field, but also consciously think about postures and movements. Without proprioceptive and tactile information he neither knows where his limbs are nor controls his posture unless he looks at his body. Maintaining posture is, for him, an activity rather than an automatic process. His movement requires constant visual and mental concentration. In darkness he is unable to control movement; when he walks he cannot daydream, but must concentrate constantly on his movement. When he writes he has to concentrate on holding the pen, and on his body posture. Ian learned through trial and error the amount of force needed to pick up and hold an egg without breaking it. If his attention is directed toward a different task while holding an egg, his hand crushes the egg.

Jonathan Cole has been Ian's neurophysiologist and co-experimenter for several years. Together with a number of researchers around the world they have been investigating basic bodily movement. I had a detailed discussion with Jonathan Cole about Ian's condition.

SG: You are here in Chicago conducting experiments with Ian Waterman. Ian is someone you wrote about in *Pride and a Daily Marathon* and he continues to be the subject of much study, by you and other scientists. He lost proprioception and the sense of touch below the neckline and has profound difficulties with movement. Specifically his control of movement is almost entirely conscious, in a way that is quite different from normal. You are still finding things out about Ian. What is the latest?

Cole: I've known Ian, IW, for over twelve years now, and the work we did was neurophysiological to start with. Some more philosophically influenced studies, as you know, came later. And then, partly because he was busy with his own work, for a while we did little, although I meet Ian frequently. But then it just happened that one or two other projects came up. One of them is how Ian orders and perceives his action in various different ways.

The general question is when you make a movement, how do you know that you made it. You need feedback, but what forms of this are available? One is visual. The other is feedback of movement and position sense, which we get from the moving part itself.[1]

Ian does not have movement or position sense. So when he orders a movement, how does he know that it has occurred? Most of the time he uses vision, but vision is insufficient for several reasons. First, it is too slow to control movement. Secondly, his visual attentiveness is probably insufficient to explain how he can walk, because he is unable to think about all aspects of walking and unable to see all the joints that he uses. In everyday life vision is insufficient, and it certainly is in experiments where we turn out all the lights!

---

1   Charles Phillips, in Oxford, was always careful to talk about movement and position sense, rather than proprioception, because some people understand proprioception to be a form of conscious perception, while for others it is not necessarily solely conscious. As Henry Head said, we don't know the position of each muscle spindle in terms of its stretch or joint position. Everything is presented to consciousness in a form in which we understand it. So we know the arm position or where the thumb is; we don't know the angles and joints, etc. (Phillips 1985; Head 1920).

In a lot of experiments we are trying to look at how precisely he can order movement and then produce it without feedback. In other words the central programs of movement that Chris Frith, Dan Wolpert and Chris Miall amongst many others are investigating. With Ian's permission we can remove visual feedback and look at his movement.

SG: What do you see when you do that.

Cole: We know, from work in Howard Poizner's lab, that if we ask Ian to point to a position in mid-air, with vision he is more accurate in returning to it than controls. In some other experiments he outperforms control subjects, because he has to be so accurate in daily life.

In an experiment with Chris Miall (Miall and Cole 2007), which is somewhat similar to an experiment that we did publish with the Quebec group at Laval (Nougier et al. 1996), we asked Ian to hold a gearstick in his fist and move the wrist backwards and forwards in nine positions. He did not see these positions, and there was no friction in the device. We just said, 'Ian, go from one to five to seven to eight to three.' We expected that if he started at position 2, with a given error, and we asked him to go to position 4, he'd put in a command to move two positions, and reproduce the same error, since he was coding for a set amplitude of movement each time.

We found that he was using an amplitude model, which we anticipated, so he could only be accurate at the end if he was accurate at the beginning. But at the extreme positions, at 1 and 9, he was more accurate than we might have expected, and in the middle he was slightly more accurate. So Chris Miall talked of 'cardinal positions' which Ian reached slightly better than we'd anticipate on a purely amplitude model. He reached the midpoint slightly better than other positions, regardless of where he started. By recording surface EMG from the forearm muscles we showed that he knew that when he is not activating either the flexion or the extensor muscles of the wrist, then the wrist relaxes ...

SG: Your wrist goes to the midpoint.

Cole: Exactly. The anatomical position of rest will be in the middle. It's a pretty stunning thing for Ian to have discovered on his own and shows his attentiveness to movement.

Normal subjects with proprioception move in a way that requires little or no attention directed at the body itself. When I walk across the room, or sit down, or stand up, or reach for a glass, my attention is primarily directed to my surrounding environment or some object in that environment. In Ian's case, however, he has to use conscious (and primarily visual) attention to control his movements. That's why Jonathan suggests that Ian *discovered* this in a very literal sense. Ian has had to relearn movement, and conduct that movement in a way that is very different from someone who has proprioception.

What precisely is proprioception? Proprioception is a complex phenomenon and it means slightly different things in different disciplines (see Gallagher 2005).

> *Proprioceptive information (PI).* Neuroscientists understand proprioception as an entirely subpersonal, nonconscious function—the unconscious registration in the central nervous system of limb position and posture. In this sense, it results in information generated in physiological (mechanical) proprioceptors located throughout the body, sent to various parts of the brain. This information is essential for the control of movement without the subject being consciously aware of that information.

> *Proprioceptive awareness (PA):* Psychologists and many philosophers view proprioception as a form of consciousness. One is said to be proprioceptively aware of one's own body, to consciously know where one's limbs are at any particular time as one moves through the world. If I ask you to close your eyes and point to your knees, you should be able to do it, because you have some kind of awareness of where your movable body parts are by proprioception.

We can refer to both PA and PI as somatic proprioception since they are generated by the same proprioceptive peripheral mechanisms delivering signals to the brain. Since PI is nonconscious and PA is conscious, and shared neuronal resources generate both, it is clear that proprioception signifies one of the specific areas where the distinction between phenomenal consciousness and physical body gets redefined. On the model of embodied movement that we are discussing here, these two aspects of proprioception are fully integrated, and this is entirely non-mysterious given they have the same neural underpinnings.

But this is not the end of the story. Although Ian has neither PI nor PA, he does have another kind of proprioception. The term 'proprioception' is taken in a much wider sense by Gibsonian psychologists. According to this view, proprioception is generated in any modality of perception (vision, touch, hearing and so on) that delivers a corresponding sense of body position relative to the environment, or a corresponding sense of self. This is sometimes called 'ecological proprioception'. For example, when I see an object in front of me (or to my right, or to my left) the visual information contains information about where my body is located, and perhaps even whether I am standing or sitting. Ian does have this sort of proprioception, and it is something that is clearly important for his own sense of posture and movement.

The kind of information and awareness that proprioception delivers, whether we are talking about somatic proprioception or ecological proprioception, is information about the self, and a primitive form of self-awareness (see Gallagher and Meltzoff 1996). The Cornell University psychologist Ulrich Neisser (1988) calls this the 'ecological self'. In this wider sense, a primitive or minimal sense of self depends on integrating different modalities of sensory information concerning one's own body as a moving agent in the environment, with the intracorporeal information provided by an internally generated sense of posture and movement (Trevarthen 1986).

In case you are missing the philosophical significance in all of this, note again that proprioception raises questions about where or how precisely to draw the line between consciousness (proprioceptive and kinaesthetic awareness) and non-conscious (sub-personal) processes that both condition one's possible bodily movements. Not only 'where to draw the line' but how things (causally) cross that line. It also gives us some clues about where to draw the line between self and non-self. In effect, we can see in just these brief considerations about proprioception that it plays an important role in how we need to think about consciousness, embodiment, and self.

Let's also note that despite the absence of proprioception and touch, there is obviously no paralysis, and no lack of motor command in Ian. That is, Ian can decide to move his body, and then move it. This involves processes in the brain that are generally referred to as *efference* processes (proprioception, in contrast, is referred to as *afference*, i.e., information coming into the brain; efference means information that the brain is sending out through the motor system). It's also important to note that when my brain issues an efference signal to my muscles instructing them to move, there is a duplicate signal (usually referred to as 'efference copy') that is sent back to certain areas of the brain to register the fact that I am moving. On one model of motor control, efference copy is matched up with the sensory (proprioceptive, visual, etc.) feedback that we get from our actual movement (in a brain mechanism called a 'comparator') in order to confirm that we have accomplished the movement that we intended.

Let's go back to Chicago.

> **Cole:** Ian has explored movement in a way I don't think anyone else ever has.
>
> **SG:** And from the inside—well not quite from the inside, since it depends on vision rather than proprioception.

Cole: He always presumes that the movement commands he makes will lead to movements, unless some scientist comes along to stop them. But he wouldn't know without vision or without the position sense he still has in his neck, or in his inner ear [that is, the vestibular sense that is important for balance].

SG: Would you say that the efference copy of the motor command constitutes a bit of feedback to him? He generates movement, but he can't match the efference copy up with anything since he has no sensory feedback, unless its vision.

Cole: This has intrigued me for years. I am not convinced that he has any conscious knowledge of efference copy.

Here, to be very clear, no one is actually conscious of sub-personal processes that are going on in the brain. Jonathan means that Ian has no conscious way of using feedback that might have been generated by the neuronal signals that constitute efference copy. Efference copy is down stream of M1. Ian will be aware of choosing and ordering movements upstream and seems from PET experiments to use conscious visual imagery, to close the loop, which is of course conscious.

Cole: In a PET study (brain imaging study using positron emission tomography), Ian opposed thumb and fingers in turn, with and without visual feedback. When he was moving, but saw a still hand [on a video inside the PET scanner], Ian activated several areas more than control subjects. There was frontal activation, suggesting the top-down [consciously controlled] way he produced the movement with attention and a cognitive load more than say, you or I. He also activated areas of bilateral cerebellum, and a posterior parietal area. This latter area was also activated more than controls when he saw the hand being moved, or when he saw the hand being moved and he made the movement himself. It has been suggested by some PET experts at the Functioning Imaging Lab at the Institute of Cognitive Neurology in London, that this is an area for efference copy. But Ian doesn't have the comparator — that is, in the situation without vision there is no sensory feedback to compare with efference copy. So I'm not sure, and we haven't published this work because we don't know exactly how to interpret it, why an area that doesn't have the comparison going on should be more active in Ian than in controls.

SG: Could it be that the comparator area simply keeps looking for something that never arrives?

Cole: We agree with your suggestion, but do not have a more formal theory at present.

SG: What of Ian's ability to time movement?

Cole: We are looking at timing in various ways. Pierre Fourneret in Lyon, with Marc Jeannerod, has two nice experiments. One is relatively simple. You have a gearstick and you move it to an external command, in various directions. What you see is a virtual gearstick with a hand. You decide whether the movement seen is the one you have made, in other words, whether there's a mismatch between what you see and what you do. The mismatch can be either in the timing of movement or the direction of movement. For the timing experiment a delay is introduced between when the virtual movement occurs and when the subject moves himself. Ian's perception of the timing of action is as good as controls.

SG: Ian has a great deal of practice in regard to explicit consciousness of his movements. By the way, what you call a *gearstick* the French call a *joystick.* Isn't this a telling difference between British neuroscience and French neuroscience? British neuroscience likes to test mechanisms and the French like to think they are testing life itself, no?

Cole: [who seems to take my remark seriously] I think this was fairer a few years ago than now. I was taught to isolate what one was testing, by say immobilizing a single joint and looking at responses to movement at that level only. In France they might look at the whole organism more. Now I hope each of these approaches has learnt from the other. More prosaically and personally I don't play computer games and so have never used a joystick!

SG: Sorry for the digression. Back to the experiments.

Cole: The other experiment was to trace a line by hand on a flat digitized screen with visual feedback given by a cursor moving across a computer screen. Subjects were led to believe that the cursor corresponded to their real movement. In fact we introduced a directional perturbation so that to move the cursor straight ahead they actually had to move to one side. The subject has to say how he moved, and this is compared with his actual movement.

SG: Yes I've tried a version of this experiment as a subject myself.[2] It sets up a conflict between vision and proprioception, and vision tends to win out over proprioception. Fourneret and Jeannerod (1998), I know, used this paradigm to test schizophrenics. But you used it to test Ian and another deafferented person, GL. So I assume they experienced no conflict.

---

2   It's based on an original experiment designed by T. I. Nielsen (1963). The apparatus he used is still in Copenhagen and Jesper Brosted Sørensen has designed some new experiments using it (see Sørensen 2005). For more on the Fourneret and Jeannerod (1998) experiment, see below.

Cole: In GL the results suggest that she is less aware of where she's gone than control subjects, who realize that they are being deceived, although they perceive only about half the bias that the are actually given (Fourneret et al. 2002). We do not have Ian's results from this yet, but I anticipate they will be different to GL's. Ian probably codes for movement position as well as timing, and he may be aware of mismatch more. Ian, on the whole, is rather better at mismatch recognition than control subjects in experiments.

SG: Part of the reason for this is that most of his movement is under conscious control.

Cole: Yes. We did an experiment using transcranial magnetic stimulation (TMS) of his brain and asked him to make a movement (Cole, et al, 1995).[3] The movement may have been one of four muscles, to move the thumb, the first finger, the little finger or to extend the wrist. If you do a TMS at high intensity it will produce a twitch movement. At threshold you will get a movement 50% of the time. But if the subject moves himself, then the TMS threshold goes dramatically down because you are facilitating motor neurons by your conscious command. We tried to find out what muscles Ian was facilitating when he tried to move the thumb. So we said, 'Ian move, 1, 2, 3, go' and just as he was moving on 'go' we would superimpose TMS. Then we looked at the twitch that was the result (at around 20 ms. or so, whereas a voluntary movement takes much longer). We were therefore looking at the focus of his cortical movement control, probably at the motor cortex level. It appears that when you or I are asked to move the thumb, we actually facilitate other muscles around the thumb although we don't move them.

SG: We are bringing them along to threshold too.

Cole: Yes, they twitched too, but less, than the target muscle. Our focus of motor command is relatively broad. When we asked Ian to move his thumb, in contrast, he facilitated just the thumb muscle movement. Ian, in relearning movements, has learned to move in a more focused way. More recently we reproduced the experiment with Ian with John Rothwell and found the same results, 10 years later, which was gratifying.

---

3   Here is a 'Copyleft' (i.e., freely available) explanation of TMS from Wikipedia (http://en. wikipedia.org/wiki/Transcranial_magnetic_stimulation): 'Transcranial magnetic stimulation (TMS) is a noninvasive method to excite neurons in the brain. The excitation is caused by weak electric currents induced in the tissue by rapidly changing magnetic fields (electromagnetic induction). This way, brain activity can be triggered or modulated without the need for surgery or external electrodes. Repetitive transcranial magnetic stimulation is known as rTMS. TMS is a powerful tool in research and diagnosis for mapping out how the brain functions, and has shown promise for noninvasive treatment of a host of disorders, including depression and auditory hallucinations.'

Then we asked him to just imagine moving the thumb. When we tried it, this was Louis Martin and I, we couldn't actually imagine moving the thumb in a way which led to reduced TMS threshold for a twitch; we couldn't imagine and selectively activate the motor cells. Ian's imagining led to facilitation of the muscle that he was asked to move alone, though at a higher TMS threshold. Sometimes we would have Ian watching the thumb and sometimes not, and we would be doing dummy runs in which we would discharge the [TMS] coil, which you can hear, over the scalp, or sometimes the dummy run would be further off, so you would hear the shock, but there would be no TMS current induced in the brain. When we asked him to imagine moving a thumb and we actually discharged a small pulse through his brain, we got a twitch. One time he looked at his thumb and said 'I didn't do that. I didn't order a movement, I imagined the movement.' And he was very indignant that it had moved.

We have also asked Ian, without looking, whether he was aware of moving when we had produced a twitch movement with TMS (Cole and Sedgwick 1992). He was not. So we activated his motor cortex without him being aware of it. This might be an argument against efference copy reaching consciousness [i.e., generating an awareness of movement] (without there being a mismatch). But we couldn't make strong claims about that, because we don't know what the effect of magnetic stimulation is on perceptual process.

SG: It complicates your interpretation.

Cole: Yes, you don't know if TMS wipes out in the perception of motor efference or not.

Body schemas

Jonathan and I have attempted to explain Ian's condition as an impairment of his body schema (Gallagher and Cole 1995). The body schema is the system of dynamic sensory-motor capacities that function without awareness or the necessity of perceptual monitoring, to regulate posture and movement. Defined in this way, the concept is somewhat abstract and in need of some detailed explanation of how it works. Proprioception is one major contributor to the body-schematic system, providing information about where one's limbs are. For example if you're thirsty and wanted to reach for the glass of water on the table in front of you, you would have to locate that glass, and you would normally do that by vision (although you could also haptically feel your way around to it). Once you know where it is you simply reach and pick it up. If there is no complex pathway that you have to take in order to reach the glass, you may even be able to glance at it and then reach as you look at something else. In this process the one thing that you don't have to do at the conscious level is locate your hand. That's because proprioception is telling your brain where your hand is—or less metaphorically, your brain is constantly registering proprioceptive information about how your body is positioned. This registration is an important part of the body schema system since somewhere in the organism the whereabouts of the organism's parts have to be 'known'. If that were not the case (as is the case with Ian) then after I located the glass, I would then have to locate my hand consciously and make a plan to get it from wherever it is to the glass. The consciously determined plan that Ian has to make in order to reach the glass is not something that someone with normal proprioception has to draw up. Rather, again at the level of the body schema, a plan, or what some theorists call a motor schema, is automatically generated or called forth to guide the trajectory of my reach, to guide the shaping of my grasp, and generally to control my movement—and all of this happens without me having to consciously attend to that movement. Although, of course, I may know and have a conscious experience of what I am doing (if you asked me, I could say that I'm reaching for my drink), in fact, I am not aware of much of the detail of that movement. For example, if I am reaching to pick up a glass my grasp shapes itself differently than if I am reaching to pick up a cup; and if I am reaching to pick up a glass to take a drink, my grasp is shaped differently than if I am reaching to pick up a glass to wash it. In these types of movement, however, I have no awareness about the different postures my fingers take, or the slight adjustments in arm trajectory that are involved.

Body-schematic processes, then, are on-line, dynamic sensory-motor processes, where 'sensory' includes intermodal sensory inputs such as proprioception, vision, touch, vestibular signals for balance, etc. The motor part involves motor commands, motor schemas, efference copy, forward control mechanisms to predict and adjust movement for success, and so on. Because the sensory aspects involved in movement are intermodal, that is, because proprioception communicates with vision, and vice versa, and the same for touch and vision, touch and proprioception, etc. the loss of proprioception and touch changes the way the visual system works for Ian. Ian makes the conscious visual system do most of the work, taking over the duties of proprioception and some of the duties of touch. Learned motor schemas may not persist indefinitely and it's possible that in order to maintain them they need to be refreshed by use and the resultant feedback. Thus, although Ian had built up a set of motor schemas in his life prior to his illness, even if they continued to exist, perhaps in a less robust way, the loss of proprioception means they were no longer accessible for him in the normal way. Whether he activates such schemas using vision is not clear.

Jonathan mentioned some experiments conducted in Lyon in Marc Jeannerod's lab at the *Institute de Sciences Cognitives*. Let's go there and see what Marc has to say about schemas.

> **SG:** In your work you have used the concept of a motor schema as a way to talk about very specific aspects of motor control. Such schemas are the elements of higher-order representations of action. In the transition from the level of motor schema to the level of action representation, do we somehow move from something that is automatic to something that is intentional?

> **Jeannerod:** First, I should say a few words concerning the concept of schema. This is a very old concept in neurophysiology. People in the second part of the 19th century, like Charlton Bastian, held that past actions were stored as 'conceptions of movement' in the sensori-motor cortex, ready to be used when the same actions were reinitiated. Later, the terms 'motor engrams' and finally 'motor schemas' were used. As you see, this concept comes close to what we would now consider as motor representations. More recently, in the hands of Tim Shallice (Norman and Shallice 1986) and Michael Arbib (1985; Arbib and Hesse 1986), the concept of motor schema has evolved into more elementary structures which can be assembled to form representations for actions. In other words, the concept of schema is a way of describing the lower levels of a motor representation: it is a way of breaking through the levels and going down to the most elementary one, perhaps at the level of a small neuronal population.

> I'm presently interested in characterizing the motor representation in no more than two or three levels. Below the lowest of these levels, there must still be other levels, perhaps with schemas, but this description goes beyond my present interest. The most elementary level I am investigating is that of automatic action, which allows people to make actions with fast corrections and adjustments to a target. Although we can do that very well, we remain unaware of what is happening, until the target is reached. Above this level there is another one where people are able to report what they have done. They realize that there was some difficulty in achieving the task—that they have tried to go left or right, that they had to make an effort, or that they have tried to do their best. Finally, there is a level where people try to understand the reason why that particular action was difficult. In experiencing a difficulty in completing the task, they may ask themselves if it was a difficulty on their part, or a difficulty from the machine, or a difficulty from someone else controlling their

hand. These questions are closer to the issue of self-consciousness than to that of mere consciousness of the action.

There are a number of possibilities for studying these levels, including in pathological conditions. This is how we came across Chris Frith's theory of central monitoring of action (Frith 1992), where it was stated that particular types of schizophrenic patients should be unable to consciously monitor their own actions. We've demonstrated that such patients do have a functional action monitor: they know what they do and they know how to do it. They are able to resolve rather complex visuomotor conflicts that have been intro-duced in the task to make it more difficult. However, they appear to fail at the upper level, which makes them unable to understand where the perturbation comes from—is it coming from their side, or from the external world, or from the machine? Of course, this type of information can only be obtained by posing the right questions to these patients; simply looking at their motor behavior is not suffi-cient.

Coming back to your question on the schemas, the examples above show that the levels of representation of the action, as I have outlined them here, cannot be broken down into schemas—or, at least, schemas become irrelevant in this context.

SG: Instead of schema, is there no other word that you would use? Would you just have to look at each case and ask the best way to describe it?

Jeannerod: Yes, and that's the difficulty.

SG: And it would depend on whether you are asking about an instance of agency as opposed to an instance of simply trying harder to correct action in an experimental situation.

Jeannerod: Yes. Let's discuss agency later. Let us first examine the automatic level, where the action seems to go smoothly by itself, and where there is very little consciousness of the action.

Fourneret and I designed an experiment where subjects had to reach a visual target by tracing a line on a graphic tablet. The display was such that they could not see their hand, the only information they had was vision of the line and of the target shown on a computer screen. On some trials, a bias was introduced, such that, in order to get to the target, subjects had to trace a line deviating by the same amount as the bias. When they reached the target, the line they saw on the screen was thus very different from the line they had drawn with their invisible hand (Fourneret and Jeannerod 1998). For biases up to ten degrees subjects performed very well: they reached the tar-get and did not notice any problem—they were unaware that the movements they had made with their hands were different from those of the lines they had seen. However, when the bias was increased beyond this value of 10 degrees, subjects suddenly became aware that the task was difficult, that they made errors in reaching for the target: as a consequence they consciously tried to correct for these errors. They were able to describe their attempts: 'It looks like I am going too far to the right, I have to move to the left, etc.'

This result contrasted very sharply with what we observed in a group of patients with frontal lobe lesions, whom we studied using the same apparatus. These patients had a typical frontal syndrome and were free of psychotic symptoms, like delusions, for example. The main effect was that they kept using the automatic mode as the bias increased, and never became conscious that the task was becoming more and more difficult and that they were making errors. This behavior was maintained for biases up to 40 degrees (Slachevsky et al. 2001).

At this point, it becomes tempting to make suggestions as to the brain structures involved in these mechanisms. First, one can assume, as many people would agree, that the automatic level is under the control of the parietal cortex; second, the above experiment indicates prefrontal cortex as the level where action is monitored. The question remains to know in which part of the cortex one would locate the mechanism for the third level, agency.

SG: So automatic action involves a nonconscious monitoring?

Jeannerod: We may have an experience of what we have done afterwards, but we are usually unaware of what we do when we are actually performing the action, of grasping an object, for example. In spite of being unaware of what we do, we make perfect adjustments of the fingers to the shape or the size of the object. Thus, the general idea is that part of our visual system drives our behavior automatically, with a minimal participation of the other part of the system which contributes to object recognition.[4]

SG: So when I reach for a glass, I may have an awareness of the glass, but I am not conscious of my reach or my grasp or what my fingers are doing.

Jeannerod: Yes, you are probably conscious of the fact that you want to drink, of the general purpose of the action. By contrast, you will

---

4 See Jacob and Jeannerod (2003) on the problem of two visual systems — one system for object recognition and another one for motor control. The book clarifies some of Jeannerod's claims here about what it means to act automatically, and to have no real subjective experience of the details of our actions. Also see Goodale and Milner (1992), and below for the discussion of the ventral and dorsal visual pathways.

become fully conscious of the action itself if your movement fails, or if the glass is empty. The question is how is it that the visual system can select the proper information (the shape of the glass) and transform it, unknowingly to the subject, into precisely adapted movements. Can we understand what it means to produce actions directed at a visual goal without being aware of that goal?

SG: Such actions would depend on motor representations, which are not yet motor images.

Jeannerod: It is difficult to speak of motor images at this stage, simply because an image, by definition, should be conscious. Yet, some people like Lawrence Parsons (1994) now tend to assume that there are two types of motor images. First, there are motor images that we create in our mind as conscious representations of ourselves acting. Those are the overt, conscious, images. But we may also use implicit motor image strategies for producing actions. The argument for assuming that these strategies indeed rely on some sort of motor imagery is slightly indirect: it is based on the fact that the time it takes to mentally make the action is a function of motor contingencies.

This point can be illustrated by an experimental example. Imagine that you are instructed to take a glass with marks on it where you are supposed to place your thumb and index finger. If the marks are placed in an appropriate position, the action is very easy, and the time to take the glass is short. If, on the contrary, the marks are placed in an odd position such that you have to rotate your arm in an awkward posture to grasp the glass, the action time increases. In the second part of the experiment, the glass is also presented with marks at different orientations, but, this time, you don't take it. Instead, you are instructed to tell (by pressing different keys) whether the action of grasping the glass would be easy or difficult. The time it takes to give the response is a function of the orientation of the marks, in the same way as for the real action (Frak, Paulignan & Jeannerod 2000).

The interpretation we gave to this result is that an action has to be simulated before it can be performed. This simulation process is made at a level where the contingencies of the action, like the biomechanics of the arm, are represented. The simulation will take longer in the odd condition than in the easy condition, as if the arm was mentally 'rotated' in the appropriate posture before the grasping movement is executed, or before the feasibility response is given. This rather complex process is entirely non-conscious.

In fact, our experiment expands the Parsons (1994) experiment, where subjects have to identify whether a hand shown to them at different angles of rotation is a right hand or a left hand. The time for the subject to give the response is a function of the angle of rotation of the target hand: this is because the subject mentally rotates his own hand before giving the response. In addition, the pattern of response times suggests that this mental rotation follows biomechanically compatible trajectories: obviously, we cannot rotate our hand in any direction without taking the risk of breaking our arm! Again, this process remains entirely non-conscious.

A strong argument in support of the hypothesis of mental simulation can be drawn from neuroimaging experiments: they show that the motor system of subjects is activated also when they think about a movement (a conscious process), or even when they attempt to determine the laterality of the hand they are shown.

Our discussion here raises a sticky question in the philosophy of mind. The question is whether we can describe sub-personal levels of brain function in terms that derive from the personal level of conscious experience. Here the details of mental simulation, which simply means consciously imagining something like rotating an object (without actually rotating it), are used to infer that there may be something like a sub-personal simulation involved in actual movement. It takes the same amount of time to imagine accomplishing the task as it takes to actually accomplish the task. But clearly this argument could go the other way. That is, if there is something like isomorphism between movement and the simulation (imagining) of movement, then one could certainly argue that our thought processes, our imaginings, are constrained by the sensory-motor contingencies of our embodied existence.

SG: Some of your work suggests that the hand is quicker than the eye in certain circumstances. More generally, consciousness lags behind the action. But that doesn't mean that consciousness slows down movement, or does it?

Jeannerod: Well, if you had to wait to be conscious of what you were doing, you would make your actions so slowly that you would be destroyed by the first enemy to come along. The idea is that the mechanism that generates fast and automatic actions is an adaptive one. Another example is the reaction to fearful stimuli: the body reacts, with an activation of the vegetative system, the preparation to flee, and it is only afterwards that you consciously realize what produced the emotion.

SG: Joseph LeDoux's work on fear and the amygdala (e.g., LeDoux 1998)?

Jeannerod: Yes, this is something you find in LeDoux's work. The purpose of the emotions is to activate the neurovegetative system, to warn the brain of the danger. Whatever the decision — to run away or to attack — it is taken implicitly.

SG: Yes, a good example of this occurred when I was attending a seminar at Cornell with a friend of mine. My friend got out of the passenger side of the car and found himself jumping over the car. He only then realized that he had seen a snake.

Jeannerod: That's a good example, because a snake is one of these things that we are attuned to fear. In our experiment with Castiello (Castiello and Jeannerod 1991; Castiello, Paulignan and Jeannerod 1991), the subject had to reach for an object as fast as possible. Sometimes, the object changed its location in space or its appearance (it became bigger or smaller) at the exact time where the subject was beginning his reaching movement. The subject was instructed, not only to reach for the object, but also to signal by a vocal utterance the time when he became aware that the object had changed. Even before we made the proper experiments for measuring this time to awareness, we had noticed that the people were already grasping the object when they told us that they had seen the change. When we made the experiments, we realized that subjects could report that a change had occurred only after a long delay, long after the movement had begun to adapt to that change. Indeed, this is just what your friend did when he jumped over the car before becoming aware of the presence of the snake. This is what we do when we drive a car and avoid a sudden obstacle: we become aware of the obstacle only later. We were able to measure this difference in time, which is something on the order of 350 msec. If you are driving a car and you wait until you become aware of the danger before you brake, do the calculation of the distance covered during 350 msec at 40 mph.[5] There is a great advantage of not being aware while you are doing something.

SG: Does consciousness, then, introduce something different into action? How is conscious movement different from non-conscious movement? The question I want to raise is whether this difference places qualifications on experiments when part of the paradigm is to call the subject's attention to what they are doing in regard to their movement.

Jeannerod: In regard to this distinction between doing things automatically and doing things consciously, I refer you to experiments

---

5   I did the math. 40 mph is 211,200 feet per hour. That's 3520 feet per minute, or 58.66 feet per second. That's .059 feet per millisecond, or 20.5 feet per 350 msec. So the disadvantage of consciously controlling your braking at 40 mph is that a safety margin of about 20 feet would be lost. The connection between these experiments and experiments conducted by Libet are discussed in Chapter 12 on free will. S.G.

made by Mel Goodale and his colleagues (see e.g., Goodale and Milner 1992). The typical experiment is that there is a target coming on, and you have to move your hand to that target. This is an automatic action. In a different set of trials, there is a target coming on, and you have to wait for five seconds before you move to it — time enough for consciousness to influence the movement. What they found is that the kinematics of the movement and its accuracy are very different for the two conditions. In the conscious movement, the velocity is slower and accuracy is poorer. This means that you have lost the on-line control of the movement, which works automatically: instead, you have used a system that is slower and is not adapted to doing automatic movement. The principle of the automatic movement is that it is based on a very short-lived representation. When you make a movement you have to keep track of the target to get to it, and then to erase the representation and to forget about it. You have to keep track of the target only for the duration of the movement in order to make corrections as needed. We can also use other systems, where the functions are stored for a longer time: it is possible to do movements that way, according to Goodale, by using the ventral visual pathway that indirectly reaches the motor centers through prefrontal cortex. Normally, we don't use this pathway when we do movements. As I said before, both the automaticity of the movement and the lack of consciousness of the motor process are essential attributes for behavior, because if we didn't use the regular pathway for actions (the dorsal pathway), our movements would be too slow. They would be late, and they would be delayed with respect to their expected effect. In addition, there would be a lot of useless information in the system.

We may experience this idea of moving in the wrong way (using the wrong pathway) when we learn actions that are difficult. We first try to control every bit of movement, until we learn to do it naturally and forget about how to move.

SG: The whole aim, and what we call proficiency in movement, is to move without being conscious of how one is moving.

Jeannerod: Yes to reach and grasp without paying attention to your hand, and so forth.

Representations

One of the most contentious debates in the philosophy of mind concerns the status of *representations*. This is a term used by many different theorists in many disciplines. One problem is that for every five theorists who use the term, there are at least six different definitions for that term. One is never (or almost never) sure what the word *representation* means in cognitive science or philosophy of mind. The more substantial issue is whether there are anything like representations involved in either action or cognition. There are some philosophers, like Hubert Dreyfus, who argue that one doesn't need representations at all, especially in regard to explaining skilled actions or expert behavior. Others, like Andy Clark, Michael Wheeler, and Mark Rowlands, argue for a minimalist notion of representation. The examination of the concept of representation rightly starts at the level that we are discussing here. Are there representations involved in movement? One might think from what Marc Jeannorod has just said that much of movement, when things are right, does not require anything like conscious control. But Marc goes on to talk about how representations are indeed involved in even this sort of movement.

Jeannerod: What I mean by a representation is not conscious in itself. It is built on the basis of all sorts of information. But of course when it's there, there is the possibility of accessing it consciously, although probably not all the aspects of the representation are consciously accessible. I don't see how we could become conscious of everything involved in it. I've had this discussion when I wrote my BBS paper on mental representations (Jeannerod 1994). One of the criticisms expressed in the commentaries was to question why I had called motor images what is simply motor memory. The commentators said that we can do an action, and then think about it, or reenact it: this would be nothing more than memory, and there would be nothing special about it. At this time, in 1994, I was already thinking that there is a difference between motor image and motor memory, but I did not have many arguments to defend this position. The arguments came later, when, with Jean Decety, we made neuro-imaging studies that told us that during motor images you have the same pattern of activation that you have during action. We found activation in areas like the dorsal prefrontal cortex and the anterior cingulate areas. But the most conspicuous activation was in the motor system itself, the system which is needed to really produce movements. I was thus comforted in the idea that motor imagination is more a covert action than something memorized in the classical sense. Motor imagery is just like action. When you are preparing to act or when you are about to start moving, you don't need to remember how you did it last time.

SG: You have shifted the kind of analysis you are doing away from motor schemas, but do you also want to give up this notion as a way of explaining representations? And if so, you would still want some way to describe the levels that are underneath representation. What would you substitute for the notion of schema in this regard?

Jeannerod: I think that the best way to think about this is in terms of networks. In order to implement an intention, for example, a specific neural network will be assembled, and this network will appear as a network of activation if you use neuro-imaging techniques. What has changed to motivate the theoretical shift from schemas to networks is that you never see the schemas, but you see the networks by using this technology. It is much more convenient to think of an assemblage of brain areas which will compose the network for imagining an action, or for building an intention, and so forth, because you really see these networks and then you can make sense of those ensembles. You can also elaborate further on possible overlap between networks, on possible distinctions between networks, and so forth. It is still not the final answer, of course, because those networks as we see them are static. The brain image is a snapshot of the brain at a certain time, during a certain task. What I would like now to have is a dynamic view of networks. If I could get something like this, then I think that networks would be the best answer to your question.

SG: Moving in that direction would make the problem of the explanatory gap clearer.[6] Because with schemas you had something of the same order as representations, I suspect. Intentionality was already in the schema, whereas if we refer to neural networks, we are talking about patterns of neurons firing, and there is a bigger jump to the level of representation. Is this right? Maybe, by giving up schemas, we make what we are doing more apparent, or make the problem clearer and more difficult at the same time.

Jeannerod: Yes, it may make it clear that we will never succeed in bridging the gap!

SG: So whereas schemas seemed to give us something to talk about between the level of neurons firing and the level of representation, if we do away with schemas, we get a much more complex level at the bottom, but it still doesn't add up to the representation. Unless you decide that the representation is nothing more than the neural network.

Jeannerod: That's discouraging, but I think I agree. But you know that the problem of levels of explanation is still open. As a neuro-

---

6   The 'explanatory gap', as we saw in the previous chapter, is a term coined by Levine (1983) to signify the brain-mind problem: how does something like a conscious mind get generated out of purely physical processes like neurons firing?

scientist I will try to understand how the networks are built, or how they can implement a representation, and that's it. Of course I agree that someone else should take over the explanation of the cognitive stage. I do it from time to time.

SG: And why not?

Jeannerod: The philosophers may be mad that I do it!

SG: But no one really knows how to solve that problem, so this is still a problem for everybody. Let me add that reference to schemas may lead us to think that we have an explanation where we really don't. So if we take away the schemas, and look, we see that the gap is still there, and it's not going to be filled up by schemas.

Jeannerod: It is true that the recursive property of the schemas was a way of getting closer and closer to the neuronal level, starting from the higher level of explanation. That was the message of Arbib and the philosopher Mary Hesse in their Gifford lectures (Arbib and Hesse, 1986). In their book, they explain how the schema theory can go from bottom up to explain the conceptual level.

SG: That is still just a model. One would use the vocabulary of schemas, or a different vocabulary, to formulate a cognitive model. In contrast, what you are talking about now, you can take a picture of it. The network is there in the brain, and your work is much more empirically informed.

Jeannerod: Absolutely. It is actually happening and it makes sense out of all that we know from previous studies in neurology, monkey studies, and so on, about distribution of functions in the brain. And connections between different areas. Now is there anything else to know once you have seen the network?

SG: Yes, then you have to work your way up and your way down. What is the nature of the representation? One way to explain the representation was by referring to the hierarchical integration of schemas. But now if you don't have the schemas, then what is the nature of the representation? Is representation just taking the place of the schemas?

Jeannerod: No. Perhaps it takes over part of the role of the schemas, but not everything. Now we have to find another explanation for connecting the networks into cognitive states. The schemas provided that, but in a way that was not very realistic, neurophysiologically. Even though the schemas provided the possibility of decomposing everything down to the single neuron level, and then up to the highest level, still that was a little metaphorical. In contrast, with the networks, especially if we get to the state where we see them dynamically and can see the circulation of information, this will become certainly a much better background. That's my hope.

SG: We still need models to continue the work and to explain what we're doing. But dynamic models will capture something more than can be captured in static models?

Jeannerod: There is an attempt, mostly by neurophysiologists, to understand the dynamics of the networks. This includes all this work (with electromagnetic recording techniques) showing the synchronization of different brain areas. Here in Lyon there is a group working on olfactory memory. They have shown that when a rat is presented with an odor that it can recognize, then synchronization between the olfactory bulb and the upper level of the olfactory cortex appears. This does not happen if the rat is presented with an odor that it had not experienced before. This is one of the first demonstrations that this synchronization between areas becomes effective when there is something more than a simple sensory stimulation. In this case, there is a sensory stimulation, plus storage, recognition, memory of information. So that might explain how the different areas that compose the network communicate with each other. That will not change the fundamental problem, however, since this is still the network level.

SG: Of course, at some point you have to name certain aspects of these neural networks, patterns or connections that constitute a restricted network. So why not use the term 'schema' to name some particular pattern that seems to correspond with a behavior. That would not be the same concept of schema that you were using before.

Jeannerod: No. And there is the problem of the temporal structure of nervous activity. There are no real attempts to conceive the temporal structure in the schema. The schema is a static thing, ready to be used. You take one schema, and then another, and another, and they add up to an assembly or a larger schema.

SG: So what is missing is a concept of the dynamic schema.

Jeannerod: Right. If the schemas become dynamic, as the networks begin to be, then okay, why not come back to the schema theory and try to relate schemas to the networks. Anyway, with the networks we first have to go underneath to get to see how they come to have vectors, how they change, how to understand the mechanics of the system. Of course, we also have to go higher up to understand how this network has been constructed at a certain time, and for a certain task.

SG: And also to see how one can have an effect coming from the higher level down, how an intention might activate a network. Is it a two-way causality?

Jeannerod: Yes, it is a two-way causality. And that's as far as we can go right now. We have this new concept, we have the tools to see the networks, to try to understand them. Also we have new paradigms, and this is an important point. The networks, as they can be seen through brain imaging, are associated with cognitive paradigms drawn from psychology, neuropsychology, and so on. And these are much richer than the sensory-motor paradigms that we used during the years of classical neuroscience. Now I think, having the new tools, having the new paradigms, having the new concept, this is a good time for moving forward.

Temporality and binding problems

Dynamic systems theory has been displacing good old-fashioned computational models as the *explanans* of choice in recent years. It's an attempt to capture the dynamic nature of the motor and cognitive systems that Jeannerod is talking about. Whether schema theory can incorporate a dynamic approach is an issue we will return to later (see Chapter 10). One other issue to consider here, however, is how all of these complex networks, schemas, or representations can be integrated in order to generate the smooth kind of movement that those of us with normal proprioception are capable of.

Not far from Lyon, the city of Marseille was home to another icon of French neuroscience, the late Jacques Paillard. It would have been easy to take the high speed train down to Marseille to get his views on this problem of integration. As it happens, however, my conversation with Jacques took place in Quebec where he spent some portion of the year working at the Université Laval, with GL. We've already mentioned her as a deafferented patient similar to Ian.[7]

SG: Do you think there is something like a binding problem for movement just as there is for perceptual consciousness?

Paillard: Oh yes, I believe that is so. This is a problem studied by me and some of my students. We are looking at the problem of binding in the premotor cortex to discover the significance of synchroniza-

---

7   I got to know Jacques well on my visit there, and in numerous encounters at academic conferences. I was sorry to hear of his death in 2006. We had recorded the interview but had never found the time to go over it. For that reason it was never published until now. See his website at http://jacquespaillard.apinc.org/. It contains an extensive bibliography and many papers online.

tion between different neurons associated with some kind of movement. This is the theory of the different parts of the brain operating in synchrony to generate a meaningful configuration of synchonized neurons that produce some functional output or that has an effect on the output of other processes.

SG: This would relate to motor coordination then?

Paillard: Yes. For example, we've conducted experiments to measure the capacity of people to make a synchronous movement of a hand and a foot (Blouin et al. 2001). When I asked subjects to move their hand and their foot at the same time I was surprised to see that the foot moves first, about 30 msecs. before the hand. Therefore I tried to measure reaction time for the hand only and then for the foot only. There is a difference of 30 msec between them indicating that the reaction time is shorter for the hand than for the foot. It was difficult to explain why when a subject launches a synchronous movement of foot and hand, the foot moves first. Moreover, in this situation the subject is completely unaware of this succession, because for him it is, or seems, a synchronous movement. We then made a special measure of the duration of what the subject can dissociate in terms of the difference between foot and hand, and in that case the difference is about 800 msecs where they could be sure that the foot comes first or the hand comes first. We next tried to make a synchronous reaction time of foot and hand to sound, an auditory signal, and in that case the hand comes first and the foot comes second, and in that case too the subject does not believe it or experience it as such. He has no idea that there is a difference.

So here we have a distinction and empirical differences between self-induced movement with a goal-image and pure rapid reaction to a signal. That was the beginning of many experiments on this problem of the difference between reactive and self-induced movement. The idea of the goal-image is involved here. We think that if one wants to make a synchronous movement one has to think of it and try to predict the sensory consequence of that action, and the sensory consequence that one wants to realize is a synchrony. And then we must have return afference from the foot and the hand in order that the synchrony is registered as such somewhere. We made the postulate that the cerebellum is probably the comparator for this process. We have confirmed in our imaging study, that the cerebellum reacts specifically for this situation of self-induced versus reactive movement (Blouin, Bard and Paillard 2004).

We also confirmed this with our deafferented patient, because she has no return afferent signal. In *both* situations, she reacts with her hand first and her foot second. I'll mention that just now we are testing a normal subject, vibrating the muscle of the hand, the wrist and the limb. In this case normal subjects behave like the deafferented patients. The hand always moves first and the foot second.

SG: Because the proprioception is thrown off by the vibration technique?

Paillard: Yes. Because the sensory consequence cannot be evaluated by the system. I don't know if that means that the goal-image is really built with that predicted sensory consequence of action. This is not new. Everyone says that we have this idea that the aim of a voluntary movement is to predict what we want to receive from the movement when it is executed. But this is a problem. It is probably a low level of goal, because I think that when we have an intention to do something, of course, we do not think in reafferent terms. But maybe the nervous system does. At the conscious level we want to pick up a glass, or whatever. But the motor system estimates distance and trajectory, and so forth. I mentioned the work we're doing but I also like very much what a younger British neuroscientist named Wolpert is doing (see, e.g., Wolpert, Ghahramani and Jordan 1995). He is taking a very original approach to this problem.

SG: Yes, he has developed what he calls a forward model of motor control.

Paillard: Yes, the building of feedforward units which involve this kind of prediction of sensory consequences. Before the Wolpert model we had no explanation of that. When I made this experiment for the first time, I had about 30 subjects making a simple action. And I tried with my 30 subjects to see what they were doing on the first try, and the second try, and the third, to see if there is something built and learned by this system. The answer is no. At the first trial, full accomplishment. No learning, nothing along that line. At that time we thought, and perhaps it is true, that before making the movement, some 'pre-test' would be made to the periphery, without movement of course, and this would be a testing of the pathway.

SG: Wouldn't that slow the complete process down by adding complexity to the movement?

Paillard: Yes, of course, but it is a very quick loop. We worked a lot on this issue because my chief interest in the beginning was with proprioception. I worked on this problem of physiological spindles and the gamma system, and the difference between the alpha and the gamma control of musculature. And my idea was that there is a possibility that we pre-test the state of the periphery by means of the gamma system, before the alpha system comes to work. And there are some demonstrations that this is true. Furthermore, I though at that time, that through the gamma system there is a nice test of the muscular state of the subject. I don't call it muscular tone, but physio-tone which fluctuates with the gamma innervation and is strictly dependent on your mental effort. You make a mental effort and there is some control of the activation level. All of proprioception con-verges in the reticular formation, and probably it contributes to maintaining a vigilant state. This kind of looping is involved in the problem of relaxation, and concentration, and those kinds of things. I think this gamma loop plays a role in relating the mental state to the tone of the musculature. Because actions involve a tension, and the tension is activated through that system.

SG: This is a better story than Cartesian animal spirits interacting with the pineal gland. The tension isn't necessarily conscious, is it? It is something that defines a sub-personal system. And at this level the system is prepared for action, or is vigilant, as you say.

Paillard: Yes. You know that every morning on the radio, we had in France this kind of 'l'réveil musculaire' — an awakening of the mus-cles, like an awakening of the brain. L'réveil musculaire was to make the gamma system active. Exercise would do the same thing. This was a topic that I worked on very much at the beginning of my career. Perhaps you have heard of the Hoffman reflex. I rediscovered it or reintroduced it into neurophysiology. It is called the H-reflex. Hoffman, at the beginning of the last century, made the discovery that when you stimulate a motor-sensory nerve, sensory fibers have a very low threshold compared to motor fibers. So at threshold you stimulate the high-speed sensory fibers that connect to the motor neuron monosynaptically.

SG: These are the high speed 1A sensory fibers located in various parts of the body delivering proprioceptive signals.

Paillard: Yes, coming from the spindle, transmitting the most rapid message in the nervous system, and this message directly activates the motor neuron.

SG: It seems that the coordination of movement is serving in some way our conscious awareness. In the experiment in which you ask the subject to make a finger movement in synchrony with a foot movement, then everything is ordered by the nervous system so that it consciously seems to the person that the movements are simulta-neous, even when they are not. The nervous system seems to be orga-nized to deliver the product in terms of the conscious requirements of the person.

Paillard: Yes that is true. The puzzle to me is going the other way. How is it possible for there to be a transfer between my conscious decision and the movement, from understanding the instruction to move, to this underground work of the nervous system to actualize this goal-image. I don't understand that!

SG: Yes, this was Descartes' problem too. How the willing to move accomplishes movement.

Paillard: Of course Wolpert would say that we have in the cerebellum a kind of feedforward unit, and we choose something in the repetoire. I don't know. It seems improbable that there is a table of movements waiting there.

SG: In one of your earlier papers (Paillard 1960), you talk about synthesis in the motor system, or synthesis in the brain. One hypothesis that you mention is that things do not come together in any one place, but that there is an integrative operation that results from the complex interplay between diverse functional areas of the cortex, and you talk about the richness of connections. By the way, my impression is that this is very early for a neuroscientist to be talking in this way—it've very contemporary. But then you go on to say that in experiments researchers have cut these connections and have separated the different parts of the brain from one another horizontally (not human brains I assume), and yet they still seem to integrate. In any case you suggested a vertical set of connections through subcortical pathways. Does that idea still stand?

Paillard: That was inspired by Penfield, who postulated a position different from that represented by the horizontal organization of the cortex given to us by Hughlings Jackson. Penfield took a different position and suggested that we consider the nervous system vertically, with the primitive part in the middle, and other parts developing radially out from this in a vertical organization. I found this interesting because it allows us to understand the segregation of functions, not only horizontally but vertically. I also had the idea from Colwyn Trevarthen, a good friend who spent three years in my lab in Marseille, when we worked together on the problem of focal and ambient vision (see Trevarthen 1970). I maintained contact with him, and he was very fond of this vertical organization.

SG: And this still has promise.

Paillard: Yes, I think so. Evolution is important to follow, because you can see in the evolution of the nervous system that it follows this kind of phylogenetic development. The natural part of this is motoric and is everywhere. It is involved in growth and in enthropy.

If the motoric is everywhere, so are motor theories of cognition and of language. We'll come back to these theories in later chapters. What is clear is that even if the mind is not reducible to movement, movement plays an important explanatory role in our cognitive life. Cognitive systems are not separable from motor systems.

Chapter Five

Moving into Action

Action is not reducible to movement. If movement itself is full of the complexities mentioned in the previous chapter, action is even more difficult to explain. This is especially true for cognitive neuroscientists precisely because action is not reducible to movement, or even a collection of movements, and yet in some sense the only thing that neuroscientists have to work with is movement—whether bodily movement or the movement of chemicals across a synaptic cleft. This seems clearly expressed in a position that Wolpert, Grahramani, and Flanagan (2001) have called 'motor chauvinism'.

> From the motor chauvinist's point of view the entire purpose of the human brain is to produce movement. Movement is the only way we have of interacting with the world. All communication, including speech, sign language, gestures and writing, is mediated via the motor system. (p. 493).

One cannot deny, of course, that movement plays an important role in all of this. This is one reason why it seems right to begin to think about the mind by thinking about movement. But if movement is not everything, and if an account of movement is not sufficient for an account of action, then what else is needed? The usual answer is *intention*. So what is intention?

Now from the very beginning we should be clear that there are two things that we need to distinguish: intention and intentionality. On the one hand, intention is something that seems directly implicated in action. Generally speaking, and in normal situations, if I intend an action, then I want it to happen. There are complications and exceptions to this. In some cases I may intend the consequences of an action without necessarily wanting to do the action. For example, I may want to remain in good health, and to do so I may engage in an exercise routine that I would rather not engage in, or undergo a medical test that I would rather not undergo. Still, to the extent that I voluntarily engage in such actions, I intend them. Likewise, I may want to engage in some action, and do so, but not want the consequences that come of it. Still, we can say that a movement is not an action unless it is intended, and this distinguishes it from involuntary or automatic movement such as reflex. On the other hand, the term 'intentionality' is usually reserved for the characteristic of consciousness that involves its directedness or 'aboutness', and is the sort of thing that Franz Brentano and Edmund Husserl talk about. All consciousness is consciousness *of* something — is *directed at* something or is *about* something.

John Searle indicates the importance of getting clear about these things in a 2000 interview.

> **Searle:** You've got to at some point sit down and explain what the hell is a belief, what is an intention, what is a desire. So I wrote another book, and this was the hardest book I ever wrote, *Intentionality*. It took me almost 10 years to write that book. ... 'Intentionality' doesn't just mean intending, but it means any way that the mind has of referring to objects and states of affairs in the world. So not just intending is intentionality but believing, desiring, hoping, fearing — all of those are intentional in this philosopher's sense. ... Then it seems to me you've got a lot of fascinating questions, and that's what I'm interested in. How do consciousness and intentionality work in the brain? How is it they function logically — what are the logical structures of these phenomena? How does one organism relate to the consciousness and intentionality of other organisms? (Feser and Postrel 2000, interview with Searle).

Given the distinction between intention and intentionality, we also should note that intention certainly involves intentionality. In part, any explanation of intentional action will have to involve an explanation of intentionality. Normally, when I intend to do something, and thereby engage in intentional action, I am also directed to something or, quite simply, have something in mind. So there is always an intentionality that characterizes intentional action. This is another way of saying that intentional action is goal-directed. The goal is not always an object. A simple action might be to get a book in the next room. But that may be embedded in a larger goal — for example, to show my friend a quotation from Descartes. That goal is something more than just retrieving the book. To explain how we can retrieve a book will be difficult enough. But to introduce the idea that we do it for a social purpose which guides our actions will be to introduce extra layers of complexity that cannot be reduced to a collection of simple movements. Whereas movement can be explained in purely physical, mechanistic, and sub-personal terms, action requires reference to a personal and intentional level.

One question here is whether intentional action always involves consciousness of one's intention. Of course psychology tells us that we don't always know why we do things, so that we are not always conscious of our true intention. There are many instances of self-deception, and other instances of confabulation that reinterprets our intention when in fact we are not aware that we are confabulating. Jean-Paul Sartre provides some wonderful examples of this under the heading of 'bad faith'. Let's say you are on a date with an attractive person and you decide to hold hands. Sartre describes a woman who goes on a first date with a man.

> She knows very well the intentions which the man who is speaking to her cherishes regarding her. ... But she does not want to realize the urgency; she concerns herself only with what is respectful and discrete in the attitude of her companion. ... If he says to her, 'I find you so attractive!' she disarms this phrase of its sexual background. ... But then suppose he takes her hand. This act of her companion risks changing the situation by calling for an immediate decision. To leave the hand there is to consent in herself to flirt, to engage herself. To withdraw it is to break the troubled and unstable harmony which give the hour its charm. ... We know what happens next; the young woman leaves her hand there, but she does not notice that she is leaving it. She does not notice because it happens by chance that she is at this moment all intellect. She draws her companion up to the most lofty regions of sentimental speculation; she speaks of Life, of her life ... (Sartre 1956, 55–56).

In this case, and more generally, the phenomenology of having an intention is not very clear. Normally, at any point during an action if I stop you and ask you what you intend to do you will likely be able to say what your intention is. If I ask you after you have completed an action you should also be able to say what you intended and whether you succeeded. The problem is that often the formation of the intention prior to the action is not clear. Precisely when do I form an intention, and do I do so consciously? There are times when I consciously deliberate and then decide to do something. Clearly we would want to call that a case of intention formation. But it is also possible for me to form an intention a week or a month earlier than when I act on it, and when I act on it, I may do so in an automatic way, seemingly without a current intention.

John Searle (1983) introduces an important distinction that is now frequently used in this context. He distinguishes between *prior intention* and *intention-in-action*. The former, for example, signifies an intention formation as the outcome of conscious deliberation, and this could occur just before or well before the action. Last week I decided to take a train to Paris, and today I get up thinking about what I should read on the train, and then, thinking about what I will do in Paris, walk to the station and get on the train without any further consideration of my decision. In some way my action of walking to the train station is intentional, but it's not clear that there was anything like a well-defined separate intention to walk to the train station. That seemed to be part and parcel of my prior intention to go to Paris, an intention that in terms of conscious decision was somewhat remote in time from my action, although fully informing it. Yet if you stopped me on the way to the train station and asked, 'Is your intention to go to the train station?' my response would certainly be 'Yes'. Likewise if you asked, 'Is your intention to go to Paris?' Intention-in-action is, as the phrase indicates, an intention that guides the action as I am accomplishing it. It's implicit in the action and I don't have to consciously consider my intentions as, for example, I walk to the train station.

Things are even more complicated when you think about language and thought. Some people believe that thinking is a kind of action, and that therefore one must have an intention to think (e.g., Frith 1992). But what sort of thing would that be? Elsewhere I put it this way: 'It is difficult to conceive of an intention to think prior to thinking itself, unless it is entirely a conscious preparation, as when I might decide to sit down and start thinking about this issue. In that case, however, the intention to think is itself a thinking, and an infinite regress begins to loom: do I require an intention to think in order to intend to think?' (Gallagher 2005, 180). And in regard to language, as Searle notes, 'The speech act is, above all, a conscious voluntary intentional act' (in an interview with Boulton 2007). But does this mean that we form an intention before we speak? It doesn't seem to me that we follow the rule that the nuns in my grade school used to give us: 'Think before you speak.' As Merleau-Ponty (1962, 177) suggests, speech accomplishes thought, and doesn't simply express it. That means that sometimes I don't know what I want or intend to say before I say it. At least in most conversations we don't find ourselves consciously pausing to form an intention to utter a speech act. On the other hand, we often say things like 'I didn't intend to say that', which suggests that often we do intend to say what we say.

The importance of intentionality

Back in Lyon, Marc Jeannerod's work shows the importance of the intentional level. Specifically, he shows that the goal or the intention of my action will really determine the motor specifications of the action. Goal-directedness is a primary constituent of action (Jeannerod 2001). This means not only that the most appropriate description of our actions is a pragmatic intentional one in terms of what I want to do or accomplish, but that the motor system accomplishes movement in those terms. In other words, the motor system is not simply a mechanism that organizes itself in terms of what muscles need to be moved, but it organizes itself around intentions. It designs the reaching and grasping differently if the intention is to take a drink from the glass rather than to pick it up and throw it at someone. For Jeannerod it is at that level of pragmatic intention that the system forms the motor-control representation. The representation is cast in terms of the intention or the goal. Moreover, this is something real, in the sense that it is not just that there are various levels of description that you could use to describe what is happening — although there are indeed different levels of description. Rather, the motor system is actually keyed into the intentional level.

SG: So the level of intention carries with it all the other levels, as if they were entrained by the intention.

Jeannerod: Right.

SG: So that is why it may be quite easy for the motor image to capture all of the details, to be framed in terms of intentional action, but to carry with it all of the motor details. This importance of the intention ties into what you call the 'paradigm-dependent response' (1997, p. 16), or what others might call the context-dependent response. The same stimulus might elicit different responses depending on the situation. The shaping of the grasp will depend on the intention, and simple actions are embedded in much more complex actions.

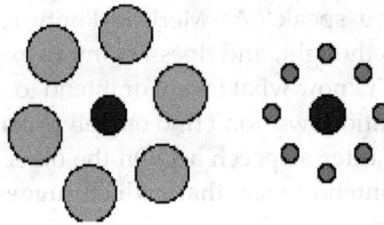

Figure 5.1 The Ebbinghaus-Titchener Illusion

Jeannerod: Yes. Complex goals or complex situations. This notion of context-dependent response could account for some of Melvin Goodale's findings on responses to optical illusions (see Aglioti, DeSouza, and Goodale 1995). Take the [Ebbinghaus]-Titchener illusion, for example (Fig. 5.1). Although the two central disks are exactly the same size you see one of them as larger than the other, because it is surrounded by smaller circles. But if you are to grasp one of those disks, you will adjust the grasp to its real size. So, when you simply look at the disks, your estimate is influenced by the visual context, but when you grasp one of them you focus on the goal of the movement, irrespective of the context, which becomes irrelevant.

SG: The context that guides the movement is pragmatic.

Jeannerod: In that case, yes.[1]

SG: I think that you in fact say that in the case of apraxic patients, their movement improves in more contextualized situations.[2] This is also something you find in Anthony Marcel's experiments where an apraxic patient will do much better at a particular movement (e.g., moving an object to her mouth) if it is contextualized in some meaningful situation (e.g., taking a drink) that they can understand. Or they do even better, Marcel says, in situations where they might have to do something with social significance. A movement that is mechanically equivalent is impossible for them in an experimental situation, but becomes possible for them in a social situation (Marcel 1992; see Gallagher and Marcel 1999).

Jeannerod: Yes, this is a common finding in neuropsychology, following the classical observations by Hughlings Jackson. There are things that patients with cortical lesions find impossible to do if you simply ask them to do a task, for example, pronounce a particular word. By contrast, this same word will be automatically uttered in the natural context of the use of this word. This 'automatic/voluntary dissociation', as it is called, is also observed in apraxic patients. If you ask them to pantomime an action like combing their hair or brushing their teeth, they will scratch their head or do funny things. But if you give them a toothbrush they will be able to perform the correct action. The idea, put forward by Marcel, that these patients are improved when the action becomes embedded in a context seems to represent a good explanation to this phenomenon. An alternative explanation is that executing an action upon request, or pantomiming that action (things that an apraxic patient cannot do) implies a *controlled* execution, in contrast to using an object in a normal situation, which implies an *automatic* execution. This difference is a rather

---

1   Note that we have just shifted the meaning of 'context' in these few lines. Jeannerod was talking about the purely perceptual context of one circle appearing to be larger than another, and so, regardless of that context the hand shapes itself appropriately. The pragmatic context that I refer to is the larger context pertaining to what I want to do with the object I reach for. Jeannerod understands the shift and agrees. From here on we are using the term 'context' in that larger sense.

2   Here is the Wikipedia definition of apraxia. 'Apraxia is a neurological disorder characterized by loss of the ability to execute or carry out learned purposeful movements, despite having the desire and the physical ability to perform the movements. It is a disorder of motor planning which may be acquired or developmental, but may not be caused by incoordination, sensory loss, or failure to comprehend simple commands (which can be tested by asking the person tested to recognize the correct movement from a series)'. (http://en.wikipedia.org/wiki/Apraxia)

radical one, if one considers that the neural systems involved in initiating the action in these two situations might not be the same, with the implication that, in apraxic patients, the neural system for initiating a controlled action might be damaged.

SG: You make a distinction between the *pragmatic* and *semantic* representations for action (Jeannerod 1994; 1997, p. 77), which is independent of the anatomical distinction between dorsal and ventral visual systems. The pragmatic representation refers to the rapid transformation between sensory input and motor commands. The semantic representation refers to the use of cognitive cues for generating actions. In the contextualized situation there is more meaning for the subject.

Jeannerod: In a certain way, yes. But let's leave aside the distinction between semantic and pragmatic for a minute. Just take the dichotomy between the ventral and the dorsal visual systems. The dorsal route has been assigned a function in generating automatic execution. That would be the way by which an apraxic could correctly perform a movement that is embedded into a sequence and a broader whole. In contrast, the request that is made to the patient to purposively do this movement detached from any other context, would be where the person would have to do something that is detached from this automatic route. In my 1997 book I am a little reluctant to map the pragmatic and semantic distinction onto the dorsal and ventral systems, respectively. There are several examples where you may find signs of perceptual, conscious manipulation of information in the dorsal system. We demonstrated this in a PET experiment where subjects were instructed to compare the shape, size or orientation of visual stimuli, without any movement involved: we found a beautiful focus of activation in the posterior parietal cortex, in addition to the activation we expected to find in the inferior temporal cortex (Faillenot, Decety and Jeannerod 1999). So, the processing of semantic information uses the resources from both pathways, it's not located exclusively in the ventral system. I have reservations about these distinctions, but it is not a serious discrepancy between Goodale and me. It is just that I would like to keep the semantic representation for action on objects free from a rigid anatomical assignment. I am very reluctant to say that we have one part of our brain which works with consciousness, and that consciousness pertains to a specific area (the ventral system), while the dorsal part would work automatically without consciousness. My distinction between pragmatic and semantic modes of processing does not compete with the model of Goodale and Milner.

SG: With this in mind, you discuss an experiment that involves people imagining that they are driving through gates of different widths. As the gates get narrower, the driver will slow down, and almost come to a stop, even when the driver knows that the car will fit. So the greater the accuracy required for driving through the gate, the slower the velocity.

Jeannerod: In fact this experiment was done with Jean Decety, in a virtual setup (Decety and Jeannerod 1996). Imagine that you are walking through a gate. We showed the subjects gates of different apparent widths placed at different apparent distances in a virtual environment, so that the subjects had no contact with reality. What they saw were virtual gates, which appeared at different apparent distances with different apparent widths. They were asked to mentally walk through the gates as fast as possible and to report the time at which they crossed the gates. In fact, mentally walking through a narrow gate placed at a relatively further distance took a longer time for the subject than walking through a wider gate. The times reported by the subjects followed Fitts' Law.[3] This is an interesting result because Fitts' Law has been demonstrated in real movements performed in visual-motor situations, but in this case we showed that it was still present in mentally simulated actions. We realized that this is indeed true in real life situations. When you drive your car into your garage, for example, you behave in the same way: you go more slowly when the gate is narrow, and you drive faster when the gate is much wider than the car. What we learned in this experiment is that this property is retained even in a mentally simulated action. Paul Fitts considered this effect as a purely visuomotor effect, which he related to the limited capacity of information transfer in the visual channel. When the difficulty of the task increases (i.e., when the amount of information to be processed increases), he said, the movement had to be slowed down to preserve accuracy: to him, this was an automatic process. Now, we find it in a situation where the action is simulated, which means that the capacity of the visual channel and the difficulty of the task are also part of the central representation which guides the action.

Jeannerod is suggesting that action is constrained not only by one's intentions but also by the sensory-motor contingencies of the situation. Action has a top-down component—'I intend to drive my car through the narrow gate in the distance'—but also a bottom-up component directly tied to motor control. I may experience the effects of the latter insofar as I may

---

3 Fitts's Law states: The time to acquire a target is a function of the distance to and size of the target.

notice that the narrower the gate the slower I go. It may also be the case that when I am learning to drive there is some instruction that I should slow down as I go through a narrow way. More likely, if I go through it too fast even without hitting anything I scare myself and make adjustments the next time. The point is that the bottom-up sensory-motor contingencies that are set up by the physical and embodied situation, and that are measurable in objective terms, also figure into my intentions. I can take ownership for the behavior of slowing down as I move through the narrow gates and say, 'Yes, of course I intended to slow down; that's what one does in such circumstances.' Still, it is likely that this aspect is not an explicit component of my intention.

Representation revisited

Just here the issue of representation arises again. When Jeannerod talks about the difficulty of the task being part of the 'central representation' which guides the action, he means a neural representation. Hubert Dreyfus is well known for criticizing this notion, especially when it comes to representation in the case of skilled intentional action.

> A phenomenology of skill acquisition confirms that, as one acquires expertise, the acquired know-how is experienced as finer and finer discriminations of situations paired with the appropriate response to each. Maximal grip [a concept Dreyfus takes from Merleau-Ponty] names the body's tendency to refine its responses so as to bring the current situation closer to an optimal gestalt. Thus, successful learning and action do not require propositional mental representations. They do not require semantically interpretable brain representations either. (Dreyfus 2002, 367).

Dreyfus's anti-representationalist stance comes from his work on the philosophy of artificial intelligence. His understanding of the concept of representation follows a traditional account of that concept which he ties to a Cartesian epistemology (here Descartes is the problem maker again). On the traditional account, representation is characterized by the following aspects (based on Rowlands 2006, 5–10).

1. Representation is internal (image, symbol, neural configuration)
2. Representation has duration (it's a discrete identifiable thing)
3. Representation bears content that is external to itself (it refers to or is about something other than itself)
4. Representation requires interpretation—it's meaning derives from a certain processing that takes place in the subject—like a word or an image its meaning gets fixed in context

5. Representation is passive (it is produced, enacted, called forth by some particular situation; or we do something with it)
6. Representation is decoupleable from its current context.

As one investigates the way that action works, each of these aspects can be challenged, and or possibly eliminated (see Gallagher 2008). Rowlands, in a way that I believe is consistent with Jeannerod's desciption, goes some distance in rejecting the traditional idea of representation in action; Dreyfus goes all the way. So do Thelen and Smith, following a dynamic systems approach:

> We are not building representations of the world by connecting temporally contingent ideas. We are not building representations at all. Mind is activity in time ... the real time of real physical causes. ... Explanations in terms of structures in the head—beliefs, rules, concepts and schemata, are not acceptable. ... Our theory has new concepts at the center—nonlinearity, re-entrance, coupling hetero-chronicity, attractors, momentum, state spaces, intrinsic dynamics, forces. These concepts are not reducible to the old ones. (1994, 338–39).

Jeannerod, Rowlands, and others such as Andy Clark (1997; Clark and Grush 1999), and Michael Wheeler (2005), however, argue for a minimal-ist concept of representation. Here are some examples of minimal representation.

1) Clark (1997) and Wheeler (2005) speak of action-oriented repre-sentations (AORs). AORs are temporary egocentric motor maps of the environment that are fully determined by the situa-tion-specific action required of the organism. On this model, it is not that the AORs re-present the pre-existing world in an inter-nal image or that they map it out in a neuronal pattern: rather, 'how the world is *is itself encoded in terms of* possibilities for action' (Wheeler 2005, 197).

2) Clark and Grush (1999) propose that the anticipatory aspect in a forward emulator involved in motor control (the sort of for-ward-model of motor control discussed by Wolpert), specifically the 'internal' neural circuitry used for predictive/anticipatory purposes in a forward emulator, involves a decoupled represen-tation, which they call a Minimal Robust Representation (MRR). The circuitry is a model, a 'decoupleable surrogate' that *stands in* for a future state of some extra-neural aspect of the move-ment—a body position (or proprioceptive feedback connected with a body position) just about to be accomplished, e.g, in the action of catching a ball. Since the emulator anticipates (repre-sents) an x that is not there—a future x—or a predicted motor

state, it is in some sense off-line, 'disengaged', or certainly decoupleable from current x or the current movement.

3) Rowlands (2006) argues that what he calls 'deeds' or pre-intentional acts (for example, the positioning of fingers in catching a ball that is flying toward you at a high rate of speed or the movement of your fingers while playing Chopin's *Fantasie Impromptu in C# Minor* on the piano—namely, the sorts of movements that Jeannerod describes as non-conscious and determined by both the action intention and the constraints of sensory-motor contingencies) are representational.

All of these aspects of action count as representational insofar as they satisfy the following requirements (as indicated by Rowlands 2006, 113–14), which constitute a definition of minimal representation:

- They *carry information* about x (the trajectory, shape, size of ball, the keyboard), and perhaps they do so simply in terms of my possible actions.
- They *track* x or function in a way that allows me to accomplish something in virtue of tracking x.
- They can *misrepresent* x.
- They *can be combined* into a more general representational structure (I catch the ball and throw it back; I continue to play the music)
- They are *decouplable* from x (x may be absent from the immediate environment—e.g., I can later remember and demonstrate how I caught the ball replicating the same act)

It may be possible to show that AORs, MRRs, or pre-intentional acts satisfy some or all of these requirements, or fail to satisfy them, in which case the concept of minimal representation might fall to a Dreyfus-like critique. We'll leave this an open question here. But let's briefly discuss the last requirement, which I take to be part of both the traditional and the minimal concepts of representation—decoupleability.

Wheeler (2005, 217–19) defines an even more minimalist concept of representation by dropping the criterion of decoupleability from the list. Without going into the details of the rather complex argument he makes, the idea is that if we adopt a dynamic systems approach and the kind of self-organizing, continuous reciprocal causation (Clark 1997; Wheeler 2006, 251) that comes along with it (for example, the sort of thing that Dreyfus and Merleau-Ponty call maximal grip), one doesn't need a representational element that is decouplable. In fact, as I read it, the idea of decoupleablity *in* action is a strange notion. Consider, for example, Clark and Grush's proposal that the anticipatory aspect of the emulator or forward-comparator involves decoupleablity.

> [O]ur suggestion is that a creature uses full-blooded internal representations if and only if it is possible to identify within the system

specific states and/or processes whose functional role is to act as *de-coupleable surrogates* for specifiable (usually extra-neural) states of affairs. (Clark and Grush 1999, 8).

Let's think about their example of a representation in action in terms of catching a ball. If I am attempting to catch a ball that is coming toward me the emulator anticipates or predicts (represents), prior to any sensory feedback from vision or proprioception, the future movement of my body that will enable me to catch the ball, given its current trajectory (which, of course, predicts where the ball will be in the very near future). As a future state of my body, tied to a future location state of the ball, the proposal is that this anticipatory representation is decoupled from the current state of my body or location state of the ball. The emulation is 'working just one step ahead of the real-world feedback' (Clark and Grush 1999, 10), and reflects what Wheeler calls a minimal decoupleability (2005, 214). But it is difficult to see how an aspect of motor control that is a constitutive part of the action itself can be decoupled from current states of the body or the ball (or from the pragmatic context). Indeed, the anticipation or prediction of the future states requires a clear reference to the current posture of my body, and the present location state of the ball, and that means it cannot be characterized as being decoupled from either of these. If one were to decouple the emulative anticipation, it would cease to be part of a forward motor control mechanism, although it may turn into part of a more tradi-tionally conceived representation process — that is, we may use this system in an 'off-line' process like memory or imagination. But it is certainly not clear in what sense this sort of anticipatory emulation *in action,* as part of the online motor-control process of action, could involve going off-line or how it might be playing the part of a stand-in for something else. Even if it is working 'just one step ahead of the real-world feedback', it is also at the same time one step behind the previous feedback, and it depends on the ongoing perception of relevant objects in the world.

Eliminating decoupleability as characteristic of a process that is pur-portedly representational and intrinsic to action, opens the way to ask what other representational characteristics might be eliminated, and then to ask what precisely is left of representation in action. Again, we leave that as an open question here. But one thing we can say is that whether action is representational, minimally representational, or non-representa-tional (following Dreyfus or the dynamical or enactive cognition approaches, see e.g., Gallagher and Varela 2003; Maturana and Varela 1980; Noë 2004; O'Regan and Noë 2001; Thelen and Smith 1994; van Gelder 1995; Varela, Thompson and Rosch 1991), the concept of represen-tation should not be understood as essential for the intentionality that defines intentional action (cf. Rowlands, 2006, 1, 27). Intentionality is a wider concept than representation; although all representation is a form of intentionality, not all intentionality is a form of representation.

This is a basic phenomenological insight. Husserl and Merleau-Ponty refer to a form of non-representational ('founding' or 'operational') intentionality which characterizes action. Action is characterized by an embodied directionality towards the world that is not mediated by mental representations. This is where the rubber meets the road, as they say; it's the relation between action and the possibilities offered by the world, mapped out not in internal representational constructs, but in dynamic affordances. Husserl allows that there are certain cognitive states that are less direct, mediated by what he calls *Vergegenwärtigung* — a re-presentation of something, for example in memory or in the imagination, that originally was or could be presented in a more immediate way. His phenomenological analysis correlates well with the neuroscientific evidence that Jeannerod and others point to, namely, that when we imagine an action or visually imagine some object, the same neuronal areas responsible for action and perception are activated. Again, however, this does not necessarily mean that action (or perception) is representational; rather it suggests that we should consider remembering and imagining to be enactive processes that re-enact action and perception. We return to this issue later in our more detailed considerations about cognition (Chapter 10).

Spatial frames of reference

Action is something that is directed to some goal or task; it is characterized by intentionality that is not necessarily representational. The phenomenologists, from Husserl to Heidegger, to Merleau-Ponty, to more recent proponents like Dreyfus, Varela, Thompson, Zahavi, and others, would say that action is always in-the-world. What this means is that it is not generated outside of a context that is defined by the agent's embodied, situated context which always involves a surrounding environment that is taken as meaningful. What 'meaning' signifies here can be understood in terms of the possible actions I may take toward the object. An object, or a state of affairs, has meaning if I can respond to it in a certain way, if I can use it, or, negatively, if I have to push it out of the way because it is an obstacle to my action, or if it imposes a limitation or liability on my action. One relation that we have to objects in the environment that allows us to sort out their meaning, and that is intricately involved in action is spatiality. Spatiality may be defined, pragmatically, not as a characteristic of the environment, but as a certain relationship that is set up by my possible actions. Let's explore this idea with Jeannerod.

SG: Reaching and grasping are two different kinds of movement. You show that reaching is dependent on an egocentric or body-centric spatial framework, whereas grasping tends to be more allocentric or object centered.

Jeannerod: Well, I've changed my mind on this distinction. Initially, the idea was that grasping is independent of the position of the object and that a grasping movement was performed in the same way whether the object was here or there. I believed that specifically because the Sakata group in Tokyo had recorded neurons in the monkey parietal cortex which encoded the shape of an object to be grasped by the animal. They clearly stated in one of their papers that the neuron activity, which was specific for a particular object and for the corresponding type of grip that the monkey made to grasp it, was independent from the position of the object in space. That seemed a good argument to say that these types of distal movements (grasping) were under the control of an allocentric framework, i.e., unrelated to the relative positions of the object and the animal's body. Since then, with my colleagues here in Lyon, we have studied the action of grasping an object located at different positions in the work field. We found that, although the shape of the hand itself was constant for all positions, the shape of the whole arm changed from one position to another. We interpreted this result by saying that grasping is not a purely distal phenomenon, it also involves the proximal segments of the upper limb: the successful grasp of an object also involves an efficient posture of the arm. And when we looked at the invariant features of all these configurations of the arm across the different spatial positions of the object, we found that the opposition axis (i.e., the position of the two fingers on the object surface) kept a fixed orientation with respect to the body axis. This means to me that the final position of the fingers on the object is coded egocentrically.

In this experiment (Paulignan et al. 1997), we used an object (a cylinder) where the fingers could be placed at any position on its surface. Of course, things may become different if the object has a complex shape which affords fixed finger positions. In that case, there must be a tradeoff between the biomechanical requirements of the arm and the requirements introduced by the object shape. Just by looking at people in such situations, I have the feeling that we prefer to change our body position with respect to the object, rather than staying at the same place and using awkward arm postures. This is an indication that the organization of the distal part of the movement (the finger grip) is not independent from the organization of the proximal part of the movement (the reach).

SG: So this kind of action is framed in a body-environment relation where when any one element varies, the others do too. This qualifies the nature of the egocentric spatial framework, doesn't it? The ego-centric framework is neither egoic nor fully centered. The frame of reference is on the body but the part of the body on which a particular movement is centered might be articulated differently from one action to the next, or from one environmental setup to the next.

Jeannerod: The trouble with studies of visual-motor transformation is that they deal with the hand movement before the object is touched. These movements are organized in a body-centered frame-work. But visuo-motor transformation is a precondition for manipu-lation. Manipulation is no longer referred to the body: you can manipulate an object in your pocket, or you can manipulate it on the table, and manipulation would be more or less the same. In that case the center of reference of the movements is the object itself.

SG: So this seems a real dialogue between the sensory-motor contin-gencies of the body and the object in question. Doesn't intention enter into it again? The intention that I have, what I intend to do with the object, will define how I will actually grasp it.

Jeannerod: The relation of intention to the frame of reference is an interesting point. What the shape of the fingers encode during the visuo-motor phase of the movement is the geometrical properties of the object, like its size or its orientation. By contrast, what is coded when you recognize or describe an object are its pictorial attributes. The difference between the geometrical attributes that trigger finger shape, and the pictorial attributes that characterize the object inde-pendently from any action directed to it, is the difference between the pragmatic and the semantic modes of operation of the system. In the pragmatic system, after all, you only need some crude coding of object shape. Accessing to the meaning of an object requires much more than its geometrical attributes. This means that the content of the intention (or the representation) for pragmatic processing or for semantic processing, respectively, must be very different.

SG: In your book, you did say that even if the pragmatic and the semantic are two distinct systems, they are tightly coordinated.

Jeannerod: Yes, it is clearly demonstrated that connections, both anatomical and conceptual, exist between these two modes of functioning.

Causality, supervenience, and agency

An account of action that emphasizes the non-representational, dynamical processes that depend on an organism engaging in online, feedback-modulated adjustments in relation to the environment may be thought of as a purely causal account. Thus Thelen and Smith's suggestion: not only action but mind 'is activity in time … the real time of real physical causes' (1994, 338). This may seem completely opposed to more phenomeno-logical approaches that emphasize that mental processes are intentional processes that cannot be reduced to causal mechanisms. Moving from movement to action, we have suggested, involves seeing how intention-ality fits into the causal story; how the intentionality of a system modu-lates the subpersonal causal mechanisms and makes them do its work so that the movement gets entrained to the intention. Of course, this seems to be the same old problem that Descartes and Elisabeth were trying to work out. Can advances in neuroscience be taken as advances on this problem?

Here I play Elisabeth to Jaak Panksepp's Descartes.

> **SG:** How do we construe the relation between subpersonal neural or neurochemical processes that seem causal in nature, and the intentionality of action or the behavior that it motivates? Does a chemical change cause a behavioral change or does a behavioral change cause a chemical change? Are these reciprocal? Do we need to talk about upward and downward causality, or does that simply land us back in a dualism of mind and body? And make it 25 words or less!

> **Panksepp:** I think that behavior and mind, and the neurodynamics of the underlying brain systems, are different facets of a harmonious process. The complexity of the interactions of feed-forward (often bottom-up) and feed-back (often top-down) within organic brain-mind systems is so large that uni-dimensional, uni-directional views of causality become troublesome and ruthless reductionism becomes simple minded if not impotent. In the intact brain, it is always useful to think about circular, two way causal systems, with interactions among all levels. Still, the devil is in the details, and sci-entific analysis is still the best way to achieve lasting knowledge on such matters. I do think that, developmentally, the bottom-up con-trols exerted by emotional arousal (i.e., intentions-in-action) are most influential in the development of behavioral control and, with men-tal maturation, the top-down controls (i.e., intentions-to-act [prior intentions]) become ever more influential in resolving complex behavioral possibilities in the real world as opposed to the prison like environments of Skinner boxes. There is no dualism involved here, and I would not call one or the other level of control 'subpersonal'. I

think self-relatedness is deeply built into the neural matrix at all levels. There is a core-self that is necessary for the rich, cognitively aware personal aspects of our lives.

Many people who enjoy thinking about the full complexity of self-related processing—with all its artistic and humanistic aspects, full of rich human imagination—find talk about causality and reductionism highly aversive ways of conceptualizing things. I myself take a bit more of the middle ground, namely, that you can't do good science on basic, evolved emotional systems by trying to capture the full complexity of human emotional life in the laboratory; but without working out mechanisms in the brain research laboratory you can't have refined and replicable knowledge about the sources of mentality. Science can never describe 'the whole' but only 'the parts', but the whole must be reconstructed from those parts. Therefore, it's okay to talk about certain things causing other things but my personal view of causality, within the context of gentle reductionism, is better captured by dual-aspect monism or the philosophical concept of supervenience[4]—that there are layers of organization in the brain-mind (Paul MacLean [1990] provided an excellent approximation) and there are linkages between these layers of organization. A worthy aim of a biologically oriented mind-scientist should be to identify the main connections among brain layers—levels of organization within the mind.

Take for example the phenomenon of separation distress. It is clearly related superveniently to what's happening in certain neural systems. CRF (Corticotrophin Releasing Factor) will increase all the indices of separation distress. Therefore, when you actually go to a laboratory and you do a causal experiment, you manipulate the system, initially in regard to just one neurochemical factor, and if you find that one factor can shift the whole organism into a new mode of emotional processing, you have some confidence of at least one basic causal influence on a complex emotional state. That's not the only factor though. With all the remaining factors being unknown, we can't even estimate what percentage of the actual real-world variance might be explained by any single known factor; but at least we have a solid and replicable piece of knowledge, with profound implications for the species, including psychiatric implications.

If one possible way to study the interrelations between causality and intentionality is by investigating correlations between changing chemicals

---

4　Supervenience is basically the idea that a certain set of properties M (e.g., mental properties) of some system supervenes upon another set P (e.g., physical properties) of the same system, just in case M-properties cannot differ without also differing with respect to their P-properties. No M-difference without a P-difference.

and changing behavior, another is to look at cases where the subject's brain has been manipulated or damaged. To understand what goes wrong is often a way to understand how a system works. If you can stand the jetlag, it's back to Quebec where I asked Jacques Paillard about specific cases where this occurs.

SG: Quebec was the home of the famous neurosurgeon Wilder Penfield, and you mentioned him before. Following in that same tradition, you probably know about an experiment by Calvin and Ojemann (1980). They stimulated a certain part of the brain of a patient who was undergoing brain surgery and the patient reported that someone other than himself was moving his hand. In this case a sense of self-agency was missing from his experience—and rightly so, since he had no intention to move his hand—the surgeons were manipulating his brain. Still, the patient knew it was his hand that was moving. Do you recognize a difference between having a sense of agency and a sense of ownership for action. The patient felt it was his own hand moving, but he was not the agent of the action.

Paillard: Yes, I know what you mean. And it is related to another kind of problem. Think of the difference between detecting a sound which comes from outside, and detecting a sound that you produce. When you produce the sound agency is there, and when you only hear the sound ownership is there. You are the one hearing the sound, but you are not producing it in the former case.

SG: Yes, the sound is in your stream of consciousness, so it is your experience, but you did not produce it.

Paillard: Yes, so the distinction between ownership and agency is clear.

SG: In intentional action, however, agency and ownership seem to be the same, or so tightly conjoined it would be difficult to distinguish them. Passive or involuntary movement is different. Accordingly, one way to think of the sense of ownership is in terms of sensory feedback. In passive movement, for example, I get the sense that I'm moving from sensory feedback—visual and proprioceptive feedback. But there is no motor or efference signal, no intention to move. Since there is also no sense of agency, doesn't this suggest that the sense of agency may depend on the efference signal? You mentioned Wolpert's notion of a forward comparator model before. Frith has suggested that the absence of efference copy in this comparator may be able to account for the lack of a sense of agency that one finds in schizophrenic symptoms of inserted thoughts and delusions of control.

Paillard: Things are not so clear, in my view. In some experiments on position sense conducted in my lab in Marseille we have shown that when we move the hand and without vision we try to indicate, by pointing with the other hand, where we feel the hand to be, there are two conditions: if I move my hand actively I point there at point A [where the hand actually is]; if my hand is moved passively, then I point at point B [just missing the hand]. If I move actively and wait for 15 seconds, where I point shifts and stabilizes at point B. We transposed that experiment into an experiment with the wrist. We place a target in a position that we can easily point to, and in pointing we make a normally shaped arrow with our fingers. I make an active movement of my hand and point, and in the process I swivel my wrist. In that case, you have pointing accuracy when you move actively, and a systematic error when you move passively. The problem: is it an efference copy that allows us to distinguish active from passive? The feeling that it is active, what you call the sense of agency, may come from a centrally generated efference copy or it may come from the peripheral gamma loop. We can test this by cooling the muscles, because we know in the cat, for instance, that when you cool the muscle the state of the the spindel decreases progressively until it stops functioning with lower temperature. When the the spindel stops, the motor system is still intact. The rest of the system is not sensitive to cold. In that case we continued to make passive/active pointing. Active pointing progressively degenerated and approached the accuracy of passive pointing. That proves that some aspect of the difference between active and passive movement depends on peripheral mechanisms. The hypothesis is that the difference would come either from efference copy centrally or through the peripheral gamma loop. When you move actively the gamma system is active and when you move passively the gamma system is silent. The activity of the gamma system is due to the internal activation of the command.

SG: So it's not the efference copy alone. Some peripheral feedback may be important for the sense of agency?

Paillard: Well, this is a limited demonstration, of course. We don't know how it is bound to the feeling we have when we produce the movement. We know that there is some difference there, and we know that there is some information coming from the muscles which is not the same information for passive and active movement. It's in the information.

Perhaps one of the most interesting pathologies that can inform us about the difference between movement and action, and about how intention

can add to — or rather, *transform* — or in the case of pathology, fail to transform — purely causal mechanisms, is apraxia. This is a neurological disorder, often caused by stroke, where patients are unable to execute learned
purposeful movements, even if they want to. They are able to move; but
they are not able to move to command. We've already mentioned some of
Tony Marcel's observations about an apraxic-like stroke patient who was
unable to move a cup-like object from the table to her face area on command in an experimental setting, but was able to serve and drink tea in a
social setting that involved expressions of hospitality (see Marcel 1992;
Gallagher and Marcel 1999). This suggests that intention has an important
effect on whatever causal mechanisms underlie action.

Apraxia can be of different kinds. *Ideational apraxia* involves a problem
in working out a plan or idea for a specific movement. With *ideomotor
apraxia* the patient is unable to carry out an instruction to act in a pretend
situation. For example, the instruction to 'act as if you were combing your
hair.' In the case of *ideokinetic apraxia* the patient is incapable of performing
simple acts, and evidence points to disruptions in cortical centers that control coordination of ideation and action. Finally, *Motor apraxia* is the inability to perform everyday kinds of tasks such as dressing, undressing, tying
shoelaces, etc. I remember when I first read a description of motor apraxia
I was struck by how complex the movements are that are required to dress
ourselves; dressing and undressing involve high degrees of balance and
coordination, as well as fine motor skills to button our buttons. And this is
the simple part, or what Rowlands calls the 'nomic' part, meaning that
such actions fall under the laws of nature. To the nomic aspects of action
we would need to add 'non-nomic' aspects, such as picking out a tie that
goes with a particular shirt. That really gets hard (really! — see Rowlands
2006, 47).

> **Paillard:** In the case of apraxia, if you give the subject a candle and a
> box of matches, well he will take the candle and the box, and may put
> the candle on the box, or he may open the box. He doesn't know how
> to organize the gesture. And he is not aware of his error. He contin-
> ues and he does not realize that it doesn't go that way.

> **SG:** So this is the kind of apraxia called ideational apraxia.

> **Paillard:** Yes. There are other levels in which there is some confu-
> sion, but now more and more we know that ideomotor apraxia is
> more parietal — caused by a lesion in the parietal lobe. Motor
> apraxias are more a matter of the premotor area. In such cases you
> can have specific agraphia [inability to write], or people talk about
> specialized apraxia. There was a famous case of a person who could
> play both piano and violin. He lost the ability to play the piano, but
> could still play the violin. It's odd like that. It can be a very specific

category of action that is lost. And the final kind, the ideokinetic apraxia is probably frontal. We know that the frontal regions are very important for organizing the sequence of thinking.

To conclude this discussion, intention is the aspect of action that makes it more than movement, and makes it irreducible to movement. Intention involves intentionality, in the sense that action is always directed toward the world, or toward some possibilities or goals. The phenomenology of intention is complicated. With Searle we can distinguish between prior intention, which can be conscious and may have a rich phenomenology, and intention-in-action, which may involve minimal consciousness, a thin phenomenology, or may even be non-conscious. Jeannerod and others have shown that all kinds of motor control processes are entrained to intention, that is, that movement is normally in the service of our actions and of what we want to accomplish. Searle's distinction between prior intention and intention-in-action is reflected in Jeannerod's distinction between semantic and pragmatic intentions, which are tightly coordinated.

As Jeannerod makes clear, the concept of representation, while not always clear, is close to ubiqutious in cognitive neuroscience. Whether we need to characterize intention and action in representational terms is an open question. A number of theorists argue for the notion of minimal rep-resentations in action (e.g., Clark, Rowlands, Wheeler), while others defend a non-representationalist view (e.g., Dreyfus, Thelen and Smith). On this latter view we are directly and dynamically in-the-world. This is reflected in the tight coordination of action with pragmatic spatiality. In this regard, an object is distant or near, not in terms of objective measurments, but in terms of my action purposes. The shape of an object is defined not in terms of geometry, but in terms of graspability. So my actions, my intentions, my projects, help to shape the world I perceive and live in. Reciprocally, the highly contextualized world I live in shapes the possibilities of my action, and as studies of apraxic patients show, have a real effect on what I can do. In this regard, when we think of questions about causality, neither supervenience (understood to be a relation between mental and physical properties of the cognitive system) nor purely physical (neuronal) cause-effect relations are sufficient for a full explanation for action and the sense of agency that comes along with action. These are topics to which we return in Chapter 12.

Chapter Six

Consciousness

Throughout our considerations of movement and action there has been a phenomenology of consciousness lurking around the edges. We have hardly brushed on the question of what consciousness is or how consciousness is possible; but we have been delineating what sorts of things we are conscious of when, for example we are engaged in action. In regard to action we have been finding out when consciousness is important and when it is not. And for the most part this has been perceptual consciousness — a perceptual intentionality that is normally directed toward things and states of affairs in the world rather than, for example, toward our own bodily movements. This is what we might call a first-order experience in contrast to something like a higher-order thought process where we may be conscious of our own thoughts and strategic cognitions, for example, when we are reflectively or metacognitively thinking about how we have just solved a mathematical or a practical problem and how we might do it better. Besides the phenomenological analysis of experience there are many other concerns about consciousness in the philosophy of mind and the cognitive sciences. One basic question is whether there are neural correlates of consciousness (NCCs) — neural processes that in some way cause or generate consciousness.

I recently participated in a debate about consciousness in San Marino. The debaters were Christopher Frith and Christof Koch (http://www.philosophy.ucf.edu/sanMarino.html). Koch was very straight forward about the whole question of consciousness depending on brain processes. Once we know the NCCs, there will not be much else to know about consciousness. Frith, on the other hand has come to think of consciousness as in some way generated in social processes. In some sense, however, Chris and Christof were answering two different questions. Christof was providing an answer to the question about how consciousness is generated *in the brain*; Chris was addressing the issue of when or in what circumstances consciousness is generated (and I'm tempted to add the phrase *in the world*). In some way this may seem to mirror the distinction we found in the analysis of action between subpersonal causal mechanisms and personal level intentionality. On the one hand, the question there was how are these two aspects integrated in action, and similarly one might think the question is the same here—how are subpersonal brain processes integrated with more personal level phenomena that may involve social or intersubjective factors so as to produce the consciousness that we know and love? And in some sense this is a question that needs to be answered. On the other hand, it would be extremely beneficial to expand our conception of causality from what is usually conceived of as the billiard-ball type of one thing banging into another with the effect of the second thing banging into something else. Put enough of these things together in a very complex way, call them neurons, and *voilà*, consciousness emerges. A rather impoverished recipe however, with no real way to account for the rich intentionality of consciousness. Isn't it possible to say that there are some contexts in the world, possibly social contexts, but not necessarily limited to social contexts, that call forth, that elicit, and in that sense cause my consciousness to emerge?

Consciousness and its neural correlates

Chris Frith is just recently retired from University College London and has taken up a distinguished research professor post at Aarhus University in Denmark. I had the opportunity to have a conversation with Chris in Aarhus several years ago, before his recent move, and before his debate with Christof. Our conversation touched on the kind of analysis that Christof was presenting in San Marino, that is, one focused on the brain.

> **SG:** How do you view the project of identifying the neural correlates of consciousness? Do you think it's possible, in principle, to carry through on this kind of project?

> **Frith:** In terms of the statistical definition of correlation the NCC project is straightforward and has already generated some robust observations. Correlation implies prediction, but says nothing about causality. We can predict something about consciousness by measuring neural activity (or vice versa). We can already predict, for example, whether someone is awake, dreaming or deeply asleep from the pattern of EEG and muscle activity. In the next few years we shall be able to predict (very crudely) what someone is dreaming about.

> **SG:** This is already more precise than I expected. Is the idea that you could predict content and not just the fact of being conscious, for example, in the visual modality?

Frith: Yes, that's right. At the moment we could probably predict that you were dreaming about a face (since we know about faces in the brain), but not whose face it was. We also have preliminary data suggesting that we can predict whether or not someone was conscious of the stimulus that was just presented to them. Activity in the relevant processing region (e.g. the fusiform face area for faces) is necessary, but not sufficient for awareness of a face. Activity also seems to be needed in parietal and frontal regions whatever the nature of the stimulus.

SG: Are we then seeking the neural underpinnings of consciousness in localizable processes, rather than in some global phenomenon. What role do imaging studies play in this quest?

Frith: Imaging studies must play a major role in this version of the NCC programme, especially if we extend imaging to refer to any method of measuring neural activity. The NCC is localisable in the sense that it does not depend upon every neuron in the brain. On the other hand it is highly likely that the NCC involves long-range cortico-cortical interactions and cortico-thalamic interactions. The key question, I think, is whether there is a qualitative difference between the neural activity associated with consciousness and the neural activity associated with non-conscious information processing and behavior.

SG: You say 'qualitative difference'. Someone might suppose that a neuron either fires or doesn't fire, or a set of neurons either instantiates a certain pattern or it doesn't, and if it does then consciousness results. If the NCC is some neural state X, and X is activated, then consciousness results. Is it possible to have X in one case with consciousness and X in another case without consciousness?

Frith: A fundamental assumption is that, if there is a change in the contents of consciousness, then there must be a change in neural activity of some kind. However, there can be a change in neural activity without a change in the contents of consciousness.

SG: But if there can be a change in neural activity without any change in consciousness, how can recording such changes tell you anything about conscious states at all?

Frith: On the contrary, I think this relation may tell us more about conscious states. It implies that only certain kinds of neural activity are associated with conscious states. So we can ask what's special about this kind of activity. And there is direct evidence that changes in neural activity do occur without changes in consciousness. For example, Change Blindness is a very good way of looking at the neural correlates of consciousness. This is a very popular demonstration with psychologists at the moment where you see two pictures that differ. In the demo I use in lectures there is an airplane, but in one version of the picture one of the engines is missing. If you show the two pictures repeatedly in alternation, but with a blank screen in between people may take minutes to find the difference even though they are desperately looking for it. In an experiment (Beck et al. 2001) you can arrange it so that roughly half the time volunteers notice the change and half the time they don't notice it. You also have occasions when there really is no change. In terms of consciousness there is no difference between the trials where you don't see the change and the trials where there is no change, but there is a change in neural activity in visual processing areas. You can also contrast the occasions where the change is consciously detected and those where it is not. In this comparison the stimulus input is the same but consciousness varies so the neural activity we see here in frontal and parietal cortex must be closely linked with consciousness.

SG: These are brain imaging studies.

Frith: Yes, these are imaging studies. Some people think this is relevant to problems of how we perceive the real world because what change blindness shows us is that we're not really aware of much of what's out there in the real world.

SG: So the brain is very selective about what we notice. With respect to gaining a scientific explanation of the mechanisms of consciousness (addressing the 'easy' problems if not the 'hard' problem, as Chalmers outlines this distinction)[1] what role do you think the study of pathologies can play?

Frith: Pathological cases can reveal dissociations which are much more difficult to see in normal volunteers. For example, a patient in a persistent vegetative state goes through sleep-wake cycle, but appears never to be conscious of anything. This observation shows that wakefulness can be dissociated from consciousness. Likewise a patient like DF or someone with blindsight shows that goal directed behavior can occur in the absence of consciousness.

SG: Goal directed behavior rather than forced choice response?

Frith: Yes. DF is the patient examined by Milner and Goodale (Milner & Goodale 1995) who has visual form agnosia. She can see light and dark and colour, but she can't see shape. For example, she

---

1   See Chalmers 1995. We mentioned the hard problem of consciousness in Chapter 3: how can physical processes generate consciousness, which seems so un-physical. The easy problems, which everyone also considers hard, are problems like memory, perception, and so on.

can't tell you what the orientation of a slot is or even adjust a pointer to have the same orientation. The surprising observation is that she can 'post' things through the slot accurately. This is not like guessing. She fluently adjusts the orientation of her hand to post something through the slot. So I think this is not a forced choice response, but goal directed. Normal people can also show goal directed movements where they are not aware of the cue eliciting the movement until after the movement is initiated, if at all. What this shows us is that just because someone shows goal directed behavior this does not mean they are conscious of what they are doing.

Frith is describing here what Jeannerod had called the difference between pragmatic and semantic representations. DF has no semantic access to shape, but she retains pragmatic access via the dorsal (motor-related) visual system. Normally these two systems work together to give us a full perception of the world. In the case of visual form agnosia they dissociate.

In experiments with blindsight patients, in contrast, forced choice tests are made. Blindsight is a form of blindness caused by damage to the primary visual cortex (V1) rather than damage to the eyes. Weiskrantz et al. (1974) showed that damage to area 17, the cortical projection from the dorsal lateral geniculate nucleus of the visual cortex, with minimal damage to the surrounding tissue of the posterior cortical areas, can cause blindsight. Usually only part of the visual field is blinded (the blind areas are called 'scotomas'). To simplify matters, assume that the patient is totally blind in this fashion. Because his eyes and optic nerves still function, when his eyes are open visual information is delivered to his brain, but he will not have conscious visual perception because of the brain damage. The information delivered by the eyes, however, may still register in other parts of the brain. For example, a route from the retina to the mid-brain, which is different from the route through the damaged area of V1, has been hypothesized as being a second pathway of visual information. Although a blindsight patient is blind, he is still able to detect and locate visual stimuli if he is made to do so, that is, if he is forced to guess or make a choice among alternatives in an experiment. If presented with visual stimuli, the patient will say that he cannot see them, because, of course, he is blind. But made to guess about where precisely the stimuli are presented, or about the nature of the stimuli — shape, position, etc. — he is above chance correct in his guesses. This may apply not only to relatively simple object discriminations, but also to emotionally salient stimuli (Hamm et al. 2003). His brain exploits the visual information that is informing his non-visual experience. Thus, blindsight patients are said to be non-consciously perceiving the visual stimuli (Marcel 1998; Weiskrantz 1986). Theorists interested in consciousness like to think about blindsight since it points to a specifically damaged area that somehow prevents visual consciousness. It's important to keep in mind, however, that blindsight patients are not unconscious in any other ways; they are simply deprived of consciousness in the visual modality.

Christof Koch worked closely with Francis Crick, who won the Nobel Prize for his work on discovering DNA. Crick and Koch teamed up to investigate the NCC. Crick died in 2004, and just around that time my friend Thomas Ramsøy conducted an interview with Koch (Ramsøy 2004). With Thomas and Christof's permission I've adjusted the tense of the verbs where reference is made to Francis Crick. Christof also provided some minor updates.

Ramsøy: Prof. Koch, could you please explain the basic assumptions you have proposed about consciousness?

Koch: 1. [The late] Francis Crick and I took consciousness seriously, as a brute fact that needs to be explained. The first-person perspective, feelings, qualia, awareness, phenomenal experiences are real phenomena that arise out of certain privileged brain processes. They make up the landscape of conscious life.

2. We put aside the question at the heart of the mind-body problem—why does phenomenal experience feel like anything? For now, scientists should focus on the search for the minimal neuronal mechanisms jointly sufficient for any one specific conscious experience, the neuronal correlates of consciousness (NCC). While it remains an open question whether discovering and characterizing the NCC will be sufficient to understand the structure, function, and origin of consciousness it is a necessary step.

3. The NCC have one, or more, functions, such as planning. Planning involves summarizing the current state of affairs in the world and the body and presenting this concise summary to a system that contemplates diverse courses of action open to the organism. It follows as a corollary that thinking about philosophical zombies is sterile.[2]

4. While the NCC are embedded within the brain, not all of the brain's myriad of neurons and regions contribute equally. Some will be much more important than others. Thus, our emphasis on local, particular properties of neurons rather than on more global, holistic aspects of the brain. In particular, Crick and I have argued that the firing activity of both retinal neurons and of cells in the primary visual cortex (V1) is not part of the NCC for conscious visual perception. The retina and V1 are important for many aspects of normal seeing (but probably not for the content of visual dreams or imagina-

---

2   Philosophical zombies, much discussed in the philosophy of mind, are hypothetical characters in thought experiments who look like humans, behave like humans in every way, speak like humans, etc., and maybe are human, but are completely non-conscious.

tion), but the representational content of conscious visual perception does not arise from activities in these structures. This is an eminently testable hypothesis (with much supporting evidence such as the fMRI study [see Lee, Blake and Heeger 2007]). This shows that in regard to consciousness, true progress is possible.

Ramsøy: But if your focus is on local processes in neurons, do you not run the risk of missing crucial events at a global scale? Consciousness might be, as some claim (e.g. Baars [1997]; Dehaene and Naccache [2001], and Tononi and Edelman [1998]), a global event in distributed parts of the brain. Specifically, how does such an approach relate to such global theories of consciousness in the brain?

Koch: The same question could also be asked about the molecular mechanisms underlying heredity. There is a loose parallel between the NCC and genes. Heredity is a property of an individual cell, much as consciousness is a property of an individual brain. One could easily argue that the mechanisms underlying inheritance of acquired properties involve the entire cell and are therefore necessarily global. Ribosomes, for instance, the machinery necessary for the synthesis of proteins from mRNA, are found throughout the cell. So, too, are many of the proteins they manufacture, such as the ionic channels that are anchored in the neuronal membrane. Incapacitating the various forms of RNA polymerase (the enzymes responsible for synthesizing the different kinds of RNA) blocks all protein synthesis globally, much as gas anesthesia knocks out a patient. Any one gene, however, encoded via its associated string of nucleic acids along the DNA molecule in the nucleus, transcribes into one or a few specific RNA molecules that are ultimately translated into proteins. This highly localized aspect of the genetic information is seemingly at odds with the fact that the synthesis or the expression of that protein occurs at many distinct locations in the cell. I believe it is likely that consciousness will also be based on such local and highly specific mechanisms, which is not to say that global properties of the brain don't play some role.

Note that by local I don't mean to imply spatial locality but that the NCC depend critically on very specific properties. An example of this may be loops of cortical pyramidal cells that are located in the high level inferior temporal visual cortex (IT) and in prefrontal cortex and that are reciprocally connected by powerful excitatory synapses close to the cell body. Once activity in this loop exceeds a threshold, it may maintain itself in a reverberatory state for quite some time, and may be crucial factor for the NCC.

Ramsøy: That should mean that it is possible to pinpoint areas of the brain that have (or not have) the potential to be part of the NCC? As you mention, V1 is not likely to have such properties. But is there a general picture? Does consciousness rely on a fixed set of modules or areas of the brain?

Koch: The honest answer is, of course, that we don't know. It is plausible that by dint of constant training, cortical regions previously inaccessible to consciousness will become accessible in the sense that the neuronal coalitions that constitute the NCC will now extend into these regions. This would explain how, as people mature, they can learn to introspect (the 'know thyself' of Western philosophy) or to experience the world in a new way. At the level of individual neurons, there is likely to be a great deal of flexibility in which neurons partake in what coalition to generate a conscious percept.

Ultimately, however, any such plasticity will be limited by the architecture and extent of the axons of projection neurons. There is now evidence from patients in the persistent vegetative state that primary auditory (A1) and primary somatosensory cortices (S1) are insufficient for sensory consciousness. That is, maybe all primary sensory cortical regions are off limit to the NCC. Francis and I [were thinking that] this will also hold for many regions in the frontal lobes.

Ramsøy: The 'normal' activity of neurons in primary sensory regions in vegetative and comatose states certainly points to these areas as non-essential to the NCC. But you have gone further than that: you claim that V1, for example, is not part of the NCC due to it's connectivity, and especially since it is not directly connected to the frontal cortex (your 1995 article with Francis Crick). But judging from what you just said, then this would only go for certain parts of the frontal lobes?

Koch: Yes, most certainly. We explicitly discuss the question of which regions of the frontal lobes are directly involved in consciousness and which are not in a long article published in *Neuro-Psychoanalysis* (Crick & Koch 2000; [also see Koch 2004]). The frontal lobes account for a very large fraction of all brain tissue. Neuroanatomists distinguish 40 different regions here with a very complex interconnectivity. It is not yet clear whether the same sort of neuroanatomical rules that give rise to the observed Felleman-Van Essen hierarchy (DeYoe et al. 1994; Felleman & Van Essen 1991; Van Essen, Anderson & Felleman 1992) in the visual cortex at the back of the brain are applicable to the front of the brain. However, there is no doubt that given the observed heterogeneity in cortical regions, the essential neuronal coalitions that underlie one or the other conscious percept or memory will only be found in some of these regions but not in others. The latter ones make up what we call the Unconscious Homunculus, the parts of the brain that are involved in high-level, cognitive functions and decisions but that are not consciously accessible.

Hard problems and the personal level

The search for NCC is going at the hard problem of consciousness in a very direct way. If we want to understand how it's possible for something like the firing of neurons, or some systematic set of neuronal processes in the brain to generate something like consciousness, then, as Christof says, discovering the NCC is an important step. Likewise, studying things like blindsight and other pathologies of consciousness can help us to know what counts and what doesn't as a solution to the hard problem. Tony Marcel who has worked for years at the Medical Research Council's Cognition and Brain Sciences Unit in Cambridge, and now in the Experimental Psychology Department at Cambridge University and at the University of Hertfordshire, has studied just such pathologies and has conducted important experiments on non-conscious perception. Some of my most enjoyable conversations about philosophy and neuropsychology, and theatre, and art, and detective novels, and so on, have been with Tony, often as we shared a meal and drank Adnams beer in and around Cambridge. On one occasion we attended a lecture by Francis Crick on consciousness at Jesus College, talked with Roger Penrose at the reception afterwards, and went on to further discussions at the local pub. On the occasion of the following conversation, however, we were moving. Tony had picked me up at the train station in London and was giving me a ride to Stansted airport where I was catching a plane. So the interview was conducted in traffic and in the airport with constant security and departure announcements blaring on the loud speaker.

SG: In much of your work [I shouted] you study individuals with brain damage of various types, but in explaining such cases you make reference not just to the specifics of brain function, but also to the patient's experience.

Marcel: Yes. Most cognitivism and cognitive neuroscience seems, without any explicit discussion of this, not only to explain at the subpersonal level, but not even to acknowledge phenomenal entities, and they miss the explananda at the personal level. This is something I find peculiar. For me, it has to start and end at the personal level. I don't eschew or reject, without good reason, explanations that are at the personal level.

SG: At the same time you don't reject sub-personal analysis. To put it in slightly different terms, it is not unusual in such discussions to distinguish between function and phenomenal consciousness. You also have made this distinction in some of your papers, and I'm thinking especially of your paper on Blindsight in *Brain* (Marcel 1998). For example, you have indicated that perceptual function and perceptual consciousness are two different things. Shape perception, for example, can be working perfectly fine at a functional, and I think that means, sub-personal level, without a corresponding experience of shape. But in distinguishing the perceptual conscious level, you talk about phenomenal aspect plus attentional differentiation, or attention.

Marcel: Yes, but actually you could treat the latter as part of the sub-personal level.

SG: To follow out this question of the functional and the personal versus sub-personal distinction, as you know, David Chalmers distinguishes between the hard problem of consciousness and the easy problems. The easy problems, which are not so easy, are what he calls the functional problems.

Marcel: Yes, but that is still not for me what I mean in that paper by functional, although it is in a sense. There is something which can be at the personal level and can still be functional in the following sense. For example, if you take an aspect of consciousness that I call 'awareness', which you can treat as my access to my knowledge, that could be treated as a kind of information processing stage. Something like this may be functional in the sense that Chalmers understands it, in distinction from the hard problem, which is the problem of phenomenology. I think that yes, the distinction that I'm making between awareness and phenomenology does correspond to his distinction between the easy and the hard problems.

SG: When you say awareness, you mean second-order access to the first-order phenomenal level, as you outlined in the emotion paper with Lambie (Lambie and Marcel 2002).

Marcel: Yes. But by second order I don't mean something that's very reflective necessarily, nor do I mean something that is necessarily reflexive in the Sartrean sense, although it is aligned to that.

SG: Is this first-order/second-order distinction, then, the same distinction as Ned Block (1995) makes between primary and access consciousness?

Marcel: Our distinction bears an affinity with Ned Block's distinction. But it is slightly different, since for us (a) the processes of second-order consciousness or 'awareness' in taking first-order consciousness as content can operate on the content of first-order consciousness to mould, shape it or change it, and (b) under certain modes of attention (especially immersion, when you are fully immersed in some task) second-order consciousness can disappear so that there is almost only first-order consciousness. In addition I am not sure to what extent what we build around our distinction would be acceptable to Ned Block.

SG: Would it be right to say that the only aspect that would qualify for the 'hard problem', in Chalmers's terms, would be the phenomenal aspect of consciousness.

Marcel: Well let me make just two remarks on this. One is that there are certain kinds of approaches, taken largely by philosophers, but actually by many psychologists too, that assume there are some special properties, sometimes described in terms of qualia or whatever. I'm not sure that there are such special properties. There are many things that people say are unanalyzable, and I'm not convinced that they are unanalyzable. The fact that someone may experience something as unanalyzable, or they can't very well articulate it, doesn't mean that it *is* unanalyzable. Secondly, about qualia, with some exceptions, like color, almost all of what people talk about when they talk about qualia can be treated as spatio-temporal information or spatio-temporal dynamics, which are tractable, or which have been broached certainly by Gibsonians but by other people as well. So I'm not convinced that there are special properties, and that seems to be one aspect of what is meant by 'hard'. There is another aspect that's considered hard, and this I do think is hard. In the emotion paper — and I have to say this is a very intuitive thing, but I'm not sorry that we mentioned it there — we gave a 'take' on a certain aspect of phenomenology. Actually, it's not entirely phenomenology, but a certain aspect is. It concerned having a certain type of attentional attitude. We drew on Nagel's notion of 'what it is like', a notion which doesn't say very much, by the way. The point is that *what it's like* is what it's like *for* somebody — we would use the dative case here. It seems to me, that to be *something it's like for* somebody or some creature, brings in the personal level, and for us, it brings in some aspect of self. Now that does seem to be hard. In another paper, this is my paper on the sense of agency (Marcel 2003), I tried to bring in a minimalist conception of selfhood that is really a geometrical perspectivalist aspect of where the source of an action is. But then I thought that that was not a thick enough entity for there to be a 'for', something it is like 'for' that entity. A point of view, a geometric point of view, or a point in space and time, an origin of a reference frame, can't be sufficient. It has to matter, when we say it's *for* somebody. One thing that is going to be hard is to unpack what the *'for'* means.

SG: This is also where emotions could fit into the picture.

Marcel: Yes, in the sense that things matter or that you take an interest.

SG: I think Chalmers would say that it is the phenomenal aspect that is the hard problem, and he would think of it in terms of qualia, and in terms of thought experiments like Nagel's bat, or Jackson's story of Mary the color scientist. The phenomenal aspect is hard because objective science seems unable to capture precisely that first-person experience, and any attempt to do so turns it into a third-person neuronal process and misses the phenomenal quality of the experience. So it's the explanatory gap that is hard to close.

Marcel: I have to say that I don't personally have a strong position worked out on this problem of there being a first-person/third-person explanatory gap. There are philosophers on both sides of that gap, and you see what they say to each other, and you find that both groups make some sense.

SG: So do you think it is simply a matter of two different discourses that cannot be translated?

Marcel: It's interesting to put it that way. I oscillate between two views. Sometimes I really think it is a matter of two discourses. But, oddly enough, it is not clear that there is any isomorphism between them, or that you can translate them. This is quite common in many disciplines. It is not clear that there is any mapping between the entities—an entity in one discourse may not have a counterpart in the other discourse, and it's not clear how you map between them. So sometimes I do think it is a matter of two discourses. Other times, what I find myself doing, is being caught in between and trying to negotiate or broker a marriage or arrangement. But certainly it is never the case that we can reduce one to the other. I find it an uncomfortable position, but the fact that it is uncomfortable doesn't mean that I would give it up. What I don't want to do is what I feel to be crass and ridiculous. Namely, there are a number of cognitive neuroscientists or cognitivists who take something to be phenomenological, and then say this is equivalent to some 'X' in a functionalist or information-processing scheme. I remain terribly unconvinced by that because these are not the kind of entities that exist in personal level or phenomenological discourse—they're just not, and it's absurd to say they're equivalent to such and such, because they're not. For example, here's a concept that emerges in

various ways — it doesn't have anything to do particularly with phenomenology, but I think it does have relevance — it's the notion of
there being relations, that some kinds of things are relational. Now
something that Freud said does bear very much on this — his notion
of cathexis — this idea that there is an investment in something. Take
the notion of desire. Desire is a thick, heavy term. And I mean that's
good. Yet, by desire they [the cognitivists] just mean that the system
needs something, or that I have a propositional attitude, namely I
perceive that woman, for example, plus whatever it is that I desire to
do or happen. But certainly there is more, and there is something
wrong about reducing desire to something purely cognitive. They've
just got it wrong. And it is not just the fact that there are two discourses, but rather that at least one of the discourses extends away to
other things. It extends to existential aspects. Existential discourse is
not just a descriptive one. If something is merely descriptive, it could
be mapped onto a *Naturwissenschaft*.

SG: So to the extent that a personal level discourse involves evalua-
tions or evaluative judgments, desires, emotions, a cathexis, and so
on, directed outward in a relation toward the world, they cannot be
reduced to a descriptive science.

Marcel: Towards the world, but also towards oneself. As you yourself know, an existentialist discourse will raise questions about all
sorts of things that simply have nothing to do with *Naturwissenschaft*,
or reductive natural science. By reductive here I don't mean to
devalue the term. And actually, such natural scientists usually want
nothing to do with those things.

SG: At least when they are doing their natural science.

Marcel: Viewed in these terms, the hard problem now seems to be
much harder than even Chalmers thinks.

SG: Viewed in these terms, a solution to the hard problem cannot be
found if you stay with just neuroscience or the natural sciences.

Marcel: I think that's right. But it doesn't mean that there is an
essence of consciousness, or a bottom to it, as it were, but the different ways in which things can seem to you. And I mean, for example,
something like this. I can be sitting in my office looking at my desk in
front of me. I can experience this desktop in front of me with papers
on it, and it's sort of a brown or grey-brown with lots of papers on
top. On the other hand, I can have exactly the same view and I can see
a sort of a rhomboid shape of a certain color with white and grey par-
allelograms. It seems to me that the way I attend, and I will call that
attending, can give me different things. I have different kinds of

experiences as of distinct objects or not. In fact, one thing you can have, and I think both William James, and oddly enough, Merleau-Ponty, both used the term, is the notion of perceptual field. It doesn't seem to me that the perceptual field is the basic consciousness, which many psychologists of the late 19th century were taking this to be — people in psychological experimental laboratories in Germany, that's what they were trying to do. But I don't think that's right. I think that that's one take you can have under one perceptual attitude.

SG: So consciousness is varied, and there is probably not *one* thing that we should call consciousness?

Marcel: Well, hang on. I'm saying that the content is not a single thing, or one basic thing. But there is even a problem with saying that. I don't want to say that there is something called consciousness, and then there is various content. What I don't want to do is to make what I consider to be a mistake that William James made. And I really do think it's a mistake. If you go down that road, then what you say is that there is something called consciousness, and that's a container, and consciousness itself is independent of the kind of content that might fill it. I don't want to say that. It seems to me that there is no such thing as a consciousness with no content. It's just not on, as far as I'm concerned. It seems to me to lead into the information process-ing black box approach. And listen, that is how I was educated, or rather, socialized. It's very difficult for me to get out of it, but I none-theless think it's an error.

SG: This leads to a slightly different question. Even if there is no consciousness independent of content, one can also talk about the formal features of consciousness.

Marcel: Yes, I think so.

SG: Although content changes, there is something there that has a relatively stable structure or formal features.

Marcel: Yes, that's difficult, but also very interesting. I don't know quite if you're saying this, but are you saying that you could abstract out, or do a technical analysis that would give you something irre-ducible to content?

SG: Yes, I think phenomenologists try to do that.

Marcel: Yes, that's right. I wanted to ask you, when you discuss such things with other people, have you gone onto that topic?

SG: Yes, these sorts of issues often come up in discussions I've had with proponents of higher order representation theory, for example,

David Rosenthal's higher-order thought model. I have found myself defending the idea that phenomenal consciousness doesn't require some kind of higher-order representation to make it self-conscious, but it has a certain implicit structure of its own that phenomenologists define in terms of pre-reflective self-awareness.

Marcel: That's very interesting. One of Chalmers' questions [at a recent conference] was about this issue. One of the questions was about emotion experience—what is it that makes emotion experience? My reply is that it involves two things. There are the kinds of content we are referring to as kinds of emotion content, and these are what we experience as emotion. And there is another aspect of consciousness, actually a certain kind of relational aspect that has a certain kind of structure. In other words, it doesn't need an extra stage of processing.

SG: Right, the two aspects are processed together, so to speak.

Marcel: There is a very interesting issue there. I could interpret my own statement in two ways. I could say, as long as the content had that structure in it, that is experiential. And that's it. But you could interpret it in a slightly different way. Does that structure give it an autonomous existence? If it has its own structure, and doesn't need a higher-order or extra stage, if it doesn't need anything else, does that mean it exists or has a certain existence on its own?

Pre-reflective consciousness

The idea that consciousness has a structure that includes an implicit self-awareness comes from phenomenologists like Husserl, Merleau-Ponty, and Sartre. Locke (1690), who was one of the first to use the English term 'consciousness' in the philosophical literature, suggested that it is 'impossible for any one to perceive without perceiving that he does perceive' (1690, Book II, Chapter 27, §9). But it's not that I have an internal perception or introspection that is running parallel to my perception of the world; nor is it, as Brentano thought, that I have an awareness of two objects at once—the object that I perceive in the world, and myself.

Brentano agrees with the later phenomenologists in this way: as I listen to a melody I am aware that I am listening to the melody. He acknowledges that I do not have two different mental states: my perception of the melody is one and the same as my awareness of perceiving it; they constitute one single psychical phenomenon. But in contrast to the phenomenologists, Brentano contends that by means of this unified mental state

I have an awareness of two objects: the melody and my perceptual experience.

> In the same mental phenomenon in which the sound is present to our minds we simultaneously apprehend the mental phenomenon itself. What is more, we apprehend it in accordance with its dual nature insofar as it has the sound as content within it, and insofar as it has itself as content at the same time. We can say that the sound is the primary object of the act of hearing, and that the act of hearing itself is the secondary object (Brentano 1973, 127–8).

Husserl disagrees on the notion of secondary object: pre-reflectively or non-reflectively (that is, prior to any kind of reflective or introspective attitude) my experience is not itself an object for me. I do not occupy the position or perspective of an observer who attends to this experience. That I am aware of my ongoing experience 'does not and cannot mean that this is the *object* of an act of consciousness, in the sense that a perception, a presentation or a judgement is directed upon it' (Husserl 2001/I, 273). In pre-reflective or non-observational self-consciousness, experience is not an object; rather, my intentional experience is lived through as my subjectivity, but it does not appear to me in an objectified manner.

David Chalmers has expressed the phenomenological view in his own terms, namely, that having an experience is automatically to stand in an intimate epistemic relation to the experience; a relation more primitive than knowledge that might be called 'acquaintance' (Chalmers 1996, 197). As pre-reflectively self-aware of my experience I am not unconscious of it, although I tend to ignore it, to push it to the recesses of awareness, in favor of the object I am conscious of. I am normally absorbed by the projects and states of affairs in the world, and as such I do not attend to my experiential life. I am nonetheless aware that I am attending to the world. This is a minimal self-consciousness that comes along with being a body engaged in action in the world. It provides what Tony Marcel has just called 'a geometrical perspectivalist aspect of where the source of an action is'. But the content of this pre-reflective self-awareness includes more than the sense that I am perceiving the things around me from a perspective. Much of this self-awareness is informed by what Gibson calls the ecological information that is implicit in posture and movement; it includes proprioception and kinaesthetic aspects that tell me that I've just moved in a certain way. It includes a sense of agency for my action, and a sense of ownership for my embodied movement. It has, as Tony says, a 'thin' phenomenology, and it is certainly non-conceptual. As such it is not equivalent to a more developed kind of self-consciousness that is associated with mirror self-recognition and conceptual identification; and, as such, it is something that many animals, and the youngest of human infants have (see Gallagher and Meltzoff 1996).

This pre-reflective structure means that we are not conscious without being conscious that we are conscious. A quite different view on this is taken by higher-order representation (HOR) theorists – sometimes referred to as HOT (higher-order thought) or HOP (higher-order perception) (Rosenthal 1986 for HOT, and Carruthers 1996; Armstrong 1968; Lycan 1997 for HOP). According to these authors there is a difference between conscious and non-conscious mental states (think of Blindsight) and this difference depends on the presence or absence of a relevant meta-mental state. Accordingly, they would say that the subjective feel of experience presupposes a capacity for higher-order awareness; 'such self-awareness is a conceptually necessary condition for an organism to be a subject of phenomenal feelings, or for there to be anything that its experiences are like' (Carruthers 1996, 152). This is not only a claim about how consciousness is structured, but a claim about what it is that makes consciousness consciousness. On the HOR view, what makes a mental state conscious rather than non-conscious is the fact that it is taken as an object by a relevant higher-order mental state. It is the occurrence of the higher-order representation that makes the first-order mental state conscious, and makes us conscious that it is so. This implies that a mental state is a conscious state only if we are conscious of it by means of a meta-mental state, or as Rosenthal puts it, 'the mental state's being intransitively conscious simply consists in one's being transitively conscious of it' (Rosenthal 1997, 739). This means that consciousness is not an intrinsic property of mental states, but a relational property (Rosenthal 1997, 736–7), that is, a property that a mental state has only in so far as it stands in the relevant relation to something else. It is thus a question of the mind directing its intentional aim upon its own states and operations.

There is a clear contrast between the HOR view and the phenomenological view. First, the phenomenologists are not trying to give an account of what makes a mental state conscious; they are describing a conscious mental state as it is experienced. Second, they explicitly deny that the primary kind of self-consciousness that belongs to the structure of any consciousness is to be understood in terms of some kind of second mental state – an introspection, or higher-order monitoring – that takes the first as an object. Rather, pre-reflective self-consciousness is to be understood as an *intrinsic* feature of primary, first-order experience.

It has also been suggested that on one reading the higher-order account of consciousness generates an infinite regress (see Gallagher and Zahavi 2007 for a discussion of this). That is, if a mental state is conscious only because it is taken as an object by a contemporary second-order mental state, then the second-order mental state is either conscious or non-conscious. If it is conscious, it must also be taken as an object by a contemporary third-order mental state, and so forth *ad infinitum*. If the second-order mental state is non-conscious (and this has been the standard reply to this argument in order to halt the regress, cf. Rosenthal 1997), then one has to explain what a non-conscious mental state is and why precisely such a state has the capacity of making another state conscious. Putting one non-conscious mental state into relation with another non-conscious mental state suddenly transforms one of the mental states into a conscious mental state. Why? Furthermore, from this relation, it is not clear how the now conscious mental state takes on the various aspects of phenomenality (the 'what it is like' of experience), perspective, and ownership (the sense that it is *my* experience) that seem to characterize first-order perceptual experience.

A larger system

On the kind of embodied, embedded, enactive approaches that we were talking about in previous chapters, perceptual consciousness is not divorced from movement and action. Perceptual consciousness is clearly a bodily process and as such it is necessarily egocentrically (soma-centrically) perspectival. The late Francisco Varela was certainly one of the most respected scientists participating in these debates about consciousness. But he comes at this topic from very different perspectives than most mainstream philosophers of mind and cognitive scientists. Dennett summarizes this difference in the following way.

> There are striking parallels between Francisco's 'Emergent Mind' and my 'Joycean Machines'. Francisco and I have a lot in common. In fact, I spent three months at CREA, in Paris, with him in 1990, and during that time I wrote much of *Consciousness Explained*. Yet though Francisco and I are friends and colleagues, I'm in one sense his worst enemy, because he's a revolutionary and I'm a reformer. He has the standard problem of any revolutionary: the establishment is—must be—nonreformable. All its thinking has to be discarded, and everything has to start from scratch. We're talking about the same issues, but I want to hold on to a great deal of what's gone before and Francisco wants to discard it. He strains at making the traditional ways of looking at things too wrong. (Interview with Dennett in Brockman 1995).

In my conversations with Varela we discussed neurophenomenological approaches to consciousness.

> **Varela:** As you know I lived through this cognitive revolution, through the displacement of the computational school, and the more recent displacement of the connectionist school. I'm a biologist and

was glad to see the influence of brain science on how we think about the mind. But more than that I think the more recent focus on embodied cognitive science, which my book with Evan Thompson and Eleanor Rosch (*The Embodied Mind* 1991) helped to initiate, is the most important. When I began my research in the 1970s, cognition was of central interest; consciousness, however, still appeared to be something mystical, the concern of philosophers, rather than scientists. It wasn't until the late eighties and nineties that the idea that one could learn many things about consciousness started to grow: then we started thinking in different ways about how movement comes about, how memory is constructed, how the emotions work, how the various capacities of cognitive life can be articulated. There is no agreement on anything, of course. Even whether consciousness is only found in humans, or can also be found in other animals. Wherever we find the right kind of cognitive apparatus, however, this unique phenomenon appears, the phenomenon of lived experience, or to use Thomas Nagel's expression, the phenomenon of 'what it is like' to be consciously in the world.

SG: It continues to be a problem with no solution.

Varela: David Chalmers caught the right phrase at the right time — the 'hard problem', which is the problem of the emergence of consciousness, which is really the deep question: What is consciousness? The problem is that many of the scientists and the philosophers embrace the reductionist program and are motivated by the desire to discover the so-called NCC circuits. Francis Crick, for example, studied the brain with the hope of identifying the precise circuits responsible for the phenomenon of consciousness. We are, he says, nothing but a bunch of neurons. Decidedly reductionistic. I don't mean to denigrate this work; science needs to be reductionistic in part. But we are certainly more than a bunch of neurons, and we need to be interested in the extra-neural aspects of consciousness. I don't deny that the concept of the NCC is an essential element in this quest. But other strategies are important.

SG: What does the NCC program fail to explain, and what other strategies do we need?

Varela: There is a minority of researchers that think that if we pose the problem purely in terms of the NCC it will have no solution, for the simple reason that lived experience is always something more and both logically and empirically non-reducible to neuronal function. What Husserl and Merleau-Ponty called lived experience cannot be explained purely in terms of the neuronal system. Of course one can find correlations between brain function and consciousness but that doesn't change the fact that there is a phenomenal aspect that is still not explained. My idea is that we have to change the terms of the discussion.

I think that I've been in a good position to do that because my philosophical background, like yours, is in the phenomenological tradition where the point of departure is lived experience and its intentional relation to the world. Intentionality is very important, because when I say that consciousness is lived experience I do not mean that this is something that exists only in the head. One doesn't find it in a piece of cerebral circuitry. Consciousness is not a property of a group of neurons; it belongs to an organism, in this case to a human, and one finds it in the particular action that one is living through. You can't explain consciousness if you ignore embodied action, because consciousness appears in an organism.

SG: This embodied approach, and really what you have called the 'enactive' approach, has a number of significant implications that take us beyond computation and even the wonderful ongoing research in brain science. It really implies a redefinition of the cognitive system to include elements that, as you say, are not simply in the head.

Varela: Absolutely. Let me mention three important ideas in this connection. First, consciousness has an enduring connected to the organism. The brain is always in an organism, and an organism is always involved in a self-regulating relationship to the environment — and this involves basic processes like nutrition and self-preservation, which means that the organism experiences hunger and thirst and the need for social relations. These experiences shape the way the brain works, and at bottom there is ultimately the feeling of existence, the feeling of just being here — but that too is tied to being a body. Consciousness, as this experience, is complex — it is tied to the vitality of the organism and interwoven in the feeling of existence, the emotions, sentiments, needs, and desires.

Second, consciousness is clearly coupled with the world, interacting with it through the entire sensory-motor interface. When I see an object, this bottle for example, this bottle is not an image in my head which I have to represent in there. My perception of the bottle is inseparable from my act of manipulating it — and there is good neuroscience to back this up. The action and the perception constitute a permanent but changeable coupling, and the world emerges as meaningful in the coupling. Interaction is the important principle here. It's evident from developmental studies, and from the way that the sensory-motor brain works.

So, when we talk about the contents of consciousness, the bottle, a face, the sky, and so forth, such things are not simply to be found in the information processing of neuronal circuitry. They are not centered in the brain, represented in the head, but are in the larger system, in the action, in the interaction among the external and the internal elements. In the same way, the feeling of existence lives in the interaction between the brain, the body, and the world.

Third, consciousness depends on intersubjectivity, and this is especially the case for humans. We are structurally designed to have relations with others, and the capacity for empathy. This is innate and reinforced in our everyday existence. The mother-child relationship manifests this empathy. And for the rest of my existence my mental life, and the acquisition and use of language, and the culture that comes along with it, are inseparable. Language and culture are not in my head; they depend entirely on others.

SG: If these various aspects contribute to the constitution of consciousness — body, world, others — that makes finding the NCC entirely problematic.

Varela: Indeed. Without the body, without the world, without others, the stimulation of a set of neurons amounts to nothing. This is not to say that the brain plays no role — it is the condition *sine qua non*. Indeed, it allows for the sensory-motor interaction that puts us in the world with others. But how we study the brain and discover its role cannot be done properly if we ignore the phenomenology which tells us that we are embodied and situated in our physical and social environments, and that consciousness is distributed across these elements.

SG: If we think of consciousness as the product of a kind of emergence, it is not something that emerges from just the neurobiology; it emerges from the interactions of brain, body, and environment.

Varela: Yes. This is important to understand. Central to the non-reductionist enactive view is the notion of emergence which goes against any simple dualism of mind-body. The concept of emergence is worked out in physics at the beginning of the 20th century. It derives from the observation of phase transitions or state transitions, and specifically how there is transition from a local level to a global level. For example, particles of air and water circulating in the atmosphere interact in a self-organizing way, and from this emerges a tornado, which on the one hand is nothing other than that self-organized system of air and water, but on the other hand causes mass destruction. The tornado has no substance, because its existence is simply the interrelations of its molecular components. But as anyone in Kansas will tell you, tornados are very real.

In biology the phenomeon of emergence is fundamental for explaining transitions from lower to higher levels, where ontologically new things emerge. Molecules become cells, which have different properties from molecules; cells become organisms, which have different properties from cells; organisms become conscious, and so on. Emergence in nature means that simple processes, governed by local rules, are drawn into small local interactions that, in appropriate conditions, generate something new with its own specific identity.

SG: Philosophers like Searle take up this concept of neurobiological emergence.

Varela: This concept of emergence is central to contemporary scientific research, even if many have failed to understand its importance. Science can even provide equations to describe these transitions from one level to another; from the local to the global. It is likely that consciousness, like life itself, is something in excess of the neuronal processes that we want to nail down as the NCC. It's a natural existence but totally unlike a Cartesian substance, and unlike neuronal substance; it is, so to speak, virtual — virtual but efficacious. Once a new identity emerges it has effects that are irreducible to the effects of its antecedent elements. With respect to consciousness, this means that we can truly speak of mental causality. Consciousness is not epiphenomenal, a byproduct of brain activity. Rather, the emergence of a mental state can have an effect on the local components, and there is indisputable evidence that experience changes the brain, that my experiences change the states of the synaptic processes in my brain.

I think this way of thinking of things changes, or ought to change the way that we do a science of consciousness. The fact that we can talk about mental causation in scientific terms should make us think differently about consciousness and the NCC project.

All of this should lead us to further considerations about the effects of intersubjectivity, language, and culture on consciousness. In his Gifford Lectures with Mary Hesse (Arbib & Hesse 1986), Michael Arbib proposed a theory of consciousness that seems to put language before consciousness. Is it possible that consciousness evolves out of linguistic practices?

Arbib: I would say that Mary Hesse and I, in the Gifford Lectures, addressed the particular human nature of consciousness, namely that we so often find ourselves articulating in words what we feel. At times, we feel that our consciousness is directing our activity, while at other times our conscious thoughts are like epiphenomena for processes that are determining our behavior. Our thesis was that it would give an evolutionary advantage to a population if each of its members could make a précis of what he was about to do and signal it to certain others to better coordinate their actions. We added that once that brain state was there, then its availability could change the way the brain itself computed, yielding changes with a further evolutionary advantage. I still think that this theory illuminates a crucial aspect of human consciousness, but I now feel dissatisfied because it tells us nothing about awareness more generally, such as we experience when admiring a beautiful face or enjoying a beautiful sunset or just basking in the warmth of the sun. I would imagine that some form of these feelings are in fact available to a huge range of animals and that a more satisfying approach to consciousness would link the Arbib-Hesse theory to a more general account of such awareness.

SG: The experience of pleasure, the avoidance of pain. These are often the forces mentioned in evolutionary theory to explain the origins of behaviors. But doesn't this already presuppose consciousness? And isn't that already a more primitive thing than language?

Arbib: To use terms like pleasure and pain when observing animal behavior begs the question as to whether in every species the feeling accompanies the behavior in the fashion that it does in most humans. Even more neutral terms like reward and punishment beg the question. If you have a bacterium moving up the food gradient is that pleasure, and if it is tumbling away from something unpleasant is that pain? Indeed, we know that there are forms of human brain damage as a result of which a person will say, 'Well I know this is a painful stimulus but I don't care'. This may be a case of the difference between having a system that can react adversely in certain situations from one that can experience pain. So to what extent, and when and where did pain really emerge? I don't know. But I think it is reasonable to believe that it emerged way back in evolution, and that understanding its emergence might be a good way to ground an account of that more primitive form of consciousness about which Hesse and I were silent.

A painful subject

I knew we wouldn't be able to get away from a discussion about consciousness without someone bringing up pain. The experience of pain (and why not pleasure?) is a basic possibility for any animal, and is often considered a measure of whether consciousness exists in the organism or not. It would be odd to say that I am in pain but I don't experience it. Pain seems to imply consciousness. Pain, more than conceptual understanding or belief seems to be essentially tied to consciousness. Wittgenstein makes us think about this. He suggests that if I believe that Lyon is south of Paris, or if I understand the concept of dark matter, and if I then go to sleep, the belief or the understanding is not affected in any way; in contrast, if I'm in pain and I go to sleep, I'm no longer in pain (see Wittgenstein, 1980 vol. II, 45; also McGinn 1989, 3, 94–109).

Even the most ancient texts of philosophy suggest that pain is a real pain in the proverbial neck. Socrates complains not about the pain he is feeling, but about the ambiguity that he feels about the distinction between pain and pleasure. Chained in his prison cell a few hours before he drinks his hemlock, Socrates has the leisure time to think about this problem.

> How singular is the thing called pleasure, and how curiously related to pain, which might be thought to be the opposite of it; for they never come to a man together, and yet he who pursues either of them is generally compelled to take the other. They are two, and yet they grow together out of one head or stem; and I cannot help thinking that if Aesop had noticed them, he would have made a fable about God trying to reconcile their strife, and when he could not, he fastened their heads together; and this is the reason why when one comes the other follows, as I find in my own case pleasure comes following after the pain in my leg, which was caused by the chain.[3]

Philosophers do tend to be a bit detached, even if it is their own pain under discussion. Let's take a look at some less detached examples. Jonathan Cole has been doing some research in this area especially in regard to spinal cord injury.

> **Cole:** One of the worst consequences of spinal cord injury is chronic pain, a phantom or deafferentation pain. This actually occurs in 60-65% of people and can be very severe in around 20%. But those in whom it is more tolerable some pain is preferred, because it gives them the illusion of connection with their bodies.
>
> **SG:** What kind of pain is it? If they actually prefer to be in pain, can it be very severe pain?
>
> **Cole:** In some of them you can say, well on a visual analog scale [e.g., 0–10], how much is the pain? Some might say two or three. They may quite like some pain rather than nothing. Incidentally I spent a long time trying to unravel the sensation of nothing and for most people it has a distinct percept.
> Others may say that their pain is higher, at seven or eight, or even

---

3   Plato, 360 BCE. Phaedo (60b). Translated by Benjamin Jowett. Available online at *The Internet Classics Archives*. http://classics.mit.edu/Plato/phaedo.html

ten, than the level, five to six, which they say they can tolerate. This is socially and emotionally, ontologically, destructive. One woman said that paralysis does not stop life but chronic pain can. The form of pain is often difficult to describe. They may say burning, tingling, gripping — it is ill defined and diffuse usually. Adjectives for pain are widely used and can be very useful, but for a richer account one needs a fuller narrative.

SG: What's the cause of the pain?

Cole: What's the cause of any central [nervous system] pain? One theory suggests that when there is an absence of sensory input to the central nervous system, pain results. Some suggest that it's analogous with tinnitus in which there is an absence of auditory input ...

SG: So it is just that nothing is happening there and the brain says something should be happening.

Cole: Exactly. It up-regulates itself to see what there is, and the consequence of that is that it starts to reach perception.

SG: Might these tetraplegic patients experience a phantom of their body, within which they experience pain? Of course they also have a real body, unlike a post-amputation phantom.

Cole: They see their bodies, but still have no feeling from them. Their pain is centrally generated but they interpret it as filling the body they can see, giving them sensation as well as visualization of their bodies.

SG: It's interesting that there is a desire to feel embodied, to feel something in their body — a desire, of course, that we who are not paralyzed or deafferented simply do not experience since the feeling of embodiment is there all the time — in the background, pre-reflectively as the phenomenologists say. We take it for granted. Is the pain localized? Do they say that it's their legs, for example, that are in pain?

Cole: Yes, it is localized. They might say that their legs feel as if on fire, or that it feels as though someone is hammering something into their fingers, or the back, or buttocks. The question then is how you treat it. As far as I'm aware there aren't many good trials on the various forms of drug and other treatments for the chronic pain in spinal cord injury. A few years ago I arranged a workshop on this in Britain, looking at research techniques. It turned out that rather than consider new techniques we didn't even know what treatments are presently being used and whether or not they are effective. People with spinal cord injury have other pains than this chronic deafferentation pain, too. They can have joint pains in the shoulder, since they have to transfer themselves from chair to bed for years and they may have arthritis. Pain is one huge problem in spinal cord injury medicine.

SG: Ramachandran has this well-known experiment with a mirror box (Ramachandran, Rogers-Ramachandran & Cobb, 1995). As you know people with phantoms often experience phantom pain because, for example, the posture of the phantom remains constant. In this case, the subject's phantom fist was clenched and unmovable. Ramachandran had him position his phantom appropriately, and then view the clenched fist of his intact arm in the mirror so that it appears to be the missing arm. He is able to unclench his intact fist, and the visual perception of his phantom fist unclenchiing relieves his serious phantom pain. Is anything of that sort possible for spinal cord patients? Is there any kind of procedure possible in which they could simulate movement, perhaps by viewing video or some such thing?

Cole: Well there are two elements to that. Firstly, people use video and virtual reality as distracters for pain. Secondly, Flor's group in Germany has done some very elegant work showing that if you use a neural prosthesis in people with amputation, and you use it a certain number of hours a day, this may reduce the phantom limb pain (Lotze et al. 1999). They also showed that if you have a stump, and have to do a tactile discrimination on the stump skin, then this may also reduce the pain (Flor et al. 2001). Both examples seem more than a simple distraction effect.

It is also intriguing that in people with a form of pain called complex regional pain syndrome, one of the most effective treatments is to *use* the part which is painful. And of course, if you are thinking of deafferentation as being the cause of the pain, in that situation, the question arises as to whether there is also a motor component to the genesis of the pain, a 'pain induced by lack-of-movement' rather than a 'lack-of-sensation induced pain'. Then the question is how you might treat it and whether you can distinguish those two.

SG: That has me thinking of the work of Marc Jeannerod (1997), Jean Decety (2001), and others on the notion of shared neural representations for movement and the imaging of movement—when one consciously *imagines* doing an action many of the same brain areas responsible for actually *doing* that same action, or *seeing* someone else do that same action, are activated. Might there be a technique that would exploit the use of the imagination of movement to address this kind of pain? Could a reflectively controlled consciousness in that regard reach down into the subpersonal mechanisms that seem to be generating this pain? I admit that sounds somewhat naïve—why don't they just think the pain away?

Cole: I understand the idea. If people with spinal cord injury for some years imagine moving their paralysed arms or legs then they activate similar areas of the brain as control subjects. If they can imagine moving, might this thought reduce their pain? If so then why haven't they, the patients, discovered it themselves?

I did have a patient who had below knee amputations with bilateral phantom limb pain, who said that when he was swimming and he imagined flicking his legs out, his pain was reduced. Another told me that if he could imagine walking around a golf course, his pain was reduced. My feeling is that that's not simply distraction, but it's difficult to be absolutely sure of that.

SG: Do you know whether the effects of brain plasticity cause any of the spinal cord pain? That is, if the brain is undergoing neural reorganization.

Cole: Yes. I divide plasticity into several aspects. When someone learns to move again after a neurological loss, then that cognitive re-training is taking advantage of plasticity; improvement needs conscious effort. Another form of plasticity occurs independently of cognitive driving and this may be what you were thinking of. Flor's hypothesis is exactly that (Grusser et al. 2001). She showed that if you look at the remapping of the sources, within the brain, of evoked potentials from an apparently insentient area, (say due to a peripheral nerve injury), by stimulating areas of skin around them, then plastic change in these evoked potential sources are correlated with pain. She suggests that pain is related to plasticity after deafferentation.

One should always be aware however that these experiments look at the sensory cortex, and many neural events related to the development of pain occur in brain areas beyond that, anterior and posterior to it.

SG: Right, but all of these things are connected, so that if you have change in the sensory cortex it's likely that other, even motor, maps of the body might be affected.

Cole: I agree. And that highly connected complexity might be why it is often so difficult to describe pain, or pleasure. I might ask tetraplegics, 'Do you remember what it was like to walk?' There's a real sense in which many of them cannot remember. Intellectually they remember walking, but not what it felt like. One guy said, 'walking along the beach, with sand on my feet—these are the sorts of memories I miss, or I would like to have again.' It was the affective, pleasurable, aspects of locomotion he missed, rather than purely the instrumental ones. But can you remember the last time you walked along a beach, feeling the pebbles between your feet, and the water on them. Intellectually, yes, but the memories of the actual experience are not easily dredged up and made fresh, and made experiential. I think we are the same in that regard. Their memories for such experiences are no different from our own.

SG: These are experiences that philosophers refer to as 'qualia' or the 'what it is like' — experiences such as the way the sand feels on one's feet. Their fleeting nature is probably the source of many of the problems that we have in explaining such experiences. Qualia are confined to present, ongoing experience; they don't seem to have a temporal 'thickness'. To remember how something felt, or how I experienced something in this qualitative sense is really difficult. One does it only intellectually, as you say, and very abstractly unless one re-lives the experience and literally has it again. Qualia are sometimes said to be ineffable. Perhaps this is why such experiences are so fleeting, because they are difficult to describe in words. After all, I could be standing on the sand for a long time, and still be standing there, and still not have a good description of how the sand feels against my feet. A poet might have a better chance. But for most of us, not only can we not remember what it *was* like, we have great difficulty describing what it *is* like, even as we experience it. So, if I ask you as we walk around the university here, what is it like to walk, you might have some difficulty answering.

Cole: Yes, and add to that that asking someone to compare what they are like now, years later, to what they were like before, is impossible too. And if they who have experienced both ways of living cannot remember, then what chance have we to empathize?

Pain is an interesting phenomenon in this context because it clearly involves consciousness and clearly shows us that both brain (as something that changes with experience) and body (standing with both feet on the sand), thought (as memory or imagination) and action (walking, swimming) are complexly related in ways that we still don't understand.

Chapter 7

Intersubjectivity

One of the most recent developments in neuroscience is the definition of a new field termed cognitive social neuroscience, marked by the launch of two new journals *Social Neuroscience* and *Social, Cognitive, and Affective Neuroscience,* both appearing in 2006. The focus on social interaction, in neuroscience, recent philosophy of mind, and other fields, like robotics, has been motivated in part by the discovery of mirror neurons (MNs) in the mid-1990s, and by further experimental and brain imaging research on resonance systems. This work, which leads to some important insights concerning intersubjectivity, is also work that is directly related to our starting point — movement.

Mirror neurons were discovered in the pre-motor cortex of macaque monkeys in the university medical school lab of Giacomo Rizzolatti and his colleagues in Parma, Italy. Using micro-electrodes they were recording from single neuronal cells and were testing what they knew to be motor neurons responsible for the planning of movement. The story is that the researchers decided to break for lunch, but they decided to eat in the lab so they didn't have to disconnect the monkey from the instruments. When they started to eat the recording instruments started to register activation of the motor neuron. They thought this odd since in fact the monkey wasn't moving but was simply staring at them as they ate. So they did further experiments and found a class of neurons that were activated both when the animal made an action, such as reaching and grasping something, and when the animal observed someone else making that action. (see, e.g., Gallese et al. 1996; Rizzolatti et al. 1996). Subsequently, good evidence has been developed to show that humans also have MNs in premotor cortex and parietal areas (Fadiga et al. 1995).

The first time I heard about MNs I was at one of the large conferences on consciousness at Tucson in 1998. Someone had cancelled out of a plenary session and Vittorio Gallese, one of the researchers from Rizzolatti's lab, was asked to step in and explain the discovery. He more or less knocked me off my seat with the data he presented. I had been working, philosophically, on a number of topics that, at the time, I thought might involve this type of mirror system, including some work with Andrew Meltzoff on neonate imitation. I was not the only one excited by this news. I couldn't get near Gallese after his talk, because there was such a crowd lined up to speak with him.

The excitement about mirror neurons has hardly diminished to this day. On the one hand the original data seemed to say simply that these neurons were activated in the presence of certain movements, and they did not discriminate on whether it was one's own movement or the other agent's movement. But subsequent testing showed that in fact these neurons were responding to intentional actions and not just the mechanical movement. For example, the neurons would fire when the monkey observed another monkey or a human reaching to pick up a piece of food; but they would not fire when the piece of food was not there and the reaching seemed to have no point. So the MNs were not registering the reaching or grasping movement; they seemed to be registering the action of intentionally reaching *for* something. In another experiment, when a monkey sees someone reaching behind a screen, the MNs fire when the monkey knows that there is something to pick up behind the screen, but they do not fire when the monkey doesn't know this or knows that there isn't something there. In more recent experiments MNs in the parietal cortex are activated in a way that shows they are keyed into the goal of the action and not necessarily the particular way or the particular movements used by the agent to obtain the goal.

Such experiments have motivated strong claims by researchers about what sorts of things MNs might be called on to explain. They have also motivated popular science reporters like Susan Blakeslee to claim in a recent *New York Times* article (January 10, 2006), entitled 'Cells that read minds', that mirror neurons explain not only how we are capable of understanding another person's actions, but also language, empathy, 'how children learn, why people respond to certain types of sports, dance, music and art, why watching media violence may be harmful and why many men like pornography'. The jury is still out on much of this, but there is currently general consensus among scientists that MNs play some role in how we understand others, or at least in how we understand their actions.

Mirror neurons and simulation theory

We're back with Marc Jeannerod in Lyon.

> **SG:** Many theorists today make reference to mirror neurons in many different contexts, for example, in explanations of language development, neonate imitation, and of how we understand others. Do you

have any reservations about their wide theoretical use across all of these different contexts?

Jeannerod: I am not working on monkeys myself. All that I know on mirror neurons is from Rizzolatti's work. Working in humans, I think that this is a useful concept, but I don't see it limited to that particular group of neurons in the ventral premotor cortex. What you see in humans is a large neural network which is activated during action observation. Thus, the idea that you get about action observation becomes very different from what you get by looking at the brain neuron by neuron. I told this to Rizzolatti and asked him why he did not look for mirror neurons in other brain areas in the monkey. What I mean is that, after all, premotor neurons don't tell us the whole story. [Note that shortly after this interview MNs were discovered in the parietal cortex (see Fogassi et al. 2005)].

SG: Gallese talks about a mirror system.

Jeannerod: Maybe it is a consequence of my advice? [laughter]. Good, because it is what you would see in the human and what you would probably see in the monkey as well, if you studied the whole brain instead of just one point. Of course, we cannot forget that the concept of mirror neurons is still very critical. It indicates that in at least one point of the brain you have the same system which is key to the relation between observing and acting.

SG: And imagining movement?

Jeannerod: Well in humans you have the same areas that are activated during doing, imagining, and observing. The question remains of the degree of overlap between activation of these areas in the three conditions. With the mirror neurons in premotor cortex, we know for sure that there is at least one point in the brain where the overlap is complete for acting and observing.

Incidentally, there is an interesting example that was chosen by Freud to illustrate the idea of empathy. This is in his book on jokes (Freud 1905). Freud tries to explain why we laugh when we see a clown or someone who is pretending to make an enormous effort to lift an apparently heavy object, and then falls on his back. We laugh because we have created within ourselves an expectation by simulating the effort of the clown, and we see something that is very different from the expectation. The effect we see is at discrepancy with respect to our internal model, and this is the source of comedy. The simulation of the action we observe does not meet the expectation. I take this as a proof for the simulation theory.

SG: Was Freud a simulation theorist?

Jeannerod: Yes, he was.

SG: A simulation theory of slapstick!

One approach to explaining how we understand others, which is gaining in importance precisely because of these discoveries in neuroscience, is called simulation theory (ST). ST is a theory developed by philosophers like Robert Gordon, Jane Heal, and Alvin Goldman. Their original proposals suggest that when we see someone else behaving in a certain way we explicitly put ourselves in their situation, and we simulate or imagine ourselves behaving in that way, and on this basis we infer what must be going on in their minds, their beliefs, desires, and intentions. In effect we 'mindread' or 'mentalize' their mental states by putting ourselves in their shoes and working out what must be going on in their head (Goldman 2005a). Here's a description of this explicit kind of simulation given by Goldman. According to him it involves three steps.

> First, the attributor creates in herself pretend states intended to match those of the target. In other words, the attributor attempts to put herself in the target's 'mental shoes'. The second step is to feed these initial pretend states [e.g., beliefs] into some mechanism of the attributor's own psychology ... and allow that mechanism to operate on the pretend states so as to generate one or more new states [e.g., decisions]. Third, the attributor assigns the output state to the target ... [e.g., we infer or project the decision to the other's mind]. (Goldman 2005b, 80-81.)

Goldman, working with Gallese, has seen the significance of the neuronal mirror system for ST. Both separately (Goldman 2006; Gallese 2001) and together (Gallese and Goldman 1998), they have developed the idea of implicit or low level simulation. Gallese puts it this way:

> Whenever we are looking at someone performing an action, beside the activation of various visual areas, there is a concurrent activation of the motor circuits that are recruited when we ourselves perform that action. ... Our motor system becomes active *as if* we were executing the very same action that we are observing ... Action observation implies action simulation ... our motor system starts to covertly simulate the actions of the observed agent (Gallese 2001, 37).

In effect, MN activation generates a kind of implicit simulation of the other person's actions. We can read this as an even stronger claim, namely, that MN activation is involved in reading not only the other person's actions, but the other person's mind. Thus, for example, Rizollatti states that 'Mirror neurons allow us to grasp the minds of others not through conceptual reasoning but through direct simulation. By feeling, not by thinking' (in Blakeslee 2006). Implicit ST understood in these or in similar terms is, in fact, the growing consensus. Indeed, use of the term 'simulation' is becoming the standard way of referring to mirror system activation. Thus, for example, Jeannerod, in an article with the philosopher Elizabeth Pacherie, writes:

> As far as the understanding of action is concerned, we regard simulation as the default procedure ... We also believe that simulation is the root form of interpersonal mentalization and that it is best conceived as a hybrid of explicit and implicit processes, with subpersonal neural simulation serving as a basis for explicit mental simulation (Jeannerod and Pacherie 2004, 129; see Jeannerod 2001b).

Since we are in Lyon we may as well ask Marc what this means.

> **SG:** I know that you and a number of people here in Lyon are interested in simulation theory, and as you mentioned, you have written about it (Jeannerod 2001; Jeannerod and Frak 1999; Jeannerod and Pacherie 2004). Also, you, Decety, and various colleagues have done some work identifying brain areas, rather than single neurons, that are activated not only when the subject performs an action, but also when the subject observes the action of another (Decety et al. 1997; Decety et al. 1994; Grezes and Decety, 2001). As your team here has discovered, the very same brain areas activated for one's own action, are activated when the subject simulates observed action, that is, when the subject imagines himself doing the action that he has observed. So there is an overlap of functions mapped onto the same brain areas. Does this neurological evidence support simulation theory?

> **Jeannerod:** Well, let me show you a diagram we are working with (Figure 1). This represents a motor cognitive situation with two people. We have agent A and agent B. The processes diagramed are represented as happening in the brain. They are based on the idea of an overlap between neural representations that you make when you observe an action or when you think of an action. Let us take an example: agent A generates a representation of a self-generated action, a motor intention. If this comes to execution, this will become a signal for agent B, such that agent B will form a representation of the action that he sees, and will simulate it. Agent B will make an estimate of the social consequences of the action he sees and will possibly change his beliefs about agent A. And then you have a cycle where these two representations interact with each other, and then the two agents. In this process I, as one of the agents, am answering the question of 'Who?' — that is, I am attributing certain actions to another person, and certain actions to myself. In fact the two representations, within an individual subject, are close to each other and

partly overlap. Determining who is acting, myself or the other, will be based on the non-overlapping part. In pathological conditions, if the overlapping area becomes greater, as it might happen in schizophrenia (on my interpretation), then you have no way of knowing who is generating the action.

SG: In this model, is there some point at which the representation of action becomes a motor image, I mean an explicit or conscious event?

Jeannerod: Well there is something that this model doesn't say. It is that probably you don't need to go through the executed action to get the social signal. You are able to disentangle intentions or states of mind, even from covert actions.

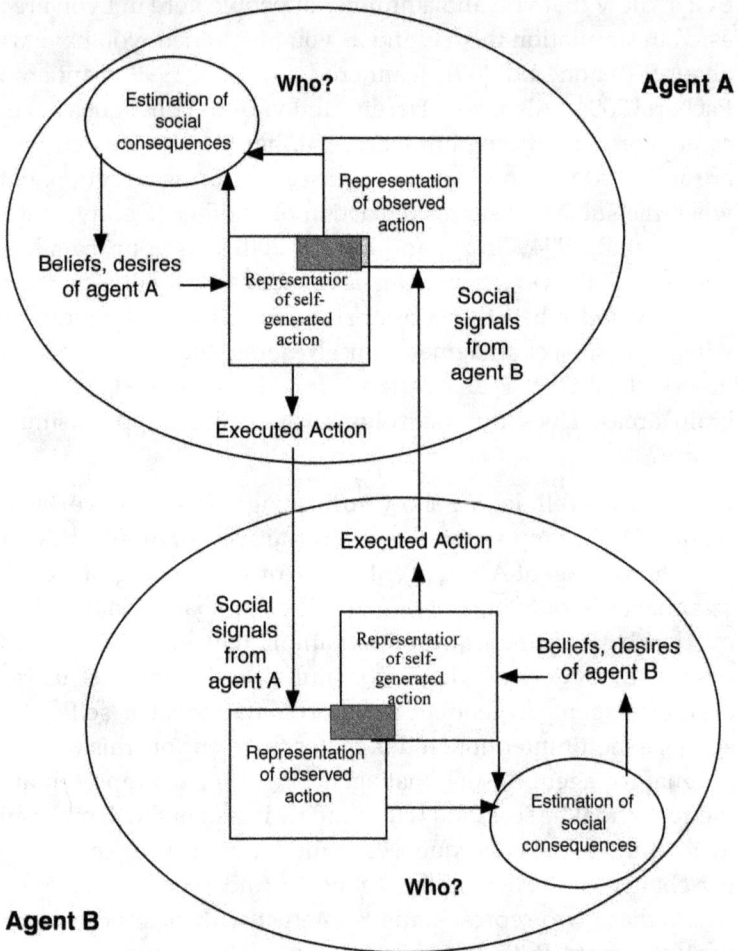

Figure 7.1 Interaction between two agents.

SG: So you can anticipate an action, or you can discern an intention in someone else.

Jeannerod: Yes, I mean that agent B may look at agent A and try to understand what his intentions are, using some form of mind reading. I think it is not necessary to execute an action to generate a signal to the other person. The signal may very well go through subliminal events like direction of gaze, posture, etc and it doesn't need to be transformed into an overt action to reach the other person.

SG: I entirely agree on this point. Let me add that, according to some simulation theorists, it is not necessary to be conscious of the simulation. The representations do not have to reach the point of overt or explicit consciousness, they can remain implicit. Simulation also leaves lots of room for misunderstanding, which it should do.

Jeannerod: Of course. In some cases it may be better to act out what we mean and avoid the misunderstanding.

SG: Let me mention that before I came here I attended the British Society for Phenomenology meeting in Oxford. Some of the phenomenologists there were convinced that neuroscientists were only interested in explaining everything in terms of neurons, and that, on this view, consciousness itself is simply a product of neuronal processes, with no causal power of its own. But your work goes in the other direction in the sense that you show that a subject's intentions will in some degree shape or determine what neurons will fire. We discussed this earlier. But here you suggest further that it may be what other people do, and how we interpret their actions, that will determine how our neurons fire, and, of course, how we will act.

Jeannerod: Yes. Here we are in the context of social neuroscience.

Simulation theorists contend that our understanding of others depends on our internal and empathetic simulation of the other person's actions and gestures. The work of Jeannerod, Decety, and their colleagues extends and complements the work of Rizzolatti, Gallese and others on MNs, and provides significant empirical support for ST. They show that neuronal patterns (and not just individual neurons) responsible for explicit action *simulation* are much the same as those activated in the *observation* and in the *performance* of action. PET and fMRI studies show significant overlap between action observation, execution, and simulation in the supplementary motor area (SMA), the dorsal premotor cortex, the supramarginal gyrus, and the superior parietal lobe (Blakemore and Decety 2001; Grezes and Decety 2001; Jeannerod 2001). Thus, some simulation theorists claim that simulation for understanding others is an implicit (non-conscious) rather than an explicit (conscious) process. In this regard, the important fact is that the simple *observation* of others (without any explicit simulation) is activating most of the same brain areas as those activated by explicit simulation. Compared to activated areas for my own action, observation of another person's action is associated with additional activation in the temporal pathway, consistent with visual processing. Explicit simulation, that is, consciously imagining the action, is associated with additional activation in the ventral premotor cortex, which may indicate a linguistic contribution. The shared activation, however, suggests that what is referred to as implicit simulation is not a separate process from our perception of others. Rather it implies that our perception of others is implicitly a simulating process. It is not that I see the other's action, and then simulate it, and then use the simulation to interpret what I see. Rather, to see the other person in action is already to understand how it is with that person. Furthermore, there is good behavioral evidence to suggest that this kind of implicit understanding of the other's intentions and actions occurs much earlier in infant development than most theory of mind and simulation approaches admit.

It should be noted that MN activation is 'neutral' in regard to agent attribution. That is, MNs fire whether I make the action or you make the action. So in themselves they cannot account for our ability to discriminate between my action and your action. Jeannerod and his colleagues (Georgieff and Jeannerod 1998; Jeannerod 1997; Jeannerod 2001a) suggest that the non-overlapping neuronal areas, that is, the areas of neuronal contrast between action execution, action observation, and explicit simulation, may be responsible for distinguishing self-agency from the agency of others. They refer to this as the 'Who system'. This suggests that an important element of self-consciousness is intrinsically tied to consciousness of others. And again, there is good behavioral evidence that a primitive or primary sense of self (and specifically, a primary form of self-consciousness) emerges much earlier than many would admit (see Gallagher and Meltzoff 1996).

I have two worries about the concept of implicit simulation, however. First, it is not clear why the MN process should be called simulation, at least in the way that ST defines simulation. For example, according to ST, simulation involves pretense; to simulate I pretend to be in the other person's place, or I generate 'as if' beliefs, etc. But no such pretense is possible in the MN system. It's not just that as mechanisms MNs either fire or don't fire—they never just pretend to fire—but more importantly in terms of content, they cannot represent pretense. To do so they would have to represent slots for two agents: *I* pretend to be *you*. But as we have just noted, MNs are neutral with respect to agent attribution. There is no *I* or *you* represented in MN activation. But even if we added the Who system activation to the MN activation, what we are describing at the subpersonal level are the processes that at the personal level correspond to social perception, and it may be best to understand MN activation as in fact simply part of the underpinnings of a direct but meaningful perception of the other person's action. This idea is reinforced by my second worry.

My second worry is about the often found claims of universality made for simulation. Goldman (2002, 7–8), for example expresses this clearly:

> The strongest form of ST would say that all cases of (third-person) mentalization employ simulation. A moderate version would say, for example, that simulation is the *default* method of mentalization … I am attracted to the moderate version … Simulation is the primitive, root form of interpersonal mentalization.

And Jeannerod and Pacherie concur:

> As far as the understanding of action is concerned, we regard simulation as the default procedure. … We also believe that simulation is the root form of interpersonal mentalization and that it is best conceived as a hybrid of explicit and implicit processes, with subpersonal neural simulation serving as a basis for explicit mental simulation. (Jeannerod and Pacherie 2004, 129).

Goldman, sharing my same worry about finding pretense in MNs, suggests that perhaps one could drop the pretense aspect of simulation and still have something like a minimal simulation where the necessary aspect would simply be a matching of the simulating state with the simulated state (see, Goldman 2006, 131ff; Goldman and Sripada 2005, 208). The notion of *matching* turns up in many descriptions of simulation. For example, Jean Decety and Julie Grèzes (2006, 6), explaining Rizzolatti's position, put it this way:

> By automatically matching the agent's observed action onto its own motor repertoire without executing it, the firing of mirror neurons in the observer brain simulates the agent's observed action and thereby contributes to the understanding of the perceived action.

The problem with the suggestion that such matching may be the criterion for a minimal simulation is twofold, appearing on both the personal and subpersonal level respectively. On the person level it is often the case that my understanding of the actions of the other person involves just the opposite of matching their action or mental states. For instance, consider the example of the snake woman (see Gallagher 2007a&b). I see a woman in front of me enthusiastically and gleefully reaching to pick up a snake; at the same time I am experiencing revulsion and disgust about that very possibility. Her action, which I fully sense and understand from her enthusiastic and gleeful expression to be something that she likes to do, triggers in me precisely the opposite feelings. In this case, neither my neural states, nor my motor actions (I may be retreating with gestures of disgust just as she is advancing toward the snake with gestures of enthusiasm), nor my feelings/cognitions match hers. Yet I understand her actions and emotions (which are completely different from mine), indeed that is what is motivating my own actions and emotions, and, moreover, I do this without even meeting the minimal necessary condition for simulation, that is, matching my state to hers. I suggest that no simulation in any form is involved in this kind of case, and I suggest that this kind of case is not rare. So that's trouble for the universal claim made for simulation.

Furthermore, on the subpersonal level the scientific research on mirror neurons suggests good reasons to think mirror neuron activation cannot involve a precise match between motor system execution and observed action. Csibra (2005) points out that conservatively, between 21 and 45% of neurons identified as mirror neurons are sensitive to multiple types of action; of those activated by a single type of observed action, that action is not necessarily the same action defined by the motor properties of the neuron; approximately 60% of mirror neurons are 'broadly congruent', which means there may be some relation between the observed action(s) and their associated executed action, but not an exact match. Only about one-third of mirror neurons show a one-to-one congruence.[1] Newman-Norlund et al. (2007, 55) suggest that activation of the broadly congruent mirror neurons may represent a complementary action rather than a similar action. In that case they could not be simulations.

Here is a short segment of an interview Thomas Ramsøy (2006) did with me on just this issue.

> **SG:** The most interesting thing about mirror neurons, or more generally resonance systems, is that they are not just about one body but about what Merleau-Ponty called intercorporality—how one body relates to another. It's the neuroscience of intercorporality that is helping us explain how our intersubjective relations are possible, without resorting to amorphous concepts like 'universal spirituality' or 'shared human nature'. But even with this good neuroscience we need to be careful about finding the right theoretical framework for developing an account of how we understand others. Gallese has joined forces with simulation theorists, and I'm not sure this is the right way to go. I've argued, in some recent papers (e.g., Gallagher

---

1   Csibra concludes: 'With strongly unequal distribution of types of action or types of grip, one could find a relatively high proportion of good match between the [observed action vs executed action] domains even if there were no causal relation between them. Without such a statistical analysis, it remains uncertain whether the cells that satisfy the definition of "mirror neuron" (i.e., the ones that discharge both with execution and observation of actions) do indeed have "mirror properties" in the everyday use of this term (i.e., are generally activated by the same action in both domains)' (2005, 3).

2007), that the concept of simulation, as it is developed in simulation theory, signifies an activity on the part of the subject. As it is usually described, the simulating subject uses her own mind as a model for understanding the other person's mind. She introduces 'pretend' beliefs or desires into the model, and in the end makes an inference about what the other person must be experiencing. Gallese is not defending this explicit, and often introspective version of simulation theory (Goldman is someone who does defend this view). Rather he is proposing that the simulation process is subpersonal and carried out by the mirror system. But in that case, my question is: What does simulation mean? All descriptions of simulation that I have seen suggest that it is something in which the subject actively engages. But the activation of the mirror system is not something that we actively engage in; it happens automatically. It's not something that I do; it's something that happens to me. In a sense, it is something that the other person elicits in me. So it strikes me as strange to call this a simulation. I think it's better to view the activation of resonance systems as part of a perceptual process that gives us access to the other person's intentions. And I think this is clearly consistent with the idea of enactive perception.

Ramsøy: So, the notion of 'simulation' implicates a conscious agent, while the description put forth by Gallese actually points out that these processes occur at a subconscious level. From this, it seems that a distinction between conscious and unconscious processes can help both to clarify concepts like 'mirror neurons', as well as to put forth specific questions relating to the subserving mechanisms. Could such a distinction be helpful in distinguishing between processes at a neural level?

SG: I think the issue is not about conscious versus non-conscious — although there is certainly a question about how much is conscious and how much is not. The real issue has to do with how one defines simulation. Whether simulation is conscious or not, it is always defined as some kind of proactive process — I do something, or my brain does something or uses some kind of model in a controlled way to accomplish something. If you look at the way simulation is described, it is always this kind of proactive engagement. Goldman's (2002; 2005a&b) descriptions of a mindreader trying to predict or 'retrodict' someone else's mental states pictures the subject as engaged in stepwise activity. The idea is that I, as subject, first deliberately create some pretend beliefs. I then, as Goldman describes it, 'feed' these beliefs into some kind of routine mechanism, and then I assign the result to the other person. Pierre Jacob (2002), for another example, characterizes simulation as engaging in an 'activity', a 'heuristic', or 'methodology' in order to compare and predict mental states. If this is what we mean by simulation, what happens to the concept when we attribute simulation to subpersonal brain processes? According to Gallese, we still get descriptions of proactive processes. He still considers it a process of modeling in a stepwise fashion in which the second step is simulative modeling of the other's intentional actions. What we know is that when I see another person's action there is, among other things, sensory activation in the visual system followed by activation in the pre-motor cortex. Moreover, it's agreed that this is something that takes place automatically. But to call it simulation is to suggest a controlled, proactive process. It would be better to call it a perceptual elicitation since the resonance is automatically generated in my system by the action of the other. If you insist that this kind of perceptual elicitation is a simulation, then, at best, you are changing the definition of simulation, and at worst, distorting our understanding of what is going on.

In denying that mirror neurons are simulating or specifically creating a match in such cases, I am not denying that mirror neurons may be involved in our interactions with others, possibly contributing to our ability to understand others or to keep track of ongoing intersubjective relations. Moreover, I do not want to deny that in some cases we may in fact engage in explicit simulation, although I suggest these are rare cases, and that in some of these cases we may be engaged in a different kind of simulation from the standard dyadic model described by ST. Matthew Ratcliffe (2007) has proposed that as we engage with another person we may sometimes in fact simulate, not their mental states, but our interaction, for example, in an attempt to predict where our interaction is heading. One can generalize this and suggest that we may also simulate the potential interaction of agents other than ourselves. I say 'potential' interaction, because if it is a current interaction, whether between ourselves and someone else, or between other agents that we can see or overhear, etc., then there would be very little reason to try to simulate what is directly accessible (see Jacob 2008 for further discussion).

Theory of Mind

That there is much more going on, however, both on the personal and subpersonal level, comes out in the conversation I had with Jaak Panksepp. As a champion of affective neuroscience, he wants to bring emotion into play in the discussion of how we interact with others. It's not just neurons firing at the subpersonal level, it is also neurochemicals flowing; and yet this is never divorced from the personal level context that may modulate brain reaction.

> **Panksepp:** Among these neurotransmitter systems it's very easy to envision that their effects are context dependent, most especially social contexts, and how the environment and how various brain systems are generating certain sets and patterns of affective chemistries. There are a host of social neurochemistries, with opiates and oxytocin being the most well studied, each with slightly different effects. For instance, recently oxytocin has been the darling of social neuroscience, but it is really only one control among many, probably one that promotes confidence, social warmth and the feeling of a secure base, but probably not without the assistance of brain opioids. These are very 'personal' chemistries, but there are many that remain to be discovered. At present, a lot of people think that whenever oxytocin is flowing in the brain you feel good and warm and loving — we don't know that for a fact, that's a theoretical inference, perhaps an overgeneralization. Let's hope is true. There are bound to be surprises, and I do think the pure positive-loving effects of oxytocin have been exaggerated.
>
> For instance, after we discovered that vasotocin and oxytocin could dramatically reduce separation distress in the mid 1980s, we asked the following question from rats: 'Does an animal like to have oxytocin in their brain as measured by conditioned place preferences — namely, will they seek out a specific location where they had gotten oxytocin in the past?' We obtained no clean and powerful affirmative signal, as one would expect from a pure 'love-molecule'. However, when we gave the oxytocin in an environment that included other animals then the desire to return to that location was more clearly amplified by oxytocin. So oxytocin did not carry a specific affective message by itself; it only promoted an affective message that could be amplified by social context … which, I think, makes it especially nice.

We get to the topic of *theory of mind* (ToM) in an indirect way in this conversation. Before we go there, let me explain that the phrase 'theory of mind' can be taken in a wide sense to mean any theoretical approach to explaining social cognition, including ST. It can also be taken in a narrower sense to refer to a specific theoretical approach that is precisely about the use of theory in our social relations. This is sometimes called 'theory theory' (TT). Theory theorists seem to be always in a debate with simulation theorists. Rather than simulating the minds of others, the theory theorists claim that we appeal to a theory, which they, and everyone else, call 'folk psychology'. The rules of folk psychology are the rules of commonsense, and we use this commonsense approach to make sense out of the behavior of others specifically by making inferences about their beliefs, desires, and other mental states based on these rules. So whereas the simulationists feel their way into your mind, the theory theorists intellectualize their way in. In much of the following the phrase 'theory of mind' is used in the more general sense to include both ST and TT. As I indicated, in my discussion with Panksepp, we get to this rather indirectly.

SG: You argue against the likelihood of there being social biological modules at the cortical level. And you're in favor of the view that social emotional systems at the subcortical level are more likely to determine social behavior.

Panksepp: Yes, I do believe the cortex becomes specialized largely epigenetically. It has few, if any, intrinsic social abilities although some social molecules, certainly opioids, CRF and several others, directly regulate cortical tone. Perhaps they facilitate epigenetic construction of certain emotional scenarios within the cortex; this is virgin territory for inquiries. This also makes me wonder whether mirror neurons, which currently figure heavily in conceptions of mind-reading and empathy, have any intrinsic functions at birth. I expect careful analysis will eventually indicate that the functions of mirror neurons are developmentally rather than genetically derived. Once it has matured, the cortex can certainly promote many social graces, and perhaps even more frequently, various social failings, because often the emergent epigenetic functions of the cortex are as self-centered as the reptilian brain, and not harmonious with the most pro-social functions of various pro-social subcortical-limbic circuits. We must remember that neocortex, especially frontal executive areas, are adept at inhibiting primary-process emotionality. But better higher social functions can be epigenetically created by powerful sub-cortical social urges such as those of maternal nurturance and play … as well as the healthy exercise of separation-distress circuitry in the midst of a secure base.

Thus, I favor the view that in early development, the more primitive social-emotional systems rule, and with maturation the higher systems prevail, except during especially strong emotional storms. Since all human social behavior eventually comes to be regulated and controlled by higher brain functions, it is often difficult to scientifically confirm the continuing influences of the subcortical powers, but I doubt if they ever completely abandon control to the cortex. For instance, even though adult animals exhibit no intense separation distress like relatively helpless young animals, you can still make them cry like lost infants when you stimulate their subcortical separation-distress system. All the basic emotional systems continue to contribute to living, and some systems that are especially robust in youth, continue to guide daily activities of healthy human beings. I personally believe the play-urge is one of the most important forces that Mother Nature provided for the construction of a pro-social neo-cortex. And only if we parents guide this construction well, can we expect to have children that can mirror those deeply empathic responses we may need to construct better worlds.

SG: Okay. Now you emphasize the importance of play and laughter, especially in infancy and childhood, and these are intersubjective interactions that activate sub-cortical centers systems …

Panksepp: And cortical ones too. I think play is quintessentially capable of activating the very best that the cortex is capable of. The higher social brain is not encoded in our genes, but arises from our intersubjective, societal and cultural interactions.

SG: … and in this you already refer to the 'subtlety of intersubjective states', your phrase. Does this go against the established ToM approaches to inter-subjectivity, whether theory theory or stimulation theory. Can you say something about this?

Panksepp: That's a tough one. I am a fan of theory of mind. The more cognitively sophisticated the creature, because of ever more cortex, the more sophisticated their theory of mind can become … and their potential for good and evil also. Not only can one begin to worry about who is thinking about what and why, much more than other animals, but one can also appreciate how to inflict cruel and unusual punishments as well as the full measure of human empathy.

I also think there is a variant of theory of mind that has been much neglected. A primordial theory of mind may be intrinsic within the social-emotional dynamic of the core subcortical networks of pro-social emotionality. I think if one takes a little baby before they dwell, or apparently dwell, much on what his or her mother might be thinking — on what might be going on in mother's mind — the baby is already reading mother's affective presence, or lack thereof, very well. I think this reflects rather direct sub-neocortical emotional systems resonance. And the quality of maternal presence, in yet unmeasured ways, establishes an interpersonal resonance, a shared affective state, that reciprocates between the mother and child, as has been emphasized by Colwyn Trevarthen (2000). This happens spontaneously, and largely at a deep affective level, without the child dwelling on what might be on the mother's mind, but this may epigenetically create the capacity for eventual cognitive mirroring, the capacity for sympathy, within the cortex. Initially, the child simply accepts a certain goodness in the world. Thus, it seems to me that there may exist an intrinsic theory of mind that is more primitive than the way people typically conceptualize it as a local cognitive achievement of the cortex. As my friend Doug Watt (2007) envisions it, this more primitive level of social-emotional resonance may be the source of a deeper empathy than can be achieved just cortically. I suspect some autistic children have biological deficiencies or insufficiencies in these basic systems.

SG: Trevarthen and others, like Peter Hobson and Phillipp Rochat, talk about the importance of this early kind of intersubjective give and take between mother and infant.

Panksepp: This intersubjective dance between mother and infant begins when the child is just a couple of weeks old. There is an emotional psychological readiness in the system, there is a preparedness in the system and when that preparedness fails then we set the stage for developmental disorders, perhaps even autism, as you well know. Perhaps there are ways to facilitate that kind of affective theory of mind from the beginning.

SG: So those who tend to view autistic behavior as a deficiency in the more theory- or simulation-aspects of ToM, which clearly manifest themselves at around age four, are missing this earlier emotion-rich phenomenon?

Panksepp: Many of the more standard cognitive approaches give us an incomplete and potentially misleading picture. It is a powerful and useful picture but it hasn't yet incorporated what one might call the affective theory of mind — theory of mind that is more spontaneous — based on the primary-process affective dance between infant and caretaker with direct interchange of feelings, so evident in play, that might be a foundation for the development and maturation of many cognitive abilities.

Pathologies in social cognition

Both Autism and Schizophrenia are pathologies that raise questions about ToM. Autistic-spectrum disorders are complex cases involving many symptoms, but one of the central aspects of autism is that the individual lacks social interests and social capacities. It's one of the things I was thinking of when I was falling off my seat at Gallese's talk on MNs. I had been reading the literature on autism, preparing for an NEH Summer Institute at Cornell University where I met Peter Hobson for the first time. Peter's view that the social deficiencies in autism were connected to problems in developmentally-early, emotion-based aspects of experience were convincing to me, especially as I was already convinced by my discussions with Meltzoff that the youngest of infants were capable of social interaction. Infants never wait until they are four-years old to start figuring out what others are up to.[2]

Shortly after I heard about mirror neurons, I joined the over-enthusiastic MN fan club and presented a highly speculative paper on how dysfunction of MNs might be connected to autism (Gallagher 2001). I presented the paper originally in October 1998 at a conference on the island of Ischia (just off the coast of Naples). I remember this presentation well because it was for me pre-PowerPoint and someone (I don't remember whether it was me or someone else on the panel—my Who system apparently not registering this fact in long-term memory) knocked over a glass of water onto my overhead transparencies just as I was starting. So there were lots of laughs each time I put a new soggy transparency on the overhead. In any case, my wild speculations may not be far off since there has been a rash of recent work connecting autism to dysfunctional mirror neurons (see Iacoboni and Dapretto 2006; Oberman and Ramachandran 2007). There is a lot more scientific data, but I can't help but think this is still somewhat speculative.[3]

In regard to schizophrenia things are even more complex. So let's go back to Denmark and ask Christopher Frith. Frith (1992) is famous for his theory that some symptoms of schizophrenia involve a failure of self-monitoring. I was wondering where he saw the connection between this and ToM.

> **Frith:** The original idea concerned schizophrenic patients with paranoid ideas, and possibly those patients who hear other people talking about them, discussing them in the third-person. These experiences clearly have to do with representing other people's mental states, whereas self-monitoring has to do with representing your own states. It seems to me that more or less by definition a person with paranoia is incorrectly attributing mental states to other people, deciding that they are all against him, which is sometimes true, but usually in these cases it is not. There are also more subtle disorders like delusions of reference where patients incorrectly believe that people are trying to communicate with them, or they see ostensive

---

2   I'm oversimplifying what I take to be an already oversimplified connection made by theory theorists between passing false-belief tests at around 4 years of age and the capacity for intersubjective understanding. Meltzoff, by the way, defends the theory- theory camp although most of his empirical studies support a more basic, and less theory-oriented position. For Meltzoff, however, the theory-formation process begins much younger (see, Gopnick and Meltzoff 1998). Also, there is recent experimental evidence that younger infants at 15 months are able to pass false-belief tests (see Onishi and Baillargeon 2005).

3   I was trying to be clever by playing on the word 'speculative' in the title of my paper, 'Emotion and intersubjective perception: A speculative account'. 'Speculative' derives from the Latin 'speculum' which means mirror. I also meant that it was speculative in the sense that 'who knows?'

cues that are not really there. We've investigated these ideas in a very simple way, that is, by using the typical mentalizing or ToM tasks that have been used with children. We've also tried to develop versions for adults. We have shown that indeed schizophrenic patients are not very good at these tasks (e.g. Corcoran et al. 1995; Sprong et al. 2007). But it has been much more difficult to show that the problem relates to particular kinds of symptoms.

SG: Can you say something about the details of how you make such tests appropriate for the adult?

Frith: Oh, well, in some instances by changing very trivial things. In a children's version there is the famous Smarties task where you have a Smarties [candy] box that the child expects to find candies in. To make it suitable for chronic schizophrenic patients who spend most of their lives in hospitals, you use cigarette packs instead. So you say, 'Bill leaves his cigarettes on the table and while he's out someone comes and takes some of them' — which is a very realistic scenario.

SG: So it's exactly the same kind of structure as false-belief tests, with minor adjustments.

Frith: Yes, and you do your check to make sure they remember the critical details of the story, and you only use data from the people who can remember. My colleague Graham Pickup very recently published a study (Pickup and Frith 2001) where he also used a version of the false photograph task, except he used maps instead of photographs. In this task you draw a map of the ward showing where various things are. You then rearrange the objects in the ward and ask the patient where the objects will be in the map. This is equivalent to the Sally-Anne task[4] where Sally's mind (she believes falsely that her marble is still in her basket) is equivalent to the map (which shows falsely that the marble is in the basket). Graham showed that the schizophrenic patients, like people with autism, could do the false map task, but not the false belief task. The problem for me is that the patients who have the greatest difficulties are the ones who have the negative features, and the same ones who have difficulty with lots of tasks. But it is quite striking that they can still do the false map task.

---

4   A famous false-belief task based on a short narrative about Sally who leaves her marble in a basket. Anne moves Sally's marble in her absence and when she comes back she has the false belief that her marble is still where she left it. The child is presented with this scenario and then asked by the experimenter where Sally thinks the marble is. Four-year old children tend to say she thinks it's still in the basket; three-year olds, and many older autistic children will say she thinks it's in the new location. Wimmer and Perner (1983) first ran the Sally-Anne task using a dolls to represent Sally and Anne; Leslie and Uta Frith repeated the experiment using human actors.

SG: So they still have the cognitive ability to do that, but are missing something in relation to understaning others.

Frith: Yes, but the question is what is the cognitive mechanism that is needed to solve mentalising problems, like the false belief tests. Going back to the forward model [see previous discussions of Wolpert's forward motor control model in Chapter 5], what seems plausible, and what we are trying to think about now, is whether you could run forward models to solve some of these mentalizing problems. This is a bit like simulation theory, which, of course, I don't like to talk about.[5] For example, if I want to reach that tape recorder, then I first run the inverse model[6] that computes what movements I need to make in order to reach the tape recorder. However, before I actually move I also run the forward model which predicts where my hand will actually finish up if I issue the motor commands suggested by the inverse model. And that way I can test whether my hand does finish up where I want it to be. Mathematically, the inverse model is very difficult since there is no one solution to the problem, but the forward model is completely straight-forward (sic) computationally. Presumably you could apply exactly the same sort of system when you're interacting with other people. So you could be thinking, 'I want him to buy me a drink'. So that's my goal. So I run the inverse model, which suggests that I could say something like 'I feel very thirsty'. And then I can run the forward model to predict what his response would be if I did say that. So that would be a way of using this forward modeling mechanism in interaction with others. We haven't got very far with these ideas yet, but that's the kind of thinking we're doing.

SG: The move that I see you making consistently in your theoretical work is the shift from the realm of movement to the realm of cognition. You have a model developed in regard to motor control, and you ask, how can this be made to work in regard to cognition. You want to explain cognition in terms of a forward model or a sensory-feedback model, with the idea that it must work the same way in cognition as it does in motor control. You must have good reasons for taking this kind of strategy.

---

5   I'm not sure why. I thought it might be because Chris didn't want to get in trouble with his wife. He's married to Uta Frith who is a leading researcher on autism and who, I once thought, was a proponent of the theory-theory approach. Chris, however, tells me that she would deny this, thinking theory-theory and simulation-theory equally underspecified. They've worked together on these issues (see, e.g., Frith and Frith 1999). In any case, even if Chris doesn't like to talk about ST, he does so below.

6   This is a kind of reverse engineering aspect of motor control in which the brain figures out how to move my hand by starting at the goal and working back. In this case, the forward model, which normally predicts forward (hence its name) is run in reverse.

Frith: Well, that's been very much my assumption, although I guess I would agree with Rodney Cotterill (1998) when he says that movement is all we can do. So maybe the internal virtual system has to derive from this movement system. This is slightly off on a tangent, but one of my problems is I have incredibly poor imagery, very poor visual imagery, and I'm not really sure that if I haven't seen a red thing in the past ten minutes whether I can actually imagine red. So when we are thinking about imagery, I find myself saying, how on earth does this work, because redness is not something that we do. An extreme version of this motor idea is that all imagery has to be motor. Then how can you possibly have visual imagery — and that fits me very well, and I have to think that everyone else pretends to have visual imagery! Certainly, when you imagine a piece of music, you might actually be imagining playing or singing it. But I get stuck in applying this to visual imagery, like imagining red.

SG: What about imagining auditory phenomena?

Frith: Well, as I say, that might be imagining singing it.

SG: Right, so you have to run through a motor sequence.

Frith: Yes. That was partly based on an experiment that Phillip McGuire (McGuire et al. 1996) did long ago concerning imagination, which was obviously relevant to auditory hallucinations. Subjects saw a word on a screen. In one case they just looked at it; in another case they said it to themselves subvocally, which is to imagine saying it. In another condition they had to imagine someone else saying it, and for reasons which are no longer entirely clear to me, they had to imagine it being said by a Dalek — these are alien creatures that were very popular on British TV in the *Doctor Who* series. They spoke in computer type monotones. They were going to take over the universe, but the problem was that they moved around on wheels. There is a nice cartoon that portrays the bottom of a set of stairs and the Daleks are saying, 'Bang goes our attempt to take over the universe'! Anyway, what was interesting was that when you imagine subvocal speech, not surprisingly you imagine speaking, and you see activity in Broca's area and motor speech areas, and a little bit of auditory cortex. But when you imagine hearing a Dalek saying the words, the activity increased dramatically in these motor speech areas rather than what you might expect, that this would be taken over by auditory cortex.

SG: So the motor system had to work harder to get the computer accent! On the one hand, one can look for clues in how motor systems work for how cognitive systems work, as you suggest. On the other hand, it is often difficult to say how some motor problems might be connected with cognitive problems, as in the case of autism. Autists miss or misinterpret behavioral signals like another person's movements and gestures — they can't pick up the intention of the other person from their bodily comportment. Peter Hobson has some interesting videos of autistic subjects in an imitation experiment showing clear confusion between their own embodied first-person spatial perspective and the other person's embodied perspective. They seem to have problems with their own body image and subsequently in distinguishing their own body image from that of another person. Is it possible that part of the reason that autistic subjects have so much trouble with ToM tasks is rooted in problems they have with bodily comportment — both controlling their own movement and interpreting the movement of others? For example, there is evidence that infants who are later diagnosed with autism have difficulty rolling their bodies over into the crawl position (Cotterill cites Teitelbaum et al. 1998 on this point). These are motor difficulties that precede mentalistic considerations of ToM.

Frith: One aspect of motor control is the problem of co-ordinate systems or frames of reference [see Chapter 5]. In order to reach and grasp objects we have to be able to represent their position in space, but there are many ways in which we can do this. We know that in the earliest stages of visual processing such representations are in terms of retinotopic co-ordinates. This means that the representation of an object's position in these brain regions changes when ever we move our eyes. This kind of representation is useful if we want to know how to move our eyes so that the object will be in the middle of the fovea, but is not very useful if we want to reach the object with our hand or tell someone else where it is. So the brain has many other ways of representing the positions of objects. There are head-centred co-ordinate systems, shoulder-centred co-ordinate systems and even so-called allocentric representations which are in terms of absolute spatial position. Marc Jeannerod has made an interesting suggestion about the differences between the sort of co-ordinate systems that are best for controlling our movements and those that would be best for being aware of our movements. For controlling our own movements we need an egocentric system, but for being aware of our movements we need a system that is not body-centred. This kind of representation would also be useful for representing the movements of others. Perhaps people with autism and schizophrenia can never properly escape from their egocentric representations of the body.

SG: Such considerations have motivated you to say that the motor system is much more interesting than the perceptual system.

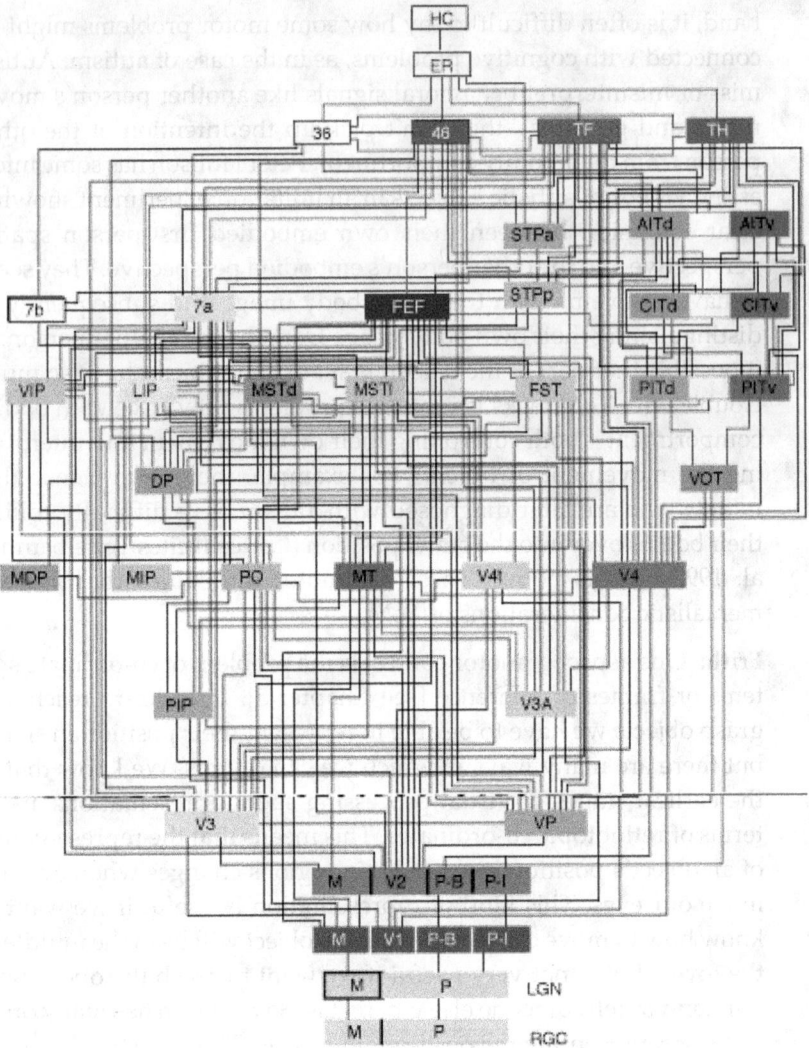

Figure 7.2. From Felleman & Van Essen 1991

Frith: The standard line in cognitive neuroscience is that we must study vision because we know so much about it. [This is the Crick and Koch strategy, see Chapter 6]. And there is the famous Van Essen diagram (fig. 7.2) showing that the visual system takes over the whole brain and involves at least 32 different areas—a face area, a color area and so on. Most of the studies on the neural correlates of consciousness are actually on vision. And I guess I think that the action system is likely to be much more relevant to understanding things like consciousness and ToM. What we do is much more important than what we see.

SG: Would you say that your group in London are proponents of the theory theory approach to the theory of mind, in contrast to Jeannerod, Gallese, and their Southern European colleagues who like the simulation account. I ask because of what seems to be the close connection between simulation theory today and the work on mirror neurons and the motor system.

Frith: I would say that our group is not completely satisfied with either theory theory or simulation theory. We certainly don't think that you are consciously putting yourself in somebody else's situation. Whatever the mechanism is it is something that happens implicitly.

SG: You have developed some evidence that the medial prefrontal paracingulate cortex is an area of the brain that is highly involved in social cognition. Knut Kampe (Kampe et al. 2000) has suggested that this area is activated when we make eye contact with another person. Would you suspect, or do you have any evidence that this is an area of the brain that malfunctions in cases of autism?

Frith: There is very little good evidence for brain abnormalities in autism because the numbers of people studied are usually too small. But we have done a study of brain structure using MRI where we found reduced gray matter in this region (Abel et al. 1999). Many studies have been done since, but no clear picture has emerged (e.g. Stanfield et al. 2007).

SG: You know my recent question to Uta Frith about false belief tests. All the false belief studies I have read test for explicit, consciously thought-out responses, and this is far from providing evidence for implicit processes, either of the simulation or the theoretical kind. Uta indicated, however, that there were studies that involve implicit processing.

Frith: Well, there are now a series of studies of false belief tasks by Wendy Garnham (Clements and Perner 1994; Garnham and Ruffman 2001; Garnham and Perner 2001) using eye gaze. She uses a version of the Sally-Anne task where Sally comes back through different doors depending on where she thinks her marble will be. So in addition to asking the child, 'Where will she look for her marble', you can see which door the child looks at just before Sally comes back. At around 3 years many children give the wrong answer, but look at the correct door. I guess this shows that they have implicit, unconscious knowledge about false beliefs. Also, of course, there is exciting new research suggesting that very young children can do false belief tasks. Is this implicit? (Onishi and Baillargeon 2005; Surian, Caldi and Sperber 2007).

The other new information about mentalising comes from brain imaging studies. What I find most interesting here is the way that the brain imaging work influences the cognitive work, and vice versa. So our imaging experiments on theory of mind, although nothing has been done with schizophrenic patients yet, were very bad experiments in the sense that we said wouldn't it be fun to do an imaging experiment on theory of mind and see what parts of the brain light up. We had no hypothesis.

SG: You did imaging studies just to see what happens.

Frith: Just to see what happens. But an interesting way of looking at imaging experiments is that they provide you more information for classifying tasks. So you can say these tasks must be similar because they activate the same brain areas. This is a completely new way of categorizing tasks. This comes out in the ToM experiments. In many experiments we see activity at the back of the superior temporal sulcus, which is exactly the same area that is activated in studies of biological motion with dot figures, where there is no mentalizing involved at all. All you see is that this is a person walking. I think that this observation makes a lot of sense because this is the sort of signal the mentalizing mechanism would need to make inferences about intentions. It also links in with the motor system again. By watching the way someone moves you can discover something about their goals and intentions. So how can you extract such information from movement? You know that there is this interesting work on computer vision showing that you can distinguish between indoor scenes and outdoor scenes by some very simple computational algorithm. There is some very simple parameter you can extract from the picture that makes the distinction. I suspect, and someone may very well have already found it, there is a fairly simple aspect of motion that allows you to distinguish the movement of biological entities from the movement of physical things blowing in the wind, or what ever. The brain has discovered how to make this distinction. The fantasy I have is that there is a special kind of movement that people with intentions make. That is the sort of direction we are be going in. My current Ph.D. student, Johannes Schultz, has developed a very nice mathematical display where you have two balls moving about, and there is a single mathematical parameter that indicates how much they are interacting with each other, in the sense that the position of one ball now (at time t) influences the position of the other ball at time t+1. You can vary this parameter. And you get very good behavioral results; as you increase this parameter it looks more and more as if one ball is following the other. This goes beyond simple biological motion. In fact, the way the individual balls move is not particularly biological. The important thing is that they appear to interact with each other. We've done some brain imaging using this paradigm and it shows, as anticipated, that posterior STS is interested in these interactive movements (Schultz et al. 2005).

I would like a model of mentalizing where you would have certain kinds of signals coming into the process in a certain kind of way. I wonder if generative neural network models might be relevant. Geof Hinton is working on these issues. You want the entity to learn about the world without having a teacher—and that strikes me as how every creature had to learn about the world until humans appeared upon the scene. For this to work, you have to have an internal model of what is outside in the world. The only information you have is what's coming through your senses. These generative models also involve a form of inverse and forward modeling. The brain asks 'If my internal model was outside in the world, what would I see through my senses'. And then it cycles around, generating a model, predicting what you should see, adjusting the model until it gets a good fit. And when you get a good fit you can say that my internal model corresponds to what's really out there. And it doesn't matter whether it does or not, as long as you survive. This approach has become almost ubiquitous in the last few years under various labels such as *generative models, predictive coding, Bayesian inference* (e.g. Yuille and Kersten 2006).

SG: It just has to get close enough for that to happen.

Frith: Yes. I used to have the idea, and I think lots of people do, that there is something deeply weird about other people's mental states and that it must be impossibly difficult to work out what they are. This was in contrast to working out what is out there in the physical world. But in terms of these generative models, there's not that much difference really. Assuming I don't have a teacher who says, 'That's a tree out there', I can never check whether my model of the physical world is correct. Now that is the same problem with other people's mental states. So if I have a mechanism for modeling things in the physical world I can also model things in other people's minds. These ideas are described in more detail in a wonderful new book (Frith 2007).

SG: Yes, I know that book and can recommend it.

Frith: As I said, I am not convinced that either simulation theory or theory theory are sufficiently well formulated for neuroscience data to help distinguish between them. We need an account that specifies what behavioral signals, like movements and gestures, are used and how they are processed. For example, faces provide cues that are used to make (unconscious) inferences about mental states. My guess is that in autism these cues are available, but not used. Studies of pragmatics might be a good way into this. With regard to mirror neurons we could certainly use imaging to see whether brain regions activated when observing actions were also activated when performing ToM tasks. Some patients with schizophrenia seem to show an over-activation of the ToM mechanism, attributing mental states when this is not appropriate. There is a growing number of studies on ToM and brain lesions (e.g. Stuss, Gallup and Alexander 2001; Samson et al. 2004; Rudebeck et al. 2006).

Intersubjectivity and empathy

My own view on questions about social cognition builds on certain things Chris Frith just mentioned — our ability to perceptually pick up cues in the other person's facial expressions, in their movements and actions, posture, gestures, vocal intonations; all of this along with learned clues from the specific context or situation in which we are interacting (Gallagher 2001; 2004; 2005). In developmental psychology Colwyn Trevarthen's concepts of primary and secondary intersubjectivity cover this ground and show that very young infants are capable of social interaction (see Trevarthen 1979; Trevarthen and Hubley 1978). Add to this, once we have acquired language capabilities, the importance of narrative and story telling from the earliest ages through all phases of adulthood (Gallagher and Hutto 2007; Hutto 2007), and it seems clear that we don't require theory or simulation as much as theory theorists and simulation theorists think we do. Much of the evidence for this view comes from developmental psychology, but also from phenomenology. To interpret the neuroscience I think that one needs genuine guidance from such personal-level sciences that can look at both the everyday experiences of most of us, and at some of the different experiences that others might have. Back in Chicago I talked about this with Jonathan Cole.

> **SG:** In much of your work you seem fascinated not only by the neurophysiological aspects of chronic neurological disease, but by what happens at the personal level.

> **Cole:** I am. I have always been interested in the two apparently opposed aspects of neurology: the intellectual understanding of the brain and nervous system, and the human aspect of the neurology,

the phenomenology or lived experience. That's why after a wonderful time studying the former at Oxford, I went for a medical elective to spend time with Oliver Sacks in New York.

SG: In some of your work you have found evidence for the idea that we use simulation to understand the actions of others.

Cole: In my work with Ian Waterman, we found that he can judge the weight someone else is picking up, but less so their anticipation of an unknown weight they are going to pick up (Bosbach et al. 2005). These two judgments are taken from viewing the same videotape. We suggested weight judgment was taken directly from observation of the movements but that judgment of anticipation — was the weight heavier or lighter than expected? — requires a simulation process, the implicit use of motor programmes, which IW does not have.

Also, as you know, I've been doing more work on Moebius Syndrome.[7] In that work we actually found a related result. People with Moebius can identify subtle facial expressions of emotion from photos (Calder et al. 2000), but are deficient in describing what parts of the face move, or how the face moves during various emotional expressions. This latter finding was suggestive rather than statistically significant on a small sample of 3. If reproduced then it suggests that imagining and describing facial expressions of emotion may require use of implicit motor programmes which people with Moebius who have never moved their faces are deficient in.

SG: Much of your work in *About Face* focused on the effects of facial pathologies on intersubjective experience, interaction with others, and so forth. Are you finding similar problems with intersubjectivity in your project on paraplegics?

Cole: Facial *differences* rather than pathologies! That's a very good question and it's a matter of dragging out people's experience. Facial disfigurement, for instance, is seen but often does not present a problem in movement or functioning. In contrast spinal cord injury is both visible and presents huge problems for functioning. People who see either may not be aware of the problems of living with them.

Those who live from wheelchairs have different perceptions of the world in terms of accessibility, and in terms of the fact that they have to look after bodily functions which previously were automatic.

Perhaps it would simplify to say that some people with spinal cord

---

7 Moebius Syndrome is a rare neurological disorder involving facial paralysis and absence of facial expression due to problems with the sixth and seventh cranial nerves, which control the face and eye muscles. At the time of writing, Jonathan's new book on Moebius was just in press at Oxford University Press.

injury[8] divide their problems into a neurological impairment (the injury), and a disability which may be socially originating. The incontinence and motor weakness may be awful, but can be tolerable. For many it is their lack of work, lack of access to public transport and public places that is more intolerable. They may feel excluded from society, not because they cannot walk—wheelchairs are efficient modes of locomotion—but because the lift is out of order, or the curbs are not cut. They are saying their disability is as much social as neurological. In a way, to describe their self in the world, as Merleau-Ponty might have put it, one has to focus on that world as well as on them.

Yet it is important not to generalize. One person told me that his spinal cord injury was the best thing that happened to them.

SG: In what sense?

Cole: He had left school with little educational achievement and was going to have a dead-end job for the rest of his life. After his spinal injury, unable to move beyond the upper arms, he had a period when he lived at home and did nothing. Then someone, completely by accident, gave him a job, and then another. Several years later he became an academic, and has had, in his view, a better and more productive and enjoyable life than he would have had if he had not sustained the injury. Other spinal cord injured people find that almost impossible to comprehend. It is so difficult to generalize.

Coming back to people with facial problems, the situation may be different because facial problems do seem to interrupt or affect interpersonal relationships in different ways.

SG: So the face is central, with respect to social interaction, in a way that full control of bodily movement is not?

Cole: I am a little concerned not to compare different conditions, but yes, the face is a unique identifier and visible area for emotional communication. The body is emotionally important, but in a different way. Some people with spinal cord injury can be quite concerned to be lumped with other impairments, say of cerebral origin. They have intact mind, intact face, intact speech—they just have problems with movement.

SG: So in terms of their own self-identity, it must be quite individualized. Perhaps if an athlete were injured in this way, they might feel the loss of their whole identity.

8 People with spinal cord injury may be termed tetraplegics [or quadriplegics] or paraplegics, if injured at the neck level or below, or people with tetraplegia etc. Some prefer to be called *people with the condition*, others are happy to be more defined by their injury. [JC]

Cole: That's an excellent example. I've seen people who are miserable and not adapted to their new situation with tetraplegia, who were athletes, and I've seen an athlete who injured his spinal cord during gymnastics, who said, well I have to say goodbye to athletics, I'll do something else now.

SG: So it would depend on one's previous sense of self.

Cole: You would think that the sort of macho man who was an athelete, and who viewed himself in those terms would not have anything left. Some remain like that, frustrated, and equally some can just let go their previous existence and do something else, become someone else.

Some say they had a period of guilt, remorse, anger, denial, depression and then found a way of living with their spinal injury. Others did not have that rite of passage into their new state, and some find the transition from one sort of life to the other just happened. They see no point in looking back and just look forward, finding new challenges. They view their new bodies as a challenge, which for those of us who are able bodied is very difficult to imagine. But that's what they do. And always, they say, they are just ordinary people in extraordinary circumstances.

The body image can be very flexible; if you break your leg you have to incorporate that into your body image, and as we grow and then age we have to incorporate those changes into our self. Some people, with severe neurological impairments, adapt too. One tetraplegic man who was very aware that he could no longer gesture 'out there', in his arms, said that he would like to inhabit his body more affectively, emotionally. He gestured more with his face and head and with his voice. Many with spinal cord injury move on from their past embodiment and seem to have, if you like, less ontological doubt than some with facial problems.

One person I have spoken to, who is a fairly vociferous worker in disability studies, considers that people with spinal cord injury do not have a problem themselves, they live in a society that gives them problems of accessibility, etc and that the best way to help are interventions in the social policy and building regulations.

SG: So change society, and that would address the disability.

Cole: Yes, he would not be disabled then. But even he has to admit that some people do badly and some better and he doesn't know why. But that doesn't invalidate his model, because if you want to improve people with neurological impairments, and make them less disabled, then you need to improve the way in which they move through the world and the choices which they have, in employment, in accessibility, in access to health care, in housing. As he said to me, 'I don't want anything that you don't have. I don't want anything special. I just want the opportunities to do what you can do.' And you can entirely respect that.

SG: On this view, the problem is not at the individual level, or a problem with the self, or a problem that has to do with what it is like to be impaired, but a problem at the social level.

Cole: He would say that his self hasn't changed. Or that he is not interested in the self. 'I'm not interested in the individual or in you understanding what it is like to be me, I just want you to give me what you have.' So although I don't view the world politically, this sort of approach to disability has to be considered.

A problem for people in a wheelchair is a lack of spontaneity and freedom of action. Yet another person, also a tetraplegic, told me that the greatest gift of all was good social skills, because then one can cope with other people and their concerns and prejudices. Those who seem to be enjoying life the most, despite their situation, are those who are most interested in other people and who can put others at ease. They make you see them as a person rather than seeing the wheelchair. That's just the same as people with facial problems. It is possible to help people with poor social skills, as the British charity *Changing Faces* is doing for facial difference.

I am not sure one can ignore or divorce the neurological condition from the person and their world. We are discussing the poles of something which is really a continuum. One could make the case that if your selfhood is limited physically, if your embodiment is limited, then you may want your immediate environment to reflect you, to be part of your extended self.

One of the things that I want to elaborate on in regard to spinal cord injury, and also in relation to Kay Toombs' work (see Toombs 1993), is imaginative transposal.[9] Our imagination is bounded by our experience. So can we imagine what it is like to be someone else? I might be able to imagine what it is like to be you, because I'm physically like you. But can I imagine what it is like to be Ian [Waterman]? Someone wrote that in writing *Pride and the Daily Marathon* (Cole 1995) I approached the unimaginable and tried to make it understandable. I think I understand what it might be like to be Ian, and I hope the reader does too.

It is in those with experiences so far from our own, with whom it is most difficult to empathize, that it is most important that we should.

9   Kay Toombs is not an arm-chair philosopher, but a wheel-chair philosopher who works on the topic of embodiment from the perspective of phenomenology and her own disability.

But how much might we ever hope to do that? In talking to people with spinal cord injury, many of them have said that you can't know what it's like to be me. You might sit in a wheelchair for a day or two, but you won't ever really be able to know what it's like to be someone else. That's something I'm puzzling over because I think that they are probably right. Kay Toombs talks about this. It's a creative act to interpret others, and that's what we do the whole time on social interaction. That's, for me, one of the origins of creativity — to exactly know the other. But can we know the other when they are so far removed from our experience?

SG: You and Ian have been involved in Peter Brook's play, *The Man Who*. This is a case where art tried to capture just that unimaginable aspect of pathological experience and present it so people could understand it.

Cole: Oh, yes. With Peter's play, based on Oliver Sacks', *The Man Who Mistook his Wife for a Hat*, it was very interesting, because they began from Oliver's writings, but then had to go back to find patients, to build the bricks upward, if you like. Actors talk about acting from the inside out. Playing Othello, everyone has a bit of them that knows what jealousy is, and they put it to work in the portrayal. Actors harness, magnify and explore this, and in doing so allow you an understanding of jealousy — there is an empathetic process going on.

SG: Yes, and we are beginning to know how that works neurologically, and what happens when we imaginatively enact what is happening in the other's behavior — you know the work of Jeannerod, Decety, and the mirror neuron group, Rizzolatti and Gallese and their colleagues. This is interesting, because much of this work focuses on movement — we see the movement of the other — and we can think of movement as expressive of some emotion, like jealousy — and there is an automatic reverberation in our own motor system that may be the basis for a direct insight into the other's experience. But what happens if our own motor system is not working in the normal way, or in the same way as the other person's motor system?

Cole: Yes. If you've got a neurological problem, which others have never experienced, then to try to understand your experience the other person has to go from the outside in. The actors studied the condition to understand it, in order to act about it. The people in Brook's play spent a year trying to do that. I would say that the performers in Brook's play are doing just the same as I am. I try to construct a life biographically, informed by science; they are doing a similar thing for artistic purposes.

SG: So in their performance they are faced with the same problem of translating, as you say, from the outside in, the same problem that the scientist faces if he or she attempts to understand their subjects in more than just an objective way. And it is related to what we might call the everyday problem that we all face when we try to understand people that we live with, except that to some extent we generally have some resources to go from the inside out.

Cole: Yes, and that just brings us back to the question about *to what extent* you can really understand another being, whose experience is beyond your own. That's part of what's puzzling me about spinal cord injury, because so many with spinal cord injury have said to me that you don't know what it's like to be me.

I guess that in trying to approach what it is to be someone else you have to do it by examples. An astronaut friend of mine is often asked what it is like in space. That's too big a question. She always answers by breaking it down into examples: how she sleeps, moves, cleans her teeth, eats. The answers to big questions are contained within the smaller answers.

So the way to try to understand what it's like to be someone with spinal cord injury is to go through and give examples of what they have to do and what their lives are like. They have to become students of their body in a way in which you or I don't. Those with spinal cord injury have to be consciously aware of those parts of the body of which we are not aware. By which I mean that if they were to sit as long as we have, without moving, in a chair, they'll get a pressure sore. They have to be aware of their bladder and their bowels, and so forth. So, if you like, the bits of the body they are aware of are the bits that you and I are not.

SG: So there is a different phenomenology of the body for them.

Cole: Yes. Their relationship to their embodiment, in terms of their body itself, without the communication aspect, is entirely different to yours and mine. They've still got the visible self, but their relation to it is very different.

SG: Merleau-Ponty (1962), as you know, addresses many of these points, including the sexual aspects. But I also think of Sidney Shoemaker (1999) who distinguishes between the sensory-motor body and the biological body. The biological body simply functions without our awareness. I'm not sure that we are more aware of the sensory-motor body, but normally we tend to live in our sensory-motor experiences, to the extent that Shoemaker suggests that the biological body doesn't have much to do with who we are. You are suggesting the spinal cord patients tend to live more in their biological experiences and that has a good deal to do with what it's like to be them.

Cole: Yes. You have written of how the body is usually absent as we are engaged in the world (Gallagher 1986). But, the limits of this become apparent in conditions like spinal cord injury.

SG: Does the wheel chair ever get incorporated into the body, as some prosthetic devices do? Or is it always experienced as distinguished?

Cole: On the whole it seems to be distinguished at one level, though it can become elaborated into a schema, like driving a car is. Then, just as for some people their cars are important and define them, so for some people their wheel chairs are important. They are even more important since a heavy wheel chair is so much more difficult than a lightweight one.

SG: There is always that proviso that it comes down to the individual. One can't generalize empathy. And I think it's clear from your work that one cannot gain anything like a total, 100% empathy with any individual. And if I get a higher degree of empathy with people who are more like me, it is still important to gain some degree of empathy with those who are not like me.

Cole: I agree entirely. Yet one person said to me, 'I don't want you to understand me, just give me the ramp [for my wheelchair].' He wanted social provision rather than empathy. But the point I make in *Still Lives* is that I may need some understanding of the problem to motivate funding the ramp. Might some sort of empathy not be necessary for giving assistance?

I was motivated by this notion of empathy and of course by interest. Tetraplegics seem almost at an extreme of an empathetic process. It is such a huge loss that I wanted to know what it is like, and to see whether I could understand it. Then most of us are never tested in the way those with neurological impairments are. To listen to their individual and differing responses to such events, whatever they are and however they adapt and live, is a great privilege. It also informs us about our own embodiment and our own society; people with neurological impairments have so much to show us about ourselves.

Chapter 8

A Short Robotic Interlude

It might seem odd to turn our attention to robots just now before we say more about other important aspects of human experience — e.g., emotion, language, self, cognition. But one could argue that this is a chapter that should have come directly after the chapter on movement. After all, robots are nothing more than intelligent moving machines, right? They don't have any real intentionality, so they don't, strictly speaking, engage in action. And surely they are not conscious, at least on most definitions of that term. The truth is that I wanted to wait until after we discussed intersubjectivity, because I think some of the most interesting work being done today is on social robotics — that is, building robots that can interact with other robots and with humans. If it turns out that the roboticists are highly successful in this project, might that change our attitudes about robots at the personal level of analysis?

Now before you start thinking that this is more or less Dennett's notion of taking an intentional stance toward a system in which there is no real intentionality, so that if we treat a robot as if it were conscious, then that's all there is to it since as far as we know that's all there is to consciousness anyway — before you start thinking that, keep in mind that my background is phenomenology and in all of our conversations so far we've been taking consciousness as something more than this. Rather, let's think of the issue this way. What if, given a certain physical system at the subpersonal level, the way this system interacts with both the physical and social environments is what allows for the emergence of something new — which may (or may not) be what we call consciousness. In fact, according to some theorists, this is the way it is with us. We have a system — the brain — the subpersonal explanation of which is never sufficient to account for consciousness; rather, for the emergence of consciousness we need embodied interaction with physical and social environments. Now it is still an open and empirical question whether the kind of system you need on the subpersonal level is precisely the system that we have — our brain — and likewise our embodiment. After all, many people are willing to attribute consciousness to certain animals, and they have different kinds of brains and different kinds of bodies. It is likely they have different kinds of worlds as well. Nonetheless, I'm convinced that we can interact with some animals in an intelligent way. Not perhaps with sheep or cattle, but certainly with the dogs that help us round them up. I don't speak Irish Gaelic, but I've always been amazed by my cousin's dogs who seem to understand more of that language than I do.

So let's call this robotics project what it is — not a set of ontological claims about robots and consciousness, but an experiment. Is it possible to design a system that moves around the world like an animal (but isn't an animal), interacts with objects, and interacts with people in a way that approaches a smooth intersubjective interaction (even if it isn't conscious — although that can be left as an open question too).

Here's a version of a subpersonal Turing Test for this experiment, as suggested by Oberman et al. (2007).[1] Currently there is good evidence to suggest that mirror neurons, which are activated when we see others engaged in intentional actions, are not activated when we see mechanical things do the things that could be done by people (see, e.g., Di Pellegrino et al. 1992; Gallese et al. 1996; Tai et al. 2004). So, if a monkey sees food being grasped by a mechanical apparatus rather than by a monkey or human hand, its MNs fail to fire. On the version of the Turing Test that would be relevant here, a robot would pass the Turing Test if in performing an action it caused our MNs to fire. That at least would signal some progress in the construction of social robots.

The robot that 'lives' in my home will not pass this test. This is a robot I bought my wife for Mother's Day — which is not a romantic holiday, so a robot is okay. Thanks to Rodney Brooks whose company, IRobot, built it, neither I nor my wife has to vacuum floors anymore. It works great, it's smart, it finds its way back to its home base if it needs charging, and it is designed in a way that prevents it from falling down stairs. But it's not much to look at and it would be difficult to start any sort of personal relation with it. If it breaks down at some point, I would have no problem throwing it out and getting a new one. Don't try doing that with a dog or a cat.

Robots, brains, and evolution

How should we think of this connection between neuroscience and robotics? Rodney Brooks (both vacuum cleaner entrepreneur and MIT professor of robotics) thinks there's not much difference in subject matter.

---

1   While checking the internet to see if anyone had thought of this, I found the Oberman et al. paper at http://bci.ucsd.edu/PAPERS/murobotpaper.pdf.

The body, this mass of biomolecules, is a machine that acts according to a set of specifiable rules ... We are machines, as are our spouses, our children, and our dogs ... I believe myself and my children all to be mere machines (Brooks 2002, 173-75).

If, contra to Brooks, we think that human bodies are not just fancy robots, and that human bodies involve something in excess of blind, automatic, even if sophisticatedly spontaneous mechanisms, we still want to know how or why that is. Movements that are, or have become hard wired in the human still can be enmeshed with an intentionality and an experiential dimension that have their own effects on behavior. Michael Arbib is someone who has thought hard about these interconnections between robotics and neuroscience.

Arbib: When Joe Ledoux (1996) studies fear conditioning, he analyzes how what we might call a painful stimulus may cause the animal to freeze or to take avoiding action. But LeDoux does not want to attribute feelings to the basic circuit for that behavior. He would suggest that it is only when that circuit is linked to hippocampus for context and to cortex that he would want to talk about feelings as distinct from fearful behavior. I don't know whether I am completely convinced, but I think one might at least say that his basic account comes close to how one should currently think about robots. Things will no doubt change in the future, but at the moment I would not be prepared to say a robot is in pain, rather than having, for example, a thermal sensor to register when and where the temperature is unduly high on part of its casing, and take appropriate action to avoid overheating. Of course, there was a time when people thought only people of their own race actually felt pain and that one need feel no constraint in what one did to people of other races, let alone animals of any kind. So we have at least moved to a stage where our understanding of pain is extended to a much greater range than it was before. Presumably, increased understanding of the brain will ground new ideas about the objective definition of what it is to experience pain, rather than just taking avoidance action.

SG: Your computational model of schemas is meant in part to be explanatory but it also has applications in artificial intelligence and robotics. And in this regard, haven't some people in robotics come around to the way you have been thinking of schemas? I know that you have studied animals and how schemas relate to the basic sensorimotor skills of perception and action. But recent work in robotics has started to look in this direction too.

Arbib: In robotics various attempts are made to explain how a computer program, or a robot, could model its world. In contrast to thinking of this purely in terms of symbol manipulation the idea is, instead, to emphasize what can be found through analogies with animal behavior or even in some cases drawing more detailed lessons from studies of the brains of behaving animals. This leads to robots which solve problems in a much more living-in-the-world kind of way, rather than abstract symbol-manipulation.

I have to say that in this regard I have been inspired by Grey Walter's book *The Living Brain* (1953/1961). He approaches an understanding of the brain from two very different perspectives. First he analyzes EEG signals of the human brain, monitored by a device (which he designed and called the Toposcope) which allows for the simultaneous recording of waveforms from many electrodes across the scalp. Second, he considers 'biologically inspired' robots, and specifically two electro-mechanical tortoises, *Machina speculatrix* and *Machina docilis*. He claims that the first robot, 'the machine that speculates', exhibits the ability to 'speculate' because, like an animal it explores the environment instead of waiting passively for something to happen. This is too behaviorist. There is nothing in *Machina speculatrix* that resembles the mental gymnastics of human speculation, whereby a human would consider possible courses of future actions. In any case, Walter presents us with two different routes: an attempt to explicate the workings of the human brain, and an attempt to design the simplest mechanisms which will yield an interesting class of robot behaviors. The latter includes a 'comparative' method in which different additions to *Machina speculatrix* yield a variety of different behaviors.

A similar kind of dual approach can be found in the work of Valentino Braitenberg. He's well-known in AI circles for his book *Vehicles* (1984; foreshadowed in Braitenberg 1965), which is very much in the spirit of *Machina speculatrix*. He is also well known in neuroscience for his work on neuroanatomy and conceptual brain modeling. Braitenberg and Onesto (1960) developed a model of the cerebellum which reconciled Braitenberg's work on neuroanatomy with the role of cerebellum in the timing of movement. This cerebellar model was influential but wrong, in part because it was developed before Ito's discovery that Purkinje cells, the output cells of the cerebellar cortex, are inhibitory (see Eccles, Ito and Szentágothai 1967).

In some way this is the difference between robotics and neuroscience. For robotics, success is defined in a technological way. If the machine works and delivers effective performance at reasonable cost, it's a success. In computational neuroscience, the measure is less straightforward. There is a continual give and take between theory and experiment. Theoretical models propose hypotheses and predictions which then stimulate new experiments; then, as new empirical data is developed, it motivates the revision of existing models — or their replacement. So in Walter and Braitenberg you can see these two approaches:

1) An incremental design of mechanisms that will deliver an interesting class of robot behaviors. In this case the biological inspiration comes from a range of externally observed animal behaviors.
2) A neuroscience approach that would explicate the workings of human and animal brains.

I want to define a 'third way' which would be a comparative computational neuroethology. This is a computational analysis of neural mechanisms that underlie animal behavior. On this approach we view homologous mechanisms as computational variants and see them as related to the different evolutionary histories or ecological niches of the animals in question. In this way, I think, we get a better understanding of human and animal brains, and an expansion of biologically-inspired robotics.

SG: So this kind of thinking can advance our understanding of biology, but also have technical applications in robotics. Some people, on hearing the term 'computational' and thinking of it as pure symbol manipulation, might be led to think of this kind of project as an abstract and somewhat disembodied approach to biology and robotics, when in fact biology and robotics are anything but disembodied. Your approach is not at all like that.

Arbib: The roots of computational neuroethology as I think of it can be found in a famous paper, 'What the frog's eye tells the frog brain' (Lettvin, Maturana, McCulloch and Pitts 1959). This is an important paper which explained the frog's visual system from an ethological perspective. It showed that you cannot divorce visual neuro-circuitry from the specifics of the animal's ecological niche. Thus, different cells in the frog's retina and tectum are specialised for detecting predators and prey. Indeed, I suggested in the late 1960s that the question is really 'What does the frog's eye tell the frog?' and this led to Rich Didday's Ph.D. thesis (Didday 1970) and the subsequent approach to action-oriented perception in the frog developed in Arbib (1972; see p. 45 and Section 7.2). I wanted to emphasize the embodied nervous system or, in other words, an action-oriented view of perception. This led me to further studies of the visuomotor co-ordination of action in the frog and toad (see Arbib 1982 for overview). The idea that my colleagues and I developed, which we called

'Rana computatrix', the frog that computes, and which was inspired by Walter's *Machina speculatrix* (although I may not have been consciously aware of this debt to him at that time), in turn inspired the names of a number of later developed 'species' of 'creatures', including Randall Beer's (1990) computational cockroach *Periplaneta computatrix,* and Dave Cliff's (1992) hoverfly *Syritta computatrix.*

SG: One might think of this as a sort of evolutionary robotics?

Arbib: Yes, I think there are varied forms of 'evolution' in the fields of biologically-inspired robotics, neural network modelling, and computational neuroethology. I've outlined this in a recent paper (Arbib 2003). First, there is the kind of *biological evolution* summarized by Darwin's theory of natural selection, and enriched by recent advances in molecular biology and genomics. Here we should note that most genes need to interact in a genetic network with many other genes in order to do what they do and to contribute to features of the phenotype.

In computational neuroethology there is something I would call *ad hoc evolution.* This is exemplified in the works of Walter and Braitenberg and the idea of adding features to a model 'to see what happens'. This approach is unconstrained by biological data, but it does result in surprisingly complex behaviors that emerge by putting together a few simple mechanisms in a pseudo-evolutionary sequence. There is another form of evolution that is connected to *genetic algorithms* (these were introduced in the pioneering book *Adaptation in Natural and Artificial Systems* by John Holland, 1975). The inspiration comes from natural selection, but delivers a method of parameter optimisation in artificial systems. You start with a population of objects with randomly assigned parameters arranged in a 'genotype'. An object's success will determine the likelihood that copies of its genotype will be used in generating the genotypes for the next generation. This plays out over a number of simulated generations in such a way that the resulting genotypes develop better and better designs to optimize function. Genetic algorithms have been used to optimize neural nets, treating connection weights as analogous to genes. Genetic algorithms also have applications in robotics where you can make the biomechanics and the neural controller subject to selection. You can also use this approach to explain social systems. The model here is biological evolution, but the result is a mathematical technique that can be applied to non-biological systems in which the 'genotype' may bear no resemblance to the biological genotype.

Finally, there is what I would call *conceptual neural evolution*. On this approach you try to understand complex neural mechanisms through an incremental process. Like ad hoc evolution, the strategy is to add features to a model 'to see what happens'. Unlike ad hoc evolution, however, the process *is* constrained by biological data, specifically data that link behavior to anatomy and neurophysiology, with no analysis of the underlying genes. The objective is to discover relations between neural circuits that implement basic schemas found in simpler species with those that underlie schemas in other more complex species.

SG: So you are not primarily interested in the real path of evolution by natural selection. Rather, you want to show how schema theory could contribute to an understanding of complex behavior, by using an 'evolution' of successively more complex models. In the end you arrive at the best approximation of the neural realization of that behavior.

Arbib: Yes and no. With the same methodology you can identify cortical functions in mammals and relate them to subcortical functions that are homologous to certain non-mammalian forms. Through such an approach we definitely get an enhanced understanding of the more complex brain. But it may also suggest hypotheses that will guide us to the genetic underpinnings of the 'real' evolution of this complexity.

Experimenting with robotics

Ezequiel Di Paolo is an evolutionary roboticist working at the University of Sussex. The idea of evolutionary robots is to design processes for passing on the right 'genetic material' (the most productive algorithms for a particular task) from one generation of robots to the next generation. Experimenting by trial and error, one discovers the designs that perform best in regard to a defined function. Di Paolo is interested in getting the best results for robot design in this way, but he is also interested in using evolutionary robotics experiments to discover the basic rules of inter-robotic, and human intersubjective communication and interaction (Di Paolo 2000). In one experiment, for example, Di Paolo found not only that his robots evolved to mutually coordinate with each other, but that they did so as an interconnected system rather than by developing individual capacities. The coordination required a mutual interaction that could not be attained if, for example, one robot was put in an environment with the right stimulus but no other robots (see De Jaegher 2006, 129ff for summary).

In another somewhat exquisite experiment Di Paolo, Rohde, and Iizuka (2007), set their robots to explore some principles of human inter-subjectivity. In some sense this is an experiment that itself evolved from two previous generations of experiments. The first generation is to be found in experiments about real intersubjective behavior in infancy. These are well-known experiments involving social contingency conducted originally by Murray and Trevarthen (1985; Trevarthen 1998; Nadel et al. 1999). Two-month-old infants interact with their mothers via a live two-way video set up. The live video image of the mother is switched to a video of her engaged in past interaction with the infant. The infant soon stops trying to engage with the mother who is obviously not responding to the present action of the infant although she still maintains her expressive behavior; the infant also becomes distressed. The principle is that interaction is a two-way street; it depends on an ongoing contingency — that is, the mother's action has to answer the infant's action and vice versa. One way to put this is to say that the infant is sensitive to social contingency (Nadel et al. 1999), but this way of putting it suggests that what is important is simply a capacity that the infant has rather than a dynamic aspect of the interaction itself. That is the issue that Di Paolo and his colleagues decided to explore.

The second-generation experiment was made by Auvray, Lenay and Stewart (2006) on the dynamics of human interaction in a shared virtual environment. Di Paolo sees this experiment as an extremely simplified variant of the Murray-Trevarthen experiment. In the virtual environment experiment, two adult subjects acting on the same system are able to move an icon left and right along a shared one-dimensional continuous (wrapped around) virtual tape. On the tape are representations of station-ary objects and moving objects, the two independent agents themselves, and a displaced 'shadow' of each agent that simply moves in the same way the agent does. As each agent moves along the tape they encounter an object, a shadow, or the other virtual agent, all of which are of the same small size. The subjects are blindfolded but receive tactile stimulations on a finger when their icon comes in contact with another entity on the tape. Their task, the same for each agent, is to indicate when they are in contact with the other agent. They are told that they will meet up with moving objects, static objects, and another agent like themselves, and they're asked to click the mouse button when they think they are scanning the other agent. You might think that this is an impossible task, but subjects do very well at it (generating approximately 70% correct responses). When they meet up with the other virtual agent, who is also looking for them, there is a kind of interaction that is missing when they meet up with an object, or with the shadow of the other agent. The shadow of the other agent is like the non-live video of the mother in the Murray and

Trevarthen experiment — the mother, and the shadow, are doing what they are doing independently of the other who tries to interact with them. Neither one responds in the right way.

> The important issue is that the scanning of an entity encountered will only stabilise in the case that both partners are in contact with each other — if interaction is only one-way, between a subject and the other's shadow, the shadow will eventually move away, because the subject it is shadowing is still engaged in searching activity. Two-way mutual scanning is the only globally stable condition. Therefore, the solution to the task does not rely on individuals performing the right kind of perceptual discrimination between different momentary sensory patterns, but emerges from the mutual perceptual activity of the experimental subjects that is oriented towards each other. (Di Paolo, Rohde and Iizuka 2008, 286).

The strategy that emerges when the agents find each other consists of a reciprocal movement of the two icons that manifests a different tempo from an agent's icon moving back and forth over the icon of an object or shadow, and the difference is due to the fact that the other agent is moving in the same back-and-forth pattern rather than in the search pattern. This actually works. The psychologist David Leavens and I tried it in Di Paolo's lab at the University of Sussex. Without vision or audition, and judging only on identical tactile stimuli that signaled the encounter of indistin-

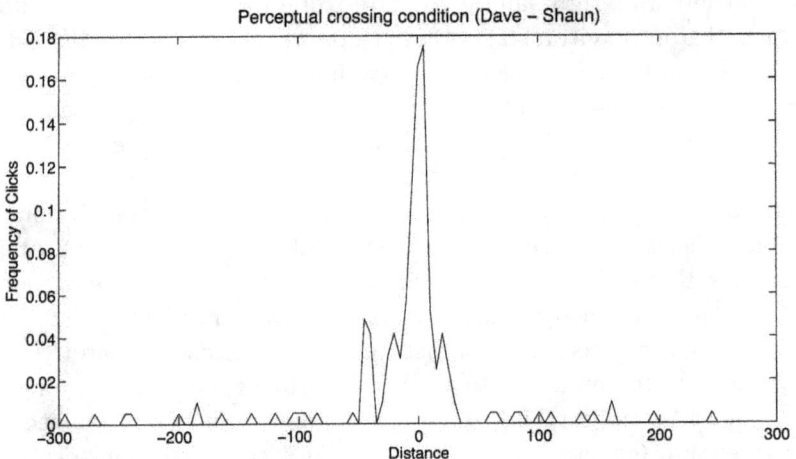

Figure 8.1 Frequency of mouse clicks are higher when one encounters (is at 0 distance from) the other's icon.

guishable icons, we were asked to click the computer mouse when we encountered and identified the other's icon. Figure 8.1 summarizes the results.

The stage is now set for the third experiment. In this experiment, however, Di Paolo, Rohde, and Iizuka get rid of the human subjects and give the same task to intelligent virtual robots, each of which have one touch sensor that activates if they touch another entity (agent, object, or shadow). The experimenters discovered something important right away.

> When we first tried to evolve agents to solve the perceptual crossing task, the evolutionary search algorithm was not able to find a satisfactory solution. The behavior that evolved was for agents to halt when crossing any object encountered on the tape, be it the partner, the fixed object or the shadow of the other. ... Only when a small time delay between a crossing on the tape and the agent's sensation was included in the model ... the evolutionary search algorithm came up with an adaptive solution. The trajectories generated by the [artificial robotic] agents are similar to those generated by some human subjects (2008, 284).

In both the second and third experiments, the humans and the robots evolved the same strategy of using an oscillating scanning movement to test whether they were meeting up with an object, a shadow, or another agent. The easiest entities to discriminate from the other agent were the moving object and the shadow, which is also moving. They keep moving in whatever direction they are moving in, so to keep oscillating across them you have to follow their motion. In contrast, when you meet up with the other agent—and it with you—you both start oscillating across each other and meet up at the middle of the oscillation trajectory, which makes it appear as if the other agent is stationary. So it turns out that it is more difficult to distinguish between the other agent and a stationary object. This discrimination is solved by considering the apparent size of the entity.

> When we inspect the duration of the stimulus upon crossing a fixed object, we realise that it lasts longer than when crossing a moving partner. This is because the fixed object does not move itself. The solution that the simulated agent adopts simply relies on integrating sensory stimulation over a longer time period, which yields a higher value for a static object, i.e., it is sensed as having a larger apparent size. This hypothesis has been tested and is supported by the fact that the agent is quite easily tricked into making the wrong decision if the size of the static object is varied, i.e. a small object is mistaken for another agent—or, likewise, the other agent is perceived as a smaller object (2008, 286).

The central point that Di Paolo, Rohde, and Iizuka want to make applies equally to all three experiments, and in that sense it tells us something about the mother-infant, or more generally, human interaction—which will also be a shared principle for human-robot interaction. The principle is this: successful coordination is not something that depends simply on individual capacities (the capacity of one agent, or the two capacities of two agents)—as suggested by the interpretation of Nadel et al. (1999), but rather on a dynamic aspect of the interaction itself. This supports an interactionist approach to the analysis of social cognition (e.g., De Jaegher 2006; Fogel 1993; Stern 2002), i.e., an approach that is clearly in contrast to the theory of mind approaches of ST or TT discussed in Chapter 7.

Social robotics

The theoretical underpinnings of social cognition have been shifting away from overly-intellectualistic conceptions based on theory of mind approaches, toward more embodied versions of simulation and interactionist theories. In ToM approaches social cognition is framed in terms of gaining access to the other person's mind; in simulation theory (especially the implicit versions) the activation of neural resonance systems (mirror neurons, shared neural representations) puts conspecifics into similar, if not the same, sensory-motor states, and this is the basis for social understanding informed by action schemas or emotion based empathy (e.g., Decety 2004; 2005; Gallese 2003). Interactionist theory appeals to the same neuroscience of resonance systems, and builds on research in developmental psychology, to show that the basis of social cognition is both perceptual and contextual (Gallagher 2001; 2005), and in many respects dependent on the dynamic aspects of interaction itself (De Jaegher 2006).

People who are communicating or interacting in pragmatic or social contexts depend to a high degree on the perception of the other's movements, postures, gestures, facial expressions (e.g., Trevarthen 1979—'primary intersubjectivity'). People also make use of pragmatic contexts (environmental features, specific objects of shared attention) to understand the actions of others (Trevarthen and Hubley 1978—'secondary intersubjectivity'). These capacities for understanding embodied, non-verbalized meanings are important mechanisms for understanding others even prior to (and preparatory to) language acquisition. They deliver very basic elements that often are sufficient (without verbal communication) for delivering meaning, but they also become integrated with linguistic communication and narrative competency in human development.

As we saw in the previous chapter, sometimes these perceptual and contextual systems fail, as in autism. Now some people might think that robots are just that—autistic. Even if I find myself taking the intentional stance toward a robot, the robot doesn't have an empathetic bone in its body. All of these issues get tied together in the work of Kerstin Dautenhahn at the University of Hertfordshire where she runs *The AuRoRA Project*. As the project's homepage states: 'Our main aim is to engage children with autism in coordinated and synchronized interactions with the environment thus helping them to develop and increase their communication and social interaction skills. ... Humans are the best models for human social behavior, but their social behavior is very subtle, elaborate, and widely unpredictable' (http://www.aurora-project.com/). Since children with autism often are fascinated by mechanical things, the idea is to create a bridge to human-human interaction through the use of sophisticated but nonetheless behaviorally simple human-robot interaction (Billard et al. 2006).

Human-robot interaction may have to follow the same rules as human-human interaction if it is going to be successful. Dautenhahn, in a news interview, follows this line.

> **Dautenhahn:** For a long time people thought the summit of human intelligence was our capacity for problem solving, IQ tests and the like. So in developing robots they designed them to do these complex tasks, like playing chess. But now people are saying that its humans' ability to deal with complex social relationships that's made us intelligent. (Interview, Dautenhahn 2006).

But this means, as Hubert Dreyfus likes to say, there are no rules. We already have computers that play chess by playing by the rules—chess is an entirely rule-governed game, and computers are completely rule-governed machines. Thus, in a *News Hour* debate on American television with Dan Dennett following the computer Deep Blue's win over Gary Kasparov in 1997, Dreyfus is keen to make this point.

> **Dreyfus:** The reason the computer could win at chess—and everybody knew that eventually computers would win at chess—is because chess is a completely isolated domain. It doesn't connect up with the rest of human life, therefore, like arithmetic, it's completely formalizable, and you could, in principle, exhaust all the possibilities. And in that case, a fast enough computer can run through enough of these calculable possibilities to see a winning strategy or to see a move toward a winning strategy. But the way our everyday life is, we don't have a formal world, and we can't exhaust the possibilities and run through them. So what this shows is in a world in which calculation is possible, brute force, meaningless calculation

[wins], the computer will always beat people; but when—in a world in which relevance and intelligence play a crucial role and meaning [depends on] concrete situations, the computer has always behaved miserably, and there's no reason to think that that will change with this victory. (Interview, Dreyfus and Dennett 1997)

Dennett, on the other hand, is not willing to turn Deep Blue's victory into a defeat for AI.

Dennett: I think that the idea that Professor Dreyfus has that there's something special about the informal world is an interesting idea, but we just have to wait and see. The idea that there's something special about human intuition that is not capturable in the computer program is a sort of illusion, I think, when people talk about intuition. It's just because they don't know how something's done. If we didn't know how Deep Blue did what it did, we'd be very impressed with its intuitive powers, and we don't know how people live in the informal world very well. And as we learn more about it, we'll probably be able to reproduce that in a computer as well.

Dreyfus, however, insists that the everyday (informal, non-rule governed) world is quite different; moreover, humans are embodied and move in a way that makes our interaction with the world quite complex, and our understanding of it implicit. This isn't a kind of propositional knowledge, but a knowledge that we gain just by doing. Dennett doesn't disagree with this and in fact this brings us back to robotics.

Dennett: [T]he most interesting work in artificial intelligence and largely for the reasons that Bert Dreyfus says … is the work that, for instance, Rodney Brooks and his colleagues and I are doing at MIT with the humanoid robot Cog, and as Dreyfus says—you've got to be embodied to live in a world, to develop real intelligence, and Cog does have a body. That's why Cog is a robot.

Cog was a project that attempted to build a human-like robot from the ground up, by focusing on basic sensory-motor capacities and the kind of capabilities that infants have, like imitation. It follows the line of thought that Rodney Brooks suggests.

The 'simple' things concerning perception and mobility in a dynamic environment … are a necessary basis for 'higher-level' intellect. … Therefore, I proposed looking at simpler animals as a bottom-up model for building intelligence. It is soon apparent, when 'reasoning' is stripped away as the prime component of a robot's intellect, that the dynamics of the interaction of the robot and its environment are primary determinants of the structure of its intelligence. (Brooks 1988, 418).

The building of such a robot is not only an engineering challenge, it's a way of doing science, and a way of testing theories. As Francisco Varela puts it in his interview with Sergio Benvenuto (2001):

> **Varela:** This constructive method is the way that science goes about its business today. This is how one proceeds at the interface between the neurosciences and artificial intelligence. Artificial intelligence involves the constructive proof of theories that originate in the neurosciences: for example, constructing robots capable of orienting themselves in the world. Scientists who construct such automata are inspired by biology, but the proof of the theory is that the robot walks.

What do you need to make a robot like Cog work in a way that would smoothly interface with our own life-world? Dennett would say you need lots more robots, and this brings us back again to a particular view on neuroscience.[2]

> **Dennett:** Kasparov's brain is a parallel-processing device composed of more than ten billion little robots. Neurons, like every other cell in a body, are robots, and the organized activity of ten billion little unthinking, uncomprehending robots IS a form of brute force computing, and surely intuition IS nothing other than such an emergent product.

> **Dreyfus:** [C]omputers will have to be embodied as we are if they are to interact with us and thus be counted as intelligent by our standards. Given this view, does Cog have a body enough like ours to have at least a modicum of human intelligence? … It need not lack intuition. The billions of dumb robot neurons in our brain properly organized and working together, somehow, I agree, [can] manifest expert intuition. … What I want to argue here is that Cog cannot manifest human-like emotions. According to neuroscience, emotions depend upon (although they are much more than) chemical changes in the brain. These changes are due to hormones, adrenaline, and the like. It may not be important that Cog's brain is silicon and ours is protein, but it might be crucial that ours is wet and Cog's is dry.

The view that Dreyfus expresses here is consistent with the interactionist approach to social cognition — one that emphasizes embodiment, emotion, an intuitive sense of meaning found in the other person's gestures, movements and facial expressions. What is clear in this is that for Dreyfus it's not just a matter of what's inside at the subpersonal level that counts if we

---

2   The following short exchange is taken from a follow up e-mail exchange between Dennett and Dreyfus published on the *Slate* website, 'Artificial Intelligence', May-June 1997. http://www.slate.com/id/3650/entry/23907/.

are looking for an emergence of cognition; rather it's also a matter of action in the world that produces meaning and is affected by the intentionality of everyday life. In contrast, Dennett takes a more theory-of-mind approach to this issue, as he indicates later in their e-mail exchange by endorsing Baron-Cohen's work. Dreyfus then takes it one step further in signaling the importance of public narrative and social roles.

> **Dennett:** [The] addition of higher-order intentionality—under-standing trickery, bluffs, and the like—has already been much dis-cussed among us [at the MIT lab]. I put a typescript copy of Simon Baron-Cohen's book, *Mindblindness* (MIT Press, 1995), in circulation in the lab several years ago; it has a handy list of suggested mecha-nisms that might rescue Cog from autism. (An automaton doesn't have to be autistic, but it will be unless rather special provisions are made for it.)

> **Dreyfus:** As you recognize in insisting that Cog be socialized, emotions such as shame, guilt, and love require an understanding of public narratives and exemplars which must be picked up not just as information but by imitating the style of peoples' behavior as they assume various social roles.[3]

---

3   Whatever happened to Cog? Perhaps as an experiment it served its purpose. Dreyfus, however, reports: 'Cog failed to achieve any of its goals and the original robot is already in a museum. But, as far as I know, neither Dennett nor anyone connected with the project has published an account of the failure and asked what mistaken assumptions underlay their absurd optimism. In a personal communication Dennett blamed the failure on a lack of graduate students' (Dreyfus 2007). The Cog website is still up and running however: (www.ai.mit.edu/projects/humanoid-robotics- group/cog/.)

Emotion and Empathy

In his 1994 book, *Descartes' Error: Emotion, Reason, and the Human Brain*, Antonio Damasio, a neuroscientist working at the University of Iowa, and now at the University of Southern California, pushed emotion onto center stage in discussions of cognitive science. From the time of Plato most mainstream philosophers had pushed emotion off to the side in favor of a conception of the mind as something primarily rational. Reason, after all, on Plato's account, was charged with keeping the unruly *pathos*, feeling and passion, under control and out of sight, and this seemed imperative if one were going to live a good (i.e., ethical, i.e., rule-governed, rational) life. Descartes, of course, followed that tradition, divorced emotion from reason, and celebrated rational thought. The emotions were something that happened in the body, so they couldn't possibly have anything to do with thinking, which was accomplished in the mind. Hence, *Descartes' Error*.

Damasio argues that what we call reason is not something that we can think of as independent from emotion, and that, in fact, without emotion we don't end up with Mr. Spock (the ultra-rationalist from Star Treck fame), but Phineas Gage, the railway worker who in an explosives accident in the mid-19th century had a tamping iron (3 feet 7 inches long and weighing 13½ pounds) blown through this brain knocking out areas that were responsible for the reciprocal modulation of reason and emotion. The resulting pathology, in this case literally a problem with *patho-logy* (literally, from *pathos* = feeling; *logos* = reason), prevented him from planning or using practical reason in his life.

> Before the accident he had been [the company's] most capable and efficient foreman, one with a well-balanced mind, and who was looked on as a shrewd smart business man. He was now fitful, irreverent, and grossly profane, showing little deference for his fellows. He was also impatient and obstinate, yet capricious and vacillating, unable to settle on any of the plans he devised for future action. (Macmillan 2000).

The frontal cortex, often thought the headquarters, or literally the head-quarter, of reason and decision, turns out to be linked in important ways to emotion centers in the mid-brain. Damage to Gage's frontal cortex thus had an effect on both his emotional and his rational life — or to put it better, his emotional-rational life suffered in every way. This is what happens with many frontal lobe injuries.

> **Damasio:** Such patients can hold their own in completely rational arguments but fail, for example, to avoid a situation involving unnecessary risk. These kinds of problems mainly occur after an injury to the forebrain. As our tests prove, the result is a lack of nor-mal emotional reactions. I continue to be fascinated by the fact that feelings are not just the shady side of reason but that they help us to reach decisions as well. (Manuela 2005, Interview, p. 14).

Damasio emphasizes the importance of embodiment and embodied emo-tions for the proper functioning of reason. Emotions are constituted by the reactions that the body has to various stimuli. Higher heart-rate, dry mouth, contracting muscles are automatic reactions to things that we fear. Damasio distinguishes such emotions from feeling, which is a conscious-ness of the physical changes that occur with emotion.

> **Damasio:** The brain is constantly receiving signals from the body, registering what is going on inside of us. It then processes the signals in neural maps, which it then compiles in the so-called somato-sensory centers. Feelings occur when the maps are read and it becomes apparent that emotional changes have been recorded — as snapshots of our physical state, so to speak. (Manuela 2005, Interview, p. 15).

Damasio goes on to qualify this description. Feelings can arise simply by changes occurring in the neural maps themselves, which happens, for example, when we simulate or empathize with another person and begin to feel their pain. Furthermore, the brain can simply ignore certain emo-tional signals, so not all emotion-body states will be felt. When an emotion is felt, however, it is a feeling of the body. He gives an example in a *New York Times* interview:

> **Damasio:** When you experience the emotion of sadness, there will be changes in facial expression and your body will be closed in, with-drawn. There are also changes in your heart, your guts: they slow down. And there are hormonal changes. The *feeling* of sadness involves your perception of these changes in your body. You may have a sense that your body has slowed down, has less energy, feels ill. Your thought processes also change. The production of new images slows down, your attention may be concentrated on a few

images. By contrast, when you experience joy and elation, you become able to create images more rapidly, and your attention can be proportionally shorter. You feel quick, not stuck. (Star 2000, Interview, p. 31).

Even if some philosophers agree with Damasio's emphasis on embodied emotion, they may find his 18th century epistemology hard to swallow — likely an emotional reaction. But we may be able to set aside the idea that the brain produces images (a production that can slow down or speed up), or reads maps; or that the feeling of emotion depends on a 'perception' of changes in your body — an idea that would make the body a perceptual object rather than the perceiving body (indeed an idea that may go back to the 17th century and 'you know who') — and setting that philosophical syntax aside, we may be able to buy the general insight that the body lives through its emotional states. Importantly, whether the perceiving subject is aware of such states or not, or in Damasio's terms, whether there is a specific feeling of them or not, such states certainly shape our perceptual experience, and more generally our cognitive life.

Fast emotions

Some of these emotional states are basic, if not simple: fear, anger, joy, disgust. Others are more complicated and may depend to some degree on social interaction: compassion, shame, jealously. Empathy, for example, may involve a basic feeling-with the other person, but also a more subtle set of cultural understandings. It furthermore seems essential for mature social interaction, and perhaps for the development of a moral sense.

> **Damasio:** For example, children who suffer brain injury in certain regions of the frontal lobe in their first year years of life develop major defects of social behavior in spite of being otherwise intelligent. They do not exhibit social emotions (compassion, shame, guilt) and they never learn social conventions and ethical rules. (Harcourt 2000, Interview).

Let's take a fast look at the fast emotions. Fear is the best-known example, and Joseph LeDoux is the best theorist on fear (not of course the most feared theorist). LeDoux discovered that the basic fear reaction is really subpersonal. It happens before you know it — before you are even conscious of what it is that you fear. He and Damasio are in agreement on the distinction between emotion and feeling, and on the importance of embodiment.

> **LeDoux:** Emotion, like cognition, is a process. Emotions are processes in the brain that detect and produce response to significant

stimuli. So, there's some kind of stimulus. The brain detects it, does some emotional processing, then some more emotional processing, then the brain produces emotional consciousness. Feelings — and sometimes people use the word interchangeably with emotion — are really the conscious consequences of emotional processing. ... Emotions often have bodily reactions connected with them — the reactions of the autonomic nervous system — such as increased heart rate, blood pressure, etc. (Robinson 2003, Interview, p. 1).

Remember I had mentioned to Marc Jeannerod about my friend who upon alighting from my car more or less jumped over the front of it before he realized why. He had seen a snake. As Marc said, 'That's a good example, because a snake is one of these things that we are attuned to fear'.[1]

LeDoux started his research, not on fear, but with Michael Gazzaniga studying the split brain in humans. When, for medical reasons, the corpus callosum of the brain is cut, the two hemispheres work independently and that produces some surprising responses in experimental settings (see Chapter 11).

> **LeDoux:** One of the questions we asked was what happens when we put information in the right hemisphere. Remember, it's the [language center in the] left hemisphere that usually does the talking, so information in the right hemisphere can't ordinarily be talked about in these patients. We put emotional information in the right hemisphere [via a visual stimulus], and the left hemisphere couldn't tell us what it saw, but it could tell us how it felt about it. That led us to the idea that emotional information and information about the content of what a stimulus is, are processed by different pathways in the brain. (Brockman 1997, Interview, p. 2).

Figuring out the emotion pathways in the days just before neuroimaging came on the scene involved a laborious series of surgical lesion studies — not on humans, but on rats (who also don't like snakes). Rather than snakes, however, LeDoux used conditioned fear with an auditory stimulus. LeDoux traced the quick working subpersonal processes responsible for jumping when you hear a loud sound (or see a snake) to the amygdala, an almond-shaped area in the forebrain, the central nucleus of which is linked to brain stem areas that control the autonomic systems involved in the fear response.

> **LeDoux:** [There is] a behavioral transition that occurs once you find yourself in danger. First, you react — evolution thinks for you. Then

---

1   See above, p. 62. My friend, James Morley, a psychologist at Ramapo University in New Jersey, recognized what sort of snake it was when he finally took a closer look. Actually, I forget what he told me, but my bet is that he remembers, because emotional memory can stay with us long after we forget other things.

you act—you're dependent on past experience and your ability to make decisions in this phase. We've shown that the transition involves the flipping of a switch in the amygdala. I don't mean this literally. What happens is that reaction involves a circuit in which information flows from the lateral amygdala to the central amygdala, which then connects with areas that control reactive bodily responses (freezing behavior; changes in autonomic nervous system responses such as blood pressure, heart rate, breathing, sweating, pupil dilation, etc; and release of stress hormones). In order to take action, you have to inhibit this 'freezing' pathway and activate a pathway in which active behaviors are controlled. This pathway involves the flow of information from the lateral to the basal amygdala. The switch flip metaphor refers to the output of the lateral amygdala, which is sent to different regions for reaction vs. action. Clinically, the reaction pathway is associated with passive coping, and the other pathway with active coping. (Ibid.).

Mapping out the subpersonal process through the amygdala was an important step in the explanation of how this one emotion, fear, could take effect even before consciousness could register danger—something very basic and evolutionarily very important. But what about other basic emotions? LeDoux first thought that he would be able to identify one system in the brain responsible for the emotions, and a likely candidate was the limbic system, of which the amygdala is a part. But he gave up on that idea.

> **LeDoux:** I think that … the idea that there is an emotion system in the brain, is misguided. I came to this conclusion empirically. Once we had outlined a neural circuit for fear responses, it was obvious that the limbic system had little to do with it. The only so-called limbic area involved was the amygdala. And the hippocampus, the centerpiece of the limbic system, had been implicated in non-emotional processes like memory and spatial behavior. (Ibid.).

It makes sense to think that emotions may be products of different systems that have evolved to address different problems involving survival. LeDoux suggests that these systems allow the organism to detect and respond to different forms of danger that require various kinds of sensory and cognitive processes, as well as different motor outputs, and feedback mechanisms.

Following the distinction between emotion and feeling mentioned by Damasio, LeDoux suggests that in evolutionary terms automatic, hard-wired, and non-conscious behavior preceded feeling, and that to understand emotion in its most basic sense one needs to study the automatic aspects of it. The more complex emotions and their conscious feelings, according to LeDoux, are likely a blend of the hard-wired basic ones. Not unlike Damasio, LeDoux would explain feeling as the result of becoming conscious of the emotion activity in the body

> **LeDoux:** So emotional feelings come about when we become consciously aware of the activity of an emotional system, which does its work for the most part outside of consciousness. (Ibid.).

LeDoux, however, is happy to stay at the subpersonal level in his explanation, and he notes that his work is compatible with Dennett's views since emotions can be treated as computational functions of the nervous system (see Brockman 1997, Interview, p. 5). It's not that LeDoux has a phobia of feelings, but he thinks all of the action that can be studied scientifically is at the subpersonal level. He writes: 'From the point of view of the lover, the only thing important about love is the feeling. But from the point of view of trying to understand what a feeling is, why it occurs, where it comes from, and why some people give and receive it more easily than others, love, the feeling, may not have much to do with it at all' (1998, 20). This view of things prompts Damasio, in his review of LeDoux's book, to say that despite a general agreement with LeDoux's position, 'I do not endorse LeDoux's general attitude toward feelings' (Damasio 1997).

Affective neuroscience and the person

In their Gifford Lectures, Michael Arbib and Mary Hesse (recall the discussion in Chapter 6) suggested that the task is not to reduce the person to mechanisms studied by cognitive sciences, but to expand or enhance the cognitive sciences in order to do justice to our humanity (Arbib and Hesse 1986, 34). Michael related this idea to emotions.

> **Arbib:** Jean-Marc Fellous and I have edited a book, *Who Needs Emotion? The Robot Meets the Brain*. The contributors come to the study of emotion either from the side of neuroscience or from artificial intelligence. People who are working on the brain tend to take a fairly reductionist view, seeing the essence of emotion in a biological system based on systems for motivations like hunger, thirst, fear, or sex, or based on particular neuromodulators like dopamine and serotonin, or based on reward and punishment. For example, LeDoux returns to the theme I mentioned above [see Chapter 8], and with Jean-Marc (Fellous & LeDoux 2005) takes fear behavior as seen in the rat and looks at the involvement of amygdala and other regions in conditioning 'fear behavior'. He and the other neuroscientists then conclude with the suggestion that once you add cerebral cortex interacting with these subcortical systems then you have consciousness and feelings, while beginning to explore the implications for robotics.

Jean-Marc and I have also co-authored an article (Arbib & Fellous 2004) where we analyze what it would mean for a robot to have emotion, distinguishing emotional expression for communication from emotion as a mechanism for the organization of behavior. Since the chemical basis of animal function differs greatly from the mechanics and computations of current machines we were led to abstract a functional characterization of emotion from biology that does not depend on physical substrate or evolutionary history. The upshot was that future robot societies might evolve with emotions very different from our own.

Although I am very impressed by the neuroscientists contributions to the study of emotions, I think that their accounts often leave out too much. I see parallels there with my current enthusiasm for studying the evolution of language where I am one of those scientists trying to show how language abilities may be grounded in basic visuomotor mechanisms in the brain. But just adding cortex and consciousness and feelings does not help us understand what distinguishes the use of language from other capacities. I thus see a danger in the neuroscience community of not looking at emotion as lived experience.

I was very struck by the recent novel by J.M. Coetzee (2003) entitled *Elizabeth Costello*, in which he has the title character giving lectures on animal rights. She speaks about Wolfgang Köhler's classic, *The Mentality of Apes*, and those classic experiments that you and I have learned from — namely the study of the chimp Sultan figuring out how to use a crate to reach the bananas. But instead of looking at the key problem-solving operations involved here, Elizabeth Costello seeks to reconstruct the other thoughts going through the chimp's mind. 'Why is he stopping me from getting bananas?' 'Does he hate me?' — and existential questions of this kind. I think of course that the character Elizabeth Costello is going too far in imputing human thoughts to the chimp, but I still think the ideas that Coetzee has her give us are worth the attention of cognitive scientists — helping us reflect on the tension between constrained behavior and its neural correlates that we can study in the lab, and the richness of lived experience. However, we do not have the luxury of ignoring the genuine insights that come from lab work. Thus in my own contribution to *Who Needs Emotion? The Robot Meets the Brain,* I try to respect what we can get from the neural and AI analyses of animal behavior and the use of emotional expression in robots that interact with people and so on, and yet remind people of that tension there with the personal reality of emotions. And one last point about the book: Just about every other chapter presents emotions as 'good things'. I thus include in my chapter a little confession about losing my temper to suggest that there are some real questions to be answered about what the place of emotion is in the economy of the modern human brain. And I title my chapter, 'Beware the Passionate Robot'.

There is some echo of this in Jaak Panksepp, who characterizes feelings as part of affect. For him the lack of study of affect or feeling in cognitive science is something of a political issue.

Panksepp: I believe one of the biggest challenges in emotion research is for us to open up discourse about the nature of affective-emotional experience, not just in humans but all mammals. I think most people in the world outside of the scientific-philosophical formal approaches to the study and discussion of emotions believe that the *experience* of affect, the valenced feeling aspect of emotions, is the defining characteristic and hence the most important dimension of emotional life. Yet it remains the least studied and the least discussed property of emotionality, with considerably more effort devoted to the autonomic arousal, behaviorally expressive, and more recently the abundant cognitive correlates. We now need a generation of scholars that are not scared to talk about the raw feeling aspects, and to fully consider the possibility that we are not the only creatures in the world that have such experiences.

It is scientifically clear that subjective feelings arise from the material dynamics of brains working in bodies that live under specific ecological constraints. I am committed to the pursuit of research that has the potential to illuminate the neural nature of affect, and the work is based on the data-supported premise that other mammals do have various basic affective experiences, from anger to hunger, that are homologous to our own.

SG: So you are suggesting that we need to use animal models to understand the emotional mind of humans.

Panksepp: All mammals have a demonstrably shared evolutionary history which is reflected in the functional similarities of their underlying brain circuits and neurochemistries. It makes little sense to remain in denial about basic mind issues just because it is such a difficult problem. Darwin himself made the assumption that other animals do have emotional experiences but his era did not have the neuroscientific tools to probe such issues; hence, he chose to restrict most of his coverage of emotions to the ethological level. Freud did talk about the nature of affect in human experience, but even during his era, neuroscience was still not sufficiently mature for a concerted empirical confrontation with the problem, a task that clearly requires appropriate animal models. Now advances in behavioral brain research allow a vigorous confrontation with such momentous issues, but the intellectual community remains reticent to pursue such questions vigorously.

For instance, prominent investigators such as Joe LeDoux (1996), who have fostered enormous advances in our understanding of how fear is learned, have also suggested that the topic of affective experience in animals may be irrelevant for understanding human emotions because feelings are just 'frosting on the cake' that arises from sophisticated higher working memory abilities that can only arise from the massively expanded human cortex. Clearly, we have more working memory space than most other species, which surely means we can think about our emotions in incredibly more subtle ways than most other animals. This allows us to be aware of our own emotional feelings, as well as potentially the feelings of other animals. But the idea that dorsolateral frontal cortical working memory mechanisms create affects, as opposed to just awareness of our affects, is simply an assumption.

For some, the idea that other animals have emotional experiences still resembles a 'ghost in the machine' argument. Edmund Rolls (1999; 2005) sustains that position by suggesting that all forms of consciousness are based on language. If language becomes the only credible arbitrator of the existence of experience then, by definition, other animals are fundamentally unconscious, and the study of animal models cannot illuminate the subjective aspects of emotions. I think the study of other behavioral outputs, especially instinctual emotional behaviors of other mammals, should suffice to clarify the raw affective varieties of experience, yielding knowledge that can be further evaluated in humans.

In contrast, Damasio (1994; 1999) has put much more stock in the neuroscientific study of emotional experience, but he has also been hesitant to ascribe emotional feelings to animals. He believes emotional feelings emerge from the neurosymbolic abilities of human somatosensory neocortex, even though more recently he recognized, because of his brain imaging results, the critical role of subcortical systems we share with other animals.

I, as a most persistent proponent of a cross-species brain systems approach to understanding emotional feelings, would claim that the affective heart of emotion research can be best advanced through studies of the brain substrates of instinctual emotional behaviors and the behavioral choices resulting from such arousals. Such studies will give us an understanding of the sources of various experiences of goodness and badness (i.e., primary process positive and negative affects). If these brain functions emerge in humans from homologous subcortical brain networks, then well-chosen animal models can clarify the basic emotional feelings of the human brain.

SG: You mentioned, just in passing, that the cortex is, of course, to some degree plastic and thus open to the influence of experience. What about subcortical plasticity?

Panksepp: Every part of the brain is plastic, and there are many types of plasticity.

SG: Is there a higher degree in the cortex?

Panksepp: Most investigators, including myself, believe that is true. The functions of subcortical regions are more genetically predetermined, while cortical functions are more epigenetically constructed. There are some remarkable subcortical plasticities as in sexual and maternal behavior circuits, but practically all neocortical functions emerge through variable epigenetic developmental landscapes, as refined through learning and memory. Most subcortical functions are more rigorously genetically prescribed. Still, I do not know of any emotional networks that do not exhibit long-term changes in arousability depending upon past experiences, but such sensitizations differ from the propositional learning based plasticity of the cortex.

There are many forms of brain plasticity. Certainly the neocortex is quintessentially plastic *in early life*. It is much closer to a general purpose learning tissue than to one that contains an abundance of genetically pre-determined functional 'modules'. For instance, one can eliminate the visual cortex of a mouse *in utero* but it still develops a fine visual cortex epigenetically in nearby neocortical regions. Although one can easily argue for evolutionarily dictated 'modules' in higher regions of the human brain, that argument is not supported by any solid neuroscientific data. Neocortex initially resembles a *tabula rasa,* but it is rapidly programmed by subcortical influences (as in the programming of sensory cortexes) and individual experiences throughout development.

Subcortical regions are more genetically dedicated to specific instinctual affective processes and intertwined body regulatory functions, but the sensitivities of these systems are changed by life experiences.

SG: Which I think leads to a philosophical issue. I wonder if you're working in the same philosophical ballpark as someone like John Searle who rejects formal and syntactical accounts of consciousness; rather, he says it's the biology that counts for consciousness. You suggest the organic properties of brain tissue have to be taken into account. Can you say what it is about the biology that is essential? Searle doesn't really say anything more than it's the biology. So one wants to know what it is about the biology.

Panksepp: I do favor the general approach that John Searle has advocated. His convictions encourage scientific work rather than just conceptual argumentation in this difficult area. Without the science, consciousness studies will remain ungrounded. For any phenomenon of consciousness, any experiential aspect of mind, there are three stages to any credible scientific analysis. First, we must identify the neural correlates of the phenomenon we wish to understand. Second, we need to fathom which are in the major chains of causality for generating experience. Third, after the major causal pathways have been sifted from correlates, we can begin to generate mechanistic conceptions of how affective experience is actually generated. I think that's where Searle becomes a bit of mysterian. He suggests that at the end of the scientific analysis there will remain an unfathomable, un-crossable gap, between the phenomenology of experience and the causal mechanisms. I think science can narrow this gap more than he does.

SG: Going back to Damasio, is it possible that this gap can get better filled in by the emphasis on the body?

Panksepp: Yes. For instance, the dynamics of instinctual emotional actions may well represent the dynamics of the corresponding emotional feelings. It is in the cognitive realm, where the explanatory gap may remain more of a chasm. However, I do not favor Damasio's William James inspired idea that emotional feelings are fundamentally linked to the bodily-sensations induced dynamics of somatosensory cortex. I think raw emotional feelings arise from primitive subcortical viscero-somatic body representations, laid out in instinctual action coordinates, which Damasio did not address in *Descartes' Error* (1994). He corrected some of those shortcomings in his following book, *The Feeling of What Happens* (1999), but he remained hesitant to ascribe any capacity for phenomenal affective experience within the neural complexities of ancient subcortical brain regions where ESB can evoked emotional behaviors along with the corresponding feelings. If the primary locus of control for emotional feelings is the somato-sensory cortex of the brain, we need to deal with a troublesome re-presentational 'read-out' process. 'Read-out' by what and how? I prefer a dual-aspect monism view where raw affect is part and parcel of primitive subcortical body schema, anchored in action coordinates.

Certainly ancient limbic cortices participate in affective experiences. We all now agree that many *sensory* affects such as disgust, pain, and other bodily states are concentrated in old paleo-cortical regions such as the insula, but those systems are well enmeshed with more ancient body representations down below. The emotional affects, which seem to ride upon viscero-somatic emotional action coordinates, seem to be organized more directly by those subcortical networks. Overall, I think the neocortical participations allow organisms to have secondary- and tertiary-process thoughts, and 'awareness' that they are having certain kinds of experiences, but those cognitive abilities do not, by themselves, generate the primary-process feelings.

One of Panksepp's most interesting ideas, in my view, is the notion that an emotional signature generated from subcortical areas reiterates itself in other parts of the brain, including the cortical areas, and so is manifested in personal-level experience. I asked Jacques Paillard about this idea.

Paillard: Emotion is clearly built into the core of this organization. It is something at the top of these primitive structures. The core, the reticular formation, the hippocampus — structures that would generate emotional states, motivations, and so on. But the whole body and not just the brain is involved. When you have an emotion you can see clearly that it has an effect on the proprioceptive attitude, and you feel your emotional state as a postural expression. There is a problem in making a dissociation between posture (*attitude* in French) which works against gravity to maintain bodily support, and attitude which expresses emotion. Posture involves both a topo-posture which locates you against gravity, and a morpho-posture which is attitude, which expresses emotion in and through the body. I think it is true that these postural aspects are of different origins than purely motor, and are different modes of driving the system. Gesture too belongs to that kind of expression.

Pursuing this concept of postural attitude, Tony Marcel suggests that one aspect of an emotion is an 'action attitude', which is a bodily state, (musculoskeletal, autonomic, and hormonal). This is neither a representation nor a plan, although, according to Marcel, there may be a nonconscious representation of the action attitude which mediates its phenomenology and through which one is aware of it. He explains this as follows: 'Bodily experience (as distinct from second-order awareness of it) is underlain by a representation of the bodily state. Such a representation can be fed in two ways, (a) as proprioceptive afferent projections from the body itself and (b) from representations of the body that themselves do not come from the body' (Lambie and Marcel 2002, p. 233). I asked him about this.

SG: As an example of the latter you mention that which underlies phantom limbs, especially in congenitally aplasic individuals, that is where individuals are born without limbs. Are you speaking of a body schema here? Does 'attitude' here, as in the French, mean posture? And if so, does this mean that we can read the emotion of another person off of their bodily posture?

Marcel: Yes. You've got it. As in the French. But 'attitude' means a bit more. It means a relation with the world (including oneself), in this case a (proto-) physical relation. When you ask if it is a body schema, I take it that you mean body schema in the sense that you yourself stipulate the term. If so, the answer is 'Yes' in the sense that it is not itself a representation. But it is not entirely equivalent to what you specifically refer to as a body schema. I suppose that phenomeno-logically speaking, it is debatable whether what we call an action atti-tude is part of non/pre-reflective experience. Clearly it is intentional (in being an attitude *to* something). But it is not a representation of one's bodily attitude; rather, one's bodily attitude itself is a form of representation, though not in the symbolic sense or in the sense that to be a representation it has to be treated as one.

SG: Is an action attitude, then, a practical stance toward the world? Not one that I take in some kind of deliberation, but one that I find myself taking because my body and my action are always situated, or, as phenomenologists say, 'in-the-world'? Isn't this at the same time a real physical stance that can be seen by others insofar as they can see my intentions and see my emotions in my posture and expression?

Marcel: I'm not sure what force or meaning your word 'practical' has, but certainly I mean that it is a stance that we take because our bodies and action are always situated. However, I do not think that we meant it to be understood as a stance that one 'finds oneself tak-ing', because it can be intended: I can take an attitude. But, yes, it is a real physical stance that can be seen by others insofar as they can see my intentions and emotions in posture and expression, though one can disguise it in the everyday sense beloved of Jacobean revenge dramatists ('I'll smile and smile, and murder while I smile.') Of course, as we know from much research, such disguised stances (as in the case of smiles) are different from 'genuine' or spontaneous ones.

As Lambie and I said in the paper, we prefer this idea to that of Nico Frijda's concept of Action Readiness because it is not just readiness, it is more embodied and nearer to action itself, and it is why it translates more easily into what may be experienced as an 'action urge'. And in my chapter on the sense of agency I review evidence of neurological stimulation that creates felt action urges; now there you have a bit of neuroscience that I think can help to get a grip on the psychology.

In classical painting one way of depicting action (which is dynamic in time as opposed to what is static in a painting) is to depict that stance just prior to the relevant movement that is impossible to maintain, like a coiled spring: this conveys a tension felt by the viewer, what Gestalt psychologists called 'pregnanz', just as in music when you have a 'hook' that is similar to a wave just before it breaks—you know where the music is going, and if it does not go there or delays one feels it.

SG: All of this helps to convey the dynamic character of an action attitude.

Practical stance or not, an action attitude is a relation toward the world. By implicating the whole body and not just the brain in the signature of emotion, both Paillard and Marcel suggest that there is not just a reiteration of subcortical patterns in cortical processes (Panksepp's idea), but that the reiterations are extra-neural as well, in the same way that body schemas are both neural and extra-neural. What gets expressed bodily, in the action attitude, is not just the outward expression of an emotion that is generated first in the brain; it may in fact run the other way: what happens in the brain may start as reiterations of one's action attitude, which is keyed to certain emotion affordances in the environment. Reiterations that reach the cortex may just as well be the end point of emotion formation as its beginning point. Moreover, this formation is often not a private matter, but very much an intersubjective matter.

SG: It is interesting that morphostasis of posture, like the morphokinesis of gesture, may be expressive of emotion. Susan Savage-Rumbaugh, who works closely with Bonobos, has said (and I have this through our mutual friend Jonathan Cole) that one needs to be careful around Bonobos, and presumably other apes, because to them posture means something (usually something sexual); you have to think about what your posture is communicating.

Paillard: Yes, we could say it has a communicative function. Animals will iterate some attitude or other without the need for explicit communication. It's a way for them all to know, to get a signal to pay attention to this individual. This seems to be a very genuine expression about the internal emotional state. I worked with baboons for fifteen years. It is quite clear that when you enter the cage of the baboon, you are not to look at the baboon and you are to take a very neutral attitude, because they look at you and interpret your posture and moves. They are very sensitive to this. That means that they bestow on us intentions.

SG: Our posture communicates what we are going to do.

Paillard: Yes, and signals are sent even with eye movements without movement of the head. On top of this, everything can be interpreted as expressing emotion. So it is very complicated.

SG: One of the main themes you developed in your writings is this idea that we won't really get a good understanding of cognition, consciousness, and experience without looking closely at the sub-cortical mechanisms for emotion and so forth. That's a theme that has been growing slowly over the last several years. The kind of question I want to put to you is this: Does this mean, in your view, that we have something like an incomplete notion of cognition? Something that we can simply add to by now considering emotional issues or is it more on the order of once we start considering these emotional dimensions that will really revolutionize our conception of what cognition is.

Paillard: I think the latter. I think the cognitive revolution was so successful because there was a large community of scholars dissatisfied with behaviorism which had tossed out all human mental activities. Human mental activity which is in the realm of thought and intellect was brought back with some gusto. But the ancient kinds of processes that we all share as creatures were marginalized once more, a second time; behaviorism marginalized them and then the cognitive revolution marginalized them. As an evolutionist as completely as I am, have been all my career, it is a no-brainer that brain/mind/emotion is an evolved process. You cannot really understand the higher reaches unless you've got a pretty good understanding as to what the lower reaches do. The lower reaches, the sub-cortical areas, have also been neglected by modern brain imaging partially because the technology doesn't highlight those systems all that well. They're tight compact systems and on top of that when you use exteroceptive stimuli and you insist upon higher cognitive processing, of course your going to see higher brain processes being aroused. Again there is a bias. People have known for pretty much the whole 20th century that the sub-cortical processes were so fundamental for so many things; then all of a sudden this knowledge is just tossed out the window because people have not been immersed intellectually in that knowledge. My heartfelt opinion based, I think, on a mountain of evidence is that until those systems are dealt with in a credible way the cognitive revolution will remain ungrounded and off in fantasy land.

SG: Now you know there is a reading of the history of philosophy starting with Plato, and even before, where rationality is the thing, and emotions are viewed as interference, something to get rid of. And Descartes, of course, as Damasio has reminded us. Is this a good reading? Historically is there any time or any place where people have actually said wait these emotions are important and we should not suppress them, or is it just now that we are coming to this?

Paillard: I think throughout human history emotions have been recognized as powerful forces and I think certainly Aristotle spent quite a bit of time on those issues as have most major philosophers. I think the problem is that aside from a little bit of surface description there is not very much you can do with it. They're not all that highly cognitively resolved; and if people carefully look at it, most of their cognitive processes revolve around their bodily needs, around the kinds of values that have emerged from social interactions positive and negative. If someone were a psychoethologist and said let us document every moment of everyone's life, they would see what percentages are devoted to those bodily needs and passions. It would be an enormous percentage; but academics sitting in their ivory towers might not see this. I also think human calamities find people addressing emotional issues.

SG: They have to face death or the death of a loved one, correct? But then they really don't know how to deal with them, personally, or academically.

Paillard: I had a colleague who was very much a behaviorist, the classic person who considered himself to be a totally intellectually creature, brighter than anyone else, which is not uncommon in our species. His relationship broke up. He came to my office and he said I'm having a strange experience. I'm sitting at my desk and tears are coming to my eyes and I don't know what it means. I said, listen, this is called sadness. It's called grief. Experience it. He didn't even know how to experience it so I think emotions can be forgotten from lack of use and I think most of our lives are devoted to making sure that our emotional concerns are taken care of and if they are taken care of then we're fine. Then we can forget them and we take each other for granted until we lose each other.

Triangulating the emotions

SG: How do you go about studying emotions?

Paillard: I think you have to have a phenomenological analysis. No questions about that. If you don't have a good analysis of the experience, which can only be done in humans, the whole issue cannot be addressed.

On this point, Tony Marcel agrees. But he offers the following qualifications.

Marcel: First, many theorists have ostensibly started out to characterise the content of emotion experience but have proceeded to give an answer to a different question. Second, if one is going to account for something, then one had better have a reasonable characterisation of it before trying to account for it. What had struck us was that several different major theorists had each characterised conscious emotion experience differently. Either there is a major problem with introspection or each of their emotion experience is different or perhaps there are both (a) different kinds of emotion experience, even for the same emotion, and (b) problems and complications in one's consciousness. Third, we do not accept that the only important aspect of psychology is process; one's experience (what we call phenomenal content and what we call referential content) is important in its own right: it is what makes up one's mental life, indeed one's life itself. For that reason I want to say that I am interested in explanation by content (as opposed to by process). Fourth, we point out with examples that the content of one's emotion experience, including its 'phenomenology', has effects, i.e. it plays a causal role (thus somewhat undermining LeDoux's stance). Now to some extent (perhaps a large extent) a more formal sense of phenomenology is implicated here as important, either in that what we were doing may be part of it or in that it may bear on what we were doing.

SG: You suggest, however, that our experience is not independent of how one attends to it, and that 'the same nonconscious state can give rise to quite different experience depending on the process that constructs the latter from the former.' If that is the case, then doesn't that qualify any claims for the importance of phenomenology, just in the sense you mean?

Marcel: I don't see why. By phenomenology I think we made clear that we meant our experience as we experience it. But you might say that what we were doing was having a go at outlining the structure of that experience and its limits. It would be within that structure or bounds that attention can have its effects. The late Robert Solomon and others have outlined how different theorists have attempted to characterise the phenomenology of emotion (or of emotion experience). They have made different proposals. It is possible that some of those different answers depend on how one attends. But further, it seems to me at least that attention is very important to phenomenology in its more formal sense. When one thinks of Brentano's emphasis on directedness, on the intentionality, it seems to me that attention may be seen as an intrinsic part of that. Indeed, when William James gives such a central place to attention, it seems to me that this is why he does so. One reason why Joint Attention between infants and carers is potentially so important is that it is the first indicator that the infant understands in a non-symbolic way that the other and itself have minds. And I do not see why laying emphasis on mental acts (attention) diminishes the importance of phenomenology—quite the opposite if one does not see them as independent.

SG: One may have an emotion because something matters, or as you put it, emotion may be relevant to a concern. In that case, does emotion depend on an appraisal or judgment consciously made by an agent?

Marcel: It may be that for many theorists of emotion who emphasise appraisal, what they mean by appraisal is a judgment. But our point is that specific things or events matter to a creature because that creature already has concerns (i.e. they matter continuously implicitly), but they may only become occurrent when there is a specific turn of events or one is asked whether they matter. Certainly we do not envisage that the only kind of judgment is one that is explicit, reflective and detached. There are judgments (if you wish to call them that) that are embedded and immediate, that are built in. What we meant by an agent is a creature whose behavior has certain characteristics and bears a certain relation to phenomenal experience rather than merely to neural information processing.

Phenomenology, behavioral analysis, and neuroscience—all of these methodologies, one correcting or supplementing the other, seem important in the study of emotion.

Paillard: That's right. My philosophy is that you cannot make real progress on emotions at simply a phenomenological level, even if that kind of analysis is necessary. You have to also have the anchor of behavioral analysis but ethological behavior much more than lever-pressing behavior. You try to link the phenomenology and the behavior. Phenomenology is collected in humans; the real ethological behavior is collected in animals, and you try to link them to common neural substrates. If there are common neural substrates, and evolution suggests the possibility of homology, then you reveal underpinnings both in humans and animals simultaneously.

Now it's obvious that the homologous processes interact with other brain mechanisms that are not shared. Other animals do not have the robust or large or complex cortex that we have, therefore, these basic processes will interact in totally unique ways. Once you start focusing on those interactions again you've got the massive layer of complexity that's very hard to deal with. Now we've known about these shared systems with animals for an incredibly long time, by inference from just neuroanatomy; but neuroanatomy was not a comfortable level of analysis because it is ultimately dead tissue. Emotions are living things and until we knew about neurochemical homologies and neurophysiological homologies one could not convince the intellectual community that you could play the homology game for certain types of things. The roots of emotional experience seems to be a subcortical phenomenon largely, but they obviously interact with the rest of the brain, and manifest themselves phenomenologially. Still, if one wants to know what emotions really are, I don't think there's any alternative but confrontation with the subcortical issues and comparison of these processes in other animals.

SG: Many emotions involve intersubjective experience.

Paillard: Absolutely. Sometimes fear and in some places anger but certainly desire, expectation for material rewards, which I think is an emotion. For instance you can't tickle yourself but another person that you have a positive social relationship with can tickle you. If you do not have that positive social relationship with that person they cannot tickle you. It is physically impossible, it's subversive; it is potentially a disgusting experience. So the nervous system is designed in regard to the social emotions to be able to filter inputs; and they change brain processing depending upon a host of other relationships that you have. Sexuality, good sexuality, emerges from people treating each other a certain way. If there is not that treatment, it is a sterile experience.

Empathy and moral feelings

There has been a new and growing interest in the concept of empathy in the last several years within the neuroscientific community, and this has led to a renewed interest in philosophical discussions of empathy (see, e.g., de Waal and Thompson 2005; Freedberg and Gallese 2007; Gallese

2001; Thompson 2001a&b; Steuber 2006). The ongoing discussion, in part, has been motivated by the discovery of mirror neurons and the idea that when we encounter another human our motor system resonates in what seems to be a natural empathic response. The debate focuses on the question of whether this kind of account is sufficient for understanding empathy.[2] Some theorists are proponents of a concept of empathy that is primitive and closely tied to immediate emotional reaction and motor resonance; others claim that empathy is *something more* than these natural and automatic processes. Although there is a growing consensus about the concept of a primitive empathic response, based on evidence from developmental psychology and the neuroscience of embodied resonance processes, it is still an open question how these processes relate to more sophisticated forms of empathy found in adult experience. When it comes to specify what the 'something more' is that is allegedly needed for empathic understanding, a second debate opens up between proponents of theory of mind (both TT and ST) and a more interactionist approach.

Empathy is sometimes used interchangeably with terms like sympathy and compassion; sometimes, however, empathy is distinguished from sympathy and compassion and treated as something more basic. Empathy is also often considered to be a moral feeling or behavior, i.e., something that is morally good; yet it is also possible to consider it as morally neutral. One could suggest that a good torturer needs empathy for his victims so that he or she can cause more pain. These are issues that we won't try to resolve here. Rather, the kind of question we are interested in applies to empathy whether it is the same or different from sympathy, or whether one considers it to have moral value or to be morally neutral. The question we will consider is the question mentioned above: is an account of empathy in terms of basic motor resonance sufficient for the concept, or is 'something more' required.

Gallese, for example, builds his theory of empathy on the mirror neuron system and the fact that

> when we observe goal-related behaviors ... specific sectors of our
> pre-motor cortex become active. These cortical sectors are those same

---

2   This debate was clearly prefigured by an older one that took place at the beginning of the 20th century, based on behavioral and phenomenological observations which suggested that embodied, sensory-motor and action-related processes were important ones for explaining our understanding of others. The central figure in this debate was Theodore Lipps. Lipps (1903), for example, discussed the concept of *Einfühlung*, which he equated with the Greek term *empatheia*. He attributed our capacity for empathy to a sensory-motor mirroring, an involuntary, 'kinesthetic' inner imitation of the observed vital activity expressed by another person. Husserl, and other phenomenologists, including Scheler, Heidegger, and Merleau-Ponty, developed phenomenological critiques of Lipps' account, contending that empathy is something more than these involuntary processes and that in some cases empathy happens as a solution or supplement to the breakdown or inadequacy of the more basic, automatic, perceptual understanding of others (see Zahavi 2001; 2005 for a good summary of these debates).

sectors that are active when we actually perform the same actions. In other words, when we observe actions performed by other individuals our motor system 'resonates' along with that of the observed agent. (Gallese 2001, 38).

For Gallese, our understanding of the other person's action relies on a neural mirroring mechanism that matches, or simulates, in the same neuronal substrate, the observed behavior with a behavior that I could execute. This lived bodily motor equivalence between what I observe others doing, and the capabilities of my own motor system allows me to use my own system as a model for understanding the other's action.

> Empathy is deeply grounded in the experience of our lived-body, and it is this experience that enables us to directly recognize others not as bodies endowed with a mind but as persons like us. ... I submit that the neural matching mechanism constituted by mirror neurons — or by equivalent neurons in humans — ... is crucial to establish an empathic link between different individuals. (Gallese 2001, 43–44).

Thus Gallese uses action understanding as a framework to define empathy. He appeals to implicit simulation theory to explain how this model can include expressive aspects of movement that give us access to the emotional states of others (Gallese and Goldman 1998).

Along this line, Tony Marcel called my attention to how observed action attitudes might generate a real feeling in a person who is observing them, and he suggests, as an example of this, Rubens's painting of *The Drunken Silenus* (Figure 9.1).

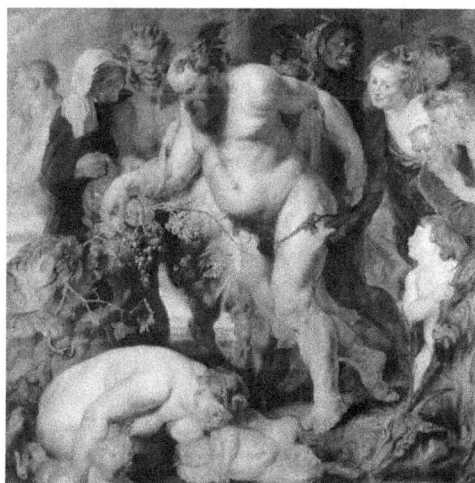

Figure 9.1 *The Drunken Silenus*
(1618: Alte Pinakothek, Munich)

Marcel: By relative angle, body posture and weight, placing of the feet relative to the specific ground and the pit, you just feel the fall that Silenus is about to have. The attitudes of all those around Silenus give the event its emotional force and poignancy. I mention all these factors because they show the 'relation with the world'. However, in this case the action attitude is one that is an expression of neither intention nor emotion. And drunkenness is not just within an individual; it is a relation with the world.

Jean Decety (2002; 2003; 2004; 2005) contends that empathy does not involve simply an emotional resonance initiated by the emotional or action state of the other. It also requires a minimal comprehension of the mental states of this person. That is, for Decety, it also requires a theory of mind (concerning which he seems to favor a more explicit ST, while others have suggested a theory theory approach). He does not deny the importance of resonance systems, especially in early infancy, and he accepts that we have an innate capacity to feel that other people are 'like us'. But we also quickly develop the capacity to put ourselves mentally in the place of others. He also emphasizes that in this process difference is just as important as similarity. Empathy is founded on our capacity to recognize that others are similar to ourselves, but to do so without confusing ourselves with the other.

Joseph LeDoux suggests something similar in regard to the feeling of trust, which seems to belong to the same family of moral feelings as empathy.

LeDoux: Trust is a social emotion. It requires the conceptualization of me, you, the prediction of what I want, of what you'll do. It's called the theory of the mind — your ability to put yourself in the mind of another and guess what they'll do. So we may be able to break trust down into separate operations. One is the individual's conception of self. Another is what he wants. A third is his ability to conceive of the existence of others. And a fourth is the ability to predict what another person will do. (Robinson 2003, Interview, p. 2).

That empathy involves primitive resonance processes in our motor system is consistent with the idea that empathy, like other moral behaviors, can be found in animals as well as humans.

Damasio: [M]oral behavior does not begin with humans. In certain circumstances numerous non-human species behave in ways that are, for all intents and purposes, comparable to the moral ways of human beings. Interestingly, the moral behaviors are emotional — compassion, shame, indignation, dominant pride or submission. As in the case of culture, the contribution of everything that is learned and created in a group plays a major role in shaping moral behaviors.

> Only humans can codify and refine rules of moral behavior. Animals can behave in moral-like ways, but only humans have ethics and write laws and design justice systems. (Harcourt 2000, interview).

Damasio here suggests that such behaviors are very basic, but also that they can become complex in humans, transformed by cultural (social, political, and legal) factors. Whether we need to bring in all of these factors to have an adequate account of empathy, Decety, LeDoux, and Damasio seem in agreement that something more is required than simply the resonance systems discussed by Gallese. Yet I think they also would agree with Gallese that these resonance systems are at the basis of empathy. The question for most theorists, however, is what the *something more* is. Is it simulation ability, or our ability to use folk psychology in a theory approach? Or is it, as Damasio suggests, something more than that; something that can link resonance systems to broader cultural contributions? In an interactionist approach, as mentioned in Chapter 7, MNs and resonance processes play an important role, interpreted as part of a direct social perception of the other's behavior, which, along with the pragmatic and social context of that behavior and our own interaction with the other, can give us a good understanding of the other's intentions, actions and emotions.

One thing that does seem important, whether you are a simulation theorist, a theory theorist, or an interaction theorist, is context. If you see someone crying, even if that activates some basic emotional mirroring on your part, one still might wonder whether empathy is called for, and that may depend on *why* the person is crying. If they are crying because they just lost the gun they were going to use to kill you, it is not clear that empathy is the best term for what your reaction may be. And that context may in fact inhibit your mirror system from generating an empathic feeling in any automatic way.

What does it take for us to grasp the intersubjective context in a way that can lead to the modulation of automatic resonance processes, and that can lead on to make connection with the larger cultural contributions that Damasio mentions? There is good evidence that sometime around the age of two years, a number of things happen that lead to a capacity for empathic understanding. Decety and Jackson (2004, 78) note:

> It is around the 2nd year that empathy may be manifested in prosocial behaviors (e.g., helping, sharing, or comforting) indicative of concern for others. Studies of children in the 2nd year of life indicate that they have the requisite cognitive, affective, and behavioral capacities to display integrated patterns of concern for others in distress ... During this period of development, children increasingly experience emotional concern 'on behalf of the victim', comprehend others' difficulties, and act constructively by providing comfort and help...

What does it take for this kind of empathy (empathic understanding) to emerge? We can point to a number of important developments in the child around this age. At 12–18 months we see the development of shared attention and secondary intersubjectivity in which children start to see things in pragmatic contexts: objects start to get their meaning from the way people interact with them. Just around the same time the ability for mirror self-recognition emerges, and this provides the child with a more objective sense of self, in contrast to an earlier, proprioceptively-based sense of self (Gallagher 2005). In addition, sometime between 15–24 months, children start to speak, or as Merleau-Ponty (1962) might put it, language starts to acquire them. Finally, between 18–24 months, children start to manifest an ability for autobiographical memory.

> By 18–24 months of age infants have a concept of themselves that is sufficiently viable to serve as a referent around which personally experienced events can be organized in memory ... the self at 18–24 months of age achieves whatever 'critical mass' is necessary to serve as an organizer and regulator of experience ... this achievement in self-awareness (recognition) is followed shortly by the onset of auto-biographical memory ... (Howe 2000, 91–2).

Along with language, autobiographical memory, and a more objective sense of self, as well as, in most cases, serious exposure to stories (an exposure that begins in early childhood and never really ends), comes the capacity for understanding narrative and generating self-narrative. But this narrative competency is multi-dimensional. First, the development of self-narrative goes hand in hand with the narrative of others. Narrative abilities are helped along when parents, for example, rehearse the child's own story for them, or elicits the story with leading questions (Howe 2000). Self-narrative requires building on our experiences of and with others and their narratives. Thus, at the beginning of this process we find that 'children of 2–4 years often "appropriate" someone else's story as their own' (Nelson 2003, 31). It may be that 2-year olds begin with scripts and with the words that others supply, rather than with full-fledged narratives. But from 2–4 years, children fine-tune their narrative competency by means of a further development of language ability, episodic memory, and the growing stability of their sense of self and others.

Narrative competency may just be the something more necessary for empathic understanding. I don't mean that empathic understanding requires an occurrent or explicit narrative story telling: but it does require the ability to frame the other person in a detailed pragmatic or social context, and to understand that context in a narrative way. My own action, and the actions of others have intelligibility and begin to make sense when I can place them in a narrative framework (see McIntyre 1981). Our understanding of others, and hence the possibility of empathizing with them, is not based on attempts to get into their heads in a mentalistic fashion (TT or ST), since we already have access to their embodied actions and the rich worldly contexts within which they act—contexts that are transformed into narratives that operate to scaffold the meaning of their actions and expressive movements.

Even if you are a simulation theorist or theory theorist, however, you need the kind of knowledge of context that comes along with narrative competency. Dan Hutto (2008), for example, has convincingly argued that narrative practice is necessary for acquiring folk psychology, which is something that the theory theorist requires. Furthermore, even to begin running a simulation routine, one requires a background knowledge of the relevant context. As Goldman describes it, 'When a mindreader tries to predict or retrodict someone else's mental state by simulation, she uses pretense or imagination to put herself in the target's "shoes" and generate the target state' (Goldman 2005a). One therefore needs to know where those shoes are and whether they are sandals, running shoes, dress shoes, high-heals, golf shoes, etc. each of which tells part of a story about the person wearing them.

An understanding of context, however, is not simply an intellectual task. It comes loaded with emotion. So much so that if you are a certain kind of professional who works with people—a physician, a homicide detective, a marriage counselor, and so on—it is often imperative that you work at detaching yourself from the emotional aspects of the case in order for you yourself to survive more or less unscathed. Abilities to detach oneself, to be apathetic in a pragmatic way, to compartmentalize certain aspects of a situation, are themselves worthy of study by the cognitive sciences. Such talents to neutralize certain emotional aspects of a situation may themselves be learned aspects of narrative competency.

Chapter 10

Language, Cognition, and Other Extras

I am not a motor chauvinist, but it is clear that our ability to move the kind of body that we have, and the ways we can do this, both constrained and enabled by the nature of that body, give us rationality. That is, reason is not a purely mental phenomenon that is given from the top down. It is not formulated in the cortex and then expressed in behavior; it is also formulated in the behavior itself, in our movements and actions, in our interactions with the environment and with others; and all of this is shaped by the emotions that are also generated in such embodied actions and interactions. If we are at certain points able to detach ourselves from our situated embodied actions, if we are able to abstract the rules of our interactions and set them down in mathematical formulae, this is a talent that emerges from the bottom up. Even abstract thinking is motivated, and to accomplish it, it requires adopting a certain emotional (or dis-emotional) attitude toward the world or toward others. So even abstract thinking is not really divorced from specific motivational and emotional aspects. Also if we think of the accomplishment of abstract thought as an 'emancipation' from our embodied engagement with the world, as that term suggests, such abstract thinking may not come easy, and may be accomplished only in a struggle to stay 'above' the dictates of feeling and action—and this struggle itself must come along with certain feelings and actions.

Language has a lot to do with this. And in all respects language starts out as movement—in a coordinated fashion we move our vocal chords, we move our tongue, we shape our mouth, we exhale our breath, and we thus speak. We not only speak, we gesture. We move our hands in coordination with our vocalizations and we thus supplement the meaning of what we are saying. Speech is for others; it is intersubjective. It's an intersubjective movement that allows us to communicate, to coordinate our actions, to learn and to teach, to organize groups, to establish institutions which are almost always organized by way of writing texts, which requires the movement of our hands with an instrument or on a keyboard. All of this movement — speaking and gesturing and writing — makes us rational. When Aristotle defined the human as the rational animal, his word for rational was a variation of *logos*, which is also the word for language. And when he declared that the human is the political animal, he was saying the same thing, because to be a political animal is to enter into the *polis* with a voice and with something reasonable to say. Short of that everything is war, and not even declared and organized war of the sort we find among nations. Without language Aristotle would be a Hobbsian.

From cortex to context: Mirror neurons and language

The connection between bodily movement and higher-order cognition has been argued for in philosophy, for example in the work of Mark Johnson (*The Body in the Mind* [1990]; also Lakoff and Johnson 1980), by appealing to metaphorical transformations of embodied postures and actions into abstract concepts. For example, Johnson suggests that our embodied sense of balance may be the basis for our concept of justice, and that, more generally, our bodily movements may shape the metaphors that we use at the more abstract levels of thought. Linguistic ability, of course, appears to be a necessary intermediary.

So how does language get its start? Mirror neurons again! Let me reiterate that I'm not convinced that MNs can explain everything. That they have some role to play in social cognition seems clear. That they have some role to play in the development of language is a topic that is very much under discussion. Part of Michael Arbib's recent enthusiasm for the study of language was rekindled by the implications of the neurophysiology of mirror neurons coming out of Rizzolatti's lab. He wants to think of the role of mirror neurons within the framework of schema theory, and here there are two issues. First, Arbib and Hesse (1986) discriminated between individual schemas (representations within the head) and social schemas (patterns of overt behavior discernible across a population). Can mirror neurons mediate between these two kinds of schemas? Second, following Arbib's paper with Rizzolatti on mirror neurons and language (Rizzolatti and Arbib 1998), can the connection be made between motor action and higher-order cognition in a way that is more direct than the appeal to metaphor that we find in Johnson and Lakoff?

> **Arbib:** With Rizzolatti I developed the Mirror System Hypothesis (MSH). This states that mirror neurons (which are activated for grasping, for example) are a missing neural link in the evolutionary development of human language. Mirror neurons were found originally in the macaque monkey and of course in contrast to humans,

monkeys do not have language. So to explore the differences and commonalities in brain mechanisms, we looked at the macaque mirror neurons for grasping and we argued for a 4-stage evolutionary progression:

1) grasping;
2) a mirror system for grasping;
3) a system of manual communications which provide an open repertoire insofar as they transcend the fixed repertoire of primate vocalizations;

4) speech, which is the result of an 'invasion' of the vocal apparatus by collaterals from the manual/oro-facial communication system

Broca's area, one of the key human speech areas in the human brain, is activated both during grasping and observation of grasping, and it's not activated in simple observation of objects. So if we think of speech as evolving out of manual communication, then it seems reasonable to postulate the evolution of Broca's area from the F5-equivalent in the common ancestry of humans and monkeys. The ability to pantomime where hand movements are recognized as standing for something else, may be an important aspect in stage (3). In stage (4) the articulation of words may be seen to parallel the grasping of objects. Others have argued for the parallelism of spoken and signed language (e.g., Stokoe 2001) but the MSH is needed to bridge from grasping in monkeys to language signs in humans. I would want to distinguish, however, speech from other vocal gestures for communication. Monkey vocalizations are related to the cingulate cortex rather than the F5 homologue of Broca's area. I think it's likely that a related system persists in humans, but as a complement to, rather than an integral part of, the speech system that includes Broca's area.

SG: This view is consistent with motor theories of language.

Arbib: Yes, at least in part MSH supports a motor theory of speech perception, the theory that perceived speech is mentally represented in terms of motor articulatory categories. We claim that a *specific* mirror system, the mirror system for grasping, is the common heritage of human and monkey. In humans it evolved to provide some basic components for the emergence of language.

SG: Back to my earlier question; can we trace a line from this kind of motor activation seen in mirror neurons from motor schemas up through language to concept formation?

Arbib: First I should note that there is no unique way of looking at mirror neurons in relation to language. Vittorio Gallese, one of the co-discoverers of mirror neurons, has written an account (Gallese & Lakoff 2005) which differs in a number of interesting ways from my own (Arbib 2008). In any case, I have tried (Arbib 2002; 2005) to trace the move from manual pragmatic actions to the pantomime of such actions, and then to the pantomime of actions that are outside of the subject's own behavioral repertoire. A good example would be flapping one's arms to mime a flying bird. From there one can imagine that conventional gestures developed in order to formalize and disambiguate pantomime (distinguishing 'bird' from 'flying', for example). These lead to more developed gestures (protosigns) and to vocal gesture (protospeech). I think that the transition to pantomime of actions outside the subject's own behavioral repertoire is essential for extending the range of communication to objects. One might begin to represent an object by representing its use. The largest step, however, comes when a community masters a set of conventional gestures, which allow them to formalize and disambiguate pantomime. Once that happens, then the community is free to invent arbitrary gestures to communicate concepts for which pantomime is inadequate.

But here I want to be careful. The concept of grasping involves a common representation of what I see when I see someone else grasp, and what I do when I grasp. One is tempted to propose mirror neuron activity in forming this sensory-motor link. However, I don't think this can hold for all concepts, or as an explanation for all concepts. This brings us back to schema theory. I distinguish between perceptual schemas and motor schemas. But I don't want to postulate on a general level any tight or necessary link between the two. A perceptual schema contributes to our understanding of what is in the environment, and can provide parameters concerning the current relationship between the organism and whatever is there. Motor schemas provide control systems required to control a wide variety of actions. Tim Shallice, for example, stresses a tight link between the perceptual and motor right here.[1] But I don't want to combine perceptual and motor schemas into a single notion of schema that integrates sensory analysis with motor control.

---

1   For Shallice (1988, 308n) the schema 'not only has the function of being an efficient description of a state of affairs [...] but also is held to produce an output that provides the immediate control of the mechanisms required in one cognitive or action operation.' For cognitive psychology, schemas are cognitive structures built up in the course of interaction with the environment to organize experience. The issue is when this is to be accomplished by a single over-learned schema, and when it is necessary to dynamically assemble a coordinated control program appropriate to the current situation.

SG: You don't want to say that a particular perceptual schema necessarily entails a particular motor schema?

Arbib: In some cases this combination might make sense, but it is also true that recognition of an object may be linked to many different courses of action. If I see an apple, I can put it in my shopping basket; place it in a bowl; peel it; cook it; eat it; discard it, throw it, and so forth. Of course, once I decide what to do with it, then specific perceptual and motor sub-schemas must be activated. Some of these actions, however, are apple-specific; others invoke generic schemas for reaching and grasping. This is important and it motivated me to separate perceptual and motor schemas. A given action may be invoked in a wide variety of circumstances; a given perception may precede many different courses of action. Schemas are very specific, and there is no one grand 'apple schema' that determines all of our apple actions.

SG: So there is no possibility of reducing the variety and particularity of schemas to a neat set of mirror neurons. And our concept of apple, for example, is much richer than can be specified by that neat set.

Arbib: And this is exactly why I reject the notion of a mirror system for concepts. Instead, I think the brain encodes a rich variety of networks of perceptual and motor schemas. It is possible that in the case of some basic actions, perceptual and motor schemas may be integrated into what we might call a 'mirror schema', but this is rare. Almost everything is context dependent, and that's precisely what makes our concepts so complex. One word or one concept may be linked to many schemas, with varying *context-dependent* activation strengths, in a complex schema network.

SG: The idea of context-dependence would point to the importance of learning, and thus to a certain level of plasticity at the neural level.

Arbib: Indeed. The Parma group has shown that some mirror neurons are activated not only by visual input but also by relevant sounds—for example, the sound of paper tearing, which goes along with the action of tearing (Kohler et al. 2002). This certainly suggests that perceptual-motor integration in mirror neurons is highly plastic. And I would suggest that it offers possible mechanisms that would facilitate the transition from manual to vocal signing. This plasticity goes from the ground up—I mean from movement all the way through conceptual formation. Studies on the mirror system for grasping in the monkey focus on such a basic repertoire of grasps that it is tempting to view them as pre-wired. But developmental studies of human infants show that it takes several months before a human infant gains the capacity for these basic grasps (e.g., the precision pinch). Erhan Oztop and Nina Bradley and I (Oztop et al. 2004) argue that, in monkey as well as in human, gaining the basic grasp repertoire depends on sensorimotor feedback.

This follows a paper I did with Oztop (Oztop and Arbib 2002; a more sophisticated model is given in Bonaiuto et al. 2007), which explains how mirror neurons organize themselves for grasp recognition as these grasps are added to the motor repertoire. It seems possible too that infants may learn through observation, so that mirror neurons develop synergistically with grasping circuitry. That the human brain can make the connections that it does, distinguishes its neural structure from that of a chimpanzee or monkey brain, although, as we know, all learning tasks are not equally amenable. Learning to speak or to sign is easier for the child than learning to read and write. This suggests that the ability to build neural connections is crucial, but also that it is not a general property shared by all areas of the human brain. Instead our human abilities involve different patterns of plasticity linked to specific brain mechanisms that have been evolved along the hominid line.

One question raised by this account is how gestures fit into the story. Does verbal language evolve out of a gestural protolanguage, as Arbib is suggesting? Is gesture 'the steppingstone for early hominid communication and, possibly, language', as Amy Pollick and Frans de Waal suggest (Tierney 2007)? Or do gestures come along with verbal language as an intrinsic part of it. David McNeill at the University of Chicago defends this latter position. According to McNeill (1992) and his research group, speech-synchronized gestures offer a new window onto language, the mental processes that are engaged by it, and insight into what protolanguage would have offered (McNeill et al. 2005; 2008; also see Tierney 2007 for a popular discussion of this point). I asked McNeill to explain.

> **McNeill:** Gestures are integral components of language, rather than something independent of it. They are synchronous and semantically and pragmatically co-expressive with speech. They are ubiquitous — they accompany about 90% of spoken utterances in descriptive discourse (Nobe 2000) — and they occur in similar form across many languages. In terms of how they relate to cognition, it's possible that thinking involves the integration of two cognitive modes at once, gestural imagery and verbal form. The integration is a temporal one, since gestures present material simultaneously while speech explicates it successively. The complex synchronous integration of gesture with speech creates a co-expressive synthesis rather than two streams of meaning.

SG: Still gestures are different from speech.

McNeill: Yes, but two points are important for the argument. First, gestures are different from speech in important ways — in their temporality as we have just mentioned, as well as in their mereological organization, that is, in terms of how their parts fit together into wholes. Speech divides the expressed event into components — first this, and then that — and this segregation of parts requires that to some extent semantic division follows syntactic division in a way that issues a composite meaning of the whole. In gesture the composite meaning is fused into unitary and simultaneous semantic wholes so there are no combinatory rules within the gesture: meaning determination moves from whole to parts, not from parts to whole. Speech and gesture are co-expressive but not redundant; they are dialectically opposed in a way that creates the conditions for what I call 'an imagery-language dialectic'. The dialectic is between speech, which can be and is conventionalized and socially constructed and carried from one place to another, and gesture, which is closely tied to the particular context at stake. The dialectic implies an opposition that gets resolved through further development. In this case the resolution comes in the form of an enriched meaning. The integrated working of the two dissimilar linguistic modes sets up an unstable relation between them that turns out to be essential for the creation of this enriched meaning. And this instability had selective advantage in evolution because it fuels thought and speech and makes communication richer and more efficient, especially in passing on knowledge in an instructional mode.

SG: So in evolutionary terms it's not gesture first, and then speech.

McNeill: That's right. What follows is that at the origin, it was not that one opposite evolved out of the other; it was not that there was fully functional gesture from which could emerge speech as on a linear development. Rather there was some kind of breakthrough to a way of combining predictable and unpredictable symbols that were integrated wholes of gesture and speech.

These predictable symbols 'could interface with individually constituted, contextually situated and essentially ephemeral imagery' (McNeill et al. 2008). This version of the story still gives a role to mirror neurons. McNeill cites George Herbert Mead: 'Gestures become significant symbols when they implicitly arouse in an individual making them the same response which they explicitly arouse in other individuals' (Mead 1974). This kind of loop may have exploited the mirror neuron circuit, generating a capacity, not found in other primate brains, for mirror neurons to respond to one's *own gestures* as if they belonged to someone else. The idea is not that we became self-conscious of our own gestures, but that mirror neuron activation added an intersubjective control that facilitated communication with others.

Moveo ergo cogito

It's not that we have to make a jump from language to higher-order cognition; the two come in one package. By 'higher-order' I mean those things we usually think about when we think about our thinking. Often they are reflective processes that go beyond perception, but also in some way depend upon perceptual processes, both phenomenologically and neurologically. We have mentioned before that both memory and imagination activate perceptual areas in the brain. Phenomenologically, this is a point often made by Husserl and his followers — that memory and imagination are (re)presentations of perceptual content; and indeed, this idea goes back to the empiricists. But there is also evidence to suggest that such cognitive processes also activate linguistic areas. It's as if movements, perceptions, thoughts, and language are all highly interconnected in the brain, as well phenomenologically embodied. Thinking is never Platonic, or never merely Platonic.

Albert Einstein's brain keeps company with a collection of brains at McMaster University in Ontario, Canada. It has an interesting history, both pre- and post-mortem, which I shall ignore here (but see http://www.pacpubserver.com/new/ news/8-4-00/einstein.html for the post-mortem history). Sandra Witelson is the neuroscientist at McMaster who did a thorough anatomical analysis of Einstein's brain. The results showed that his brain was normal in all respects but one. His parietal lobes were 15% larger than normal.

> [...] in Einstein's brain, extensive development of the posterior parietal lobes occurred early, in both longitudinal and breadth dimensions, thereby constraining the posterior expansion of the Sylvian fissure and the development of the parietal operculum, but resulting in a larger expanse of the inferior parietal lobe. ... In particular, the results predict that anatomical features of parietal cortex may be related to visuospatial intelligence (Witelson, Kigar and Harvey 1999, 2151–2).

Einstein's lateral sulcus or Sylvian fissure where it divides parietal areas from temporal areas was more or less bridged by the expanded parietal area. Phenomenological translation: Einstein had a tremendously good ability for visual imagination and spatial reasoning. The oversimplified, but nonetheless true lesson: higher-order reasoning and mathematics are not divorced from visuospatial intelligence.

This idea is reinforced by George Lakoff and Rafael Núñez (2000) who show how mathematics is grounded in concepts derived from metaphors generated in embodied experiences. As they put it:

> Human ideas are, to a large extent, grounded in sensory-motor experience. Abstract human ideas make use of precisely formulatable cognitive mechanisms such as conceptual metaphors that import modes of reasoning from sensory-motor experience. (p. xii).

Perhaps that is why, as Susan Goldin-Meadow (1999) has shown, children can solve math problems better if they are allowed to gesture while thinking; and why, as my daughter (the acting major rather than the psychology major) tells me, actors depend on stage blocking and moving around on stage for learning and delivering lines; and why, as my other daughter (the psychology major rather than the acting major) informs me, the direction you move your arm can influence your ability to make sense out of a string of words (and she even provides a reference: Glenberg and Kaschak 2002). Perhaps, in Arbib's terms, you can think of mathematical thinking as involving higher-order cognitive schemata that are ultimately traceable to the five fingers on your hand. But let's take a step back to see if schemas can do the job of moving us from simple movements, involved, for example, in drinking, up the line to thinking.

Jeannerod: What I initially liked in Arbib's schema theory (e.g., Arbib 1985) is that there was a representation or schema for every level, from the single finger movement level up to the action level which embedded lower level schemas, and so on and so forth. At the top you had the schema for the whole action, for example, getting something to drink. So, in order to drink you activated schemas to get to the kitchen; then you activated schemas to grasp the glass, to raise it to the mouth, and so on and so forth: for each sub-action you had other sub-sub-actions. That was the organizing idea of going from the higher level down to the lower one, a hierarchical organization.

What we want to have in a representation [for action] is not only the vocabulary to be assembled for producing the action (this is the static conception of the schema theory). Instead, we need the functional rules for assemblage, including the biomechanical constraints, the spatial reference frame, the initial positions, the forces to apply, etc. All these aspects form the covert part of the representation: they are present in the representation as can be demonstrated in experiments with implicit motor images of the sort that were mentioned earlier (e.g., Frak et al. 2008; Parsons et al. 1994), but they cannot be accessed consciously. The conscious part of the representation does-n't really have to include all the technicalities of the action, it just specifies the goal. But, interestingly, even if you are simply imagin-ing the action in terms of its goal, in simulating it you also rehearse all the neuronal circuitry. As we said before, if you examine the brain activity during motor imagination, you will find activation of the motor cortex, the cerebellum, etc. Even though the subject is imagin-ing a complex goal, you will observe activation in the executive areas of his brain, corresponding to motor functions which he cannot fig-ure out in his conscious experience of the image.

So even if our thought is relatively simple, such as thinking about get-ting a glass of water, there are complex activations in the brain that involve the motor system. But let's face it, most of our everyday thinking is just about such everyday practical things like getting a glass of water. Indeed, on a phenomenological analysis provided by Martin Heidegger (1966), what we call higher-order thought, or conceptual thinking is really deriva-tive from our everyday involvement with practical tasks. We encounter the world primarily on a pragmatic level of moving around and doing things. Typically it is only when something goes wrong that we start to think in what we might call an intellectual way. More about Heidegger later.[2]

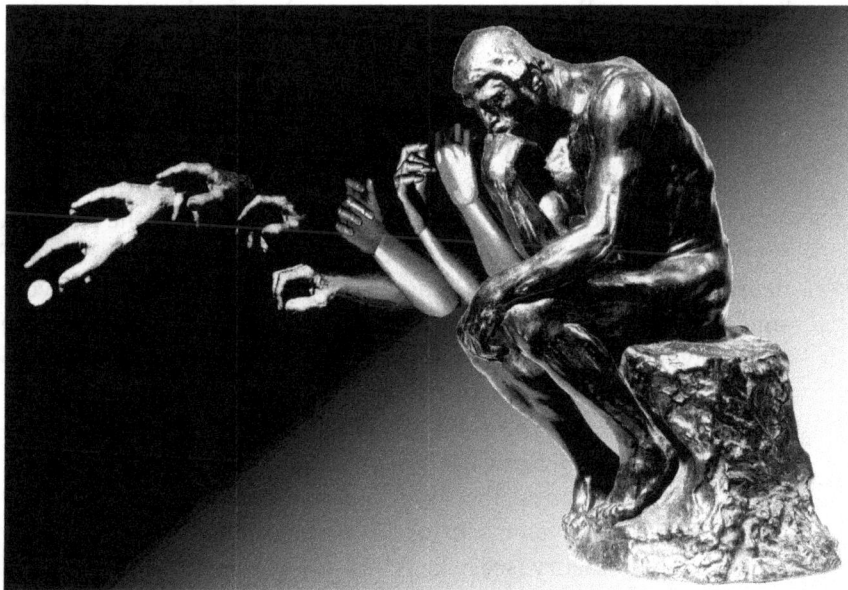

Mouvement, action et conscience: vers une physiologie de l'intention.
Colloque en l'honneur de Marc Jeannerod

---

[2] See Dreyfus (2007) and Wheeler (2005) for the most recent views of Heidegger's analysis in relation to cognitive science.

Not long after my interview with Jeannerod was published in the *Journal of Consciousness Studies*, I was back in Lyon again to attend a conference and gala event in honor of Marc Jeannerod and his accomplishments in cognitive neuroscience (see http://www.isc.cnrs.fr/colloque27-28-9.htm). People were there from all over the neuroscientific, psychological, and philosophical worlds. Michael Arbib came from the University of Southern California, for example, and having read the Jeannerod interview he was motivated to respond to the critique that Marc had raised against his schema theory — that is, that it wasn't dynamic enough. This led to the following exchange, which digs deeper into the concept of schema.

SG: In 1986 you and Mary Hesse published *The Construction of Reality*, based on your 1983 Gifford Lectures in Natural Theology. There you explored the notion of schemas and corresponding brain mechanisms. Tell me what you mean by schema. Can you say how schema theory has advanced from earlier notions of schema that one finds in Head's neurological conception of motor or body schema, and Bartlett's psychological conceptions?

Arbib: My own work on schema theory really is a confluence of neural network modeling and mathematical systems theory. On the one hand it goes back to work of Kilmer, McCulloch and Blum (1969) who modeled the reticular formation at a level above the neural level, looking both at modules and at modes of behavior, showing how networks of neurons could collaborate to commit the organism to different modes. This was one of my inspirations for developing the theory of schemas. Another came from modeling the recognition of prey and predators by the frog's brain — seeing how a perceptual schema could drive the appropriate motor schema. The actual word 'schema' came because I was describing these ideas on the frog to a friend, Richard Reiss, who had been influential in the early days of neural network modeling. He pointed out that my notion was very similar to the use of the word 'schema' by Piaget, and convinced me not to invent a new word but to use Piaget's. That of course immediately raised the challenge of trying to understand to what extent I agreed and disagreed with Piaget. But schema theory has a mathematical side as well. Ernie Manes and I expended a lot of energy to unify the mathematical theory of automata and the mathematical theory of control systems using an abstract algebraic framework called category theory (see, e.g., Arbib and Manes 1974). Within that framework, Manes and I and our student Martha Steenstrup sought to formalize a concurrent model of computation and came up with the idea of port automata (Steenstrup, Arbib and Manes 1983). An Irish student Damian Lyons then looked at my writings on schema theory from the perception and action side and my writings on port automata and combined them to advance the schema theory framework (Arbib, Iberall and Lyons 1985; 1987).

As you say, the concept of schema goes back in neurology, for example, to Henry Head. Head and his colleagues were trying to make sense of people with parietal lesions who had 'lost' awareness of half their body. In getting dressed, for example, they would put clothes on one side of the body and leave them off the other. They didn't consider it part of their body and in this respect something was wrong with their 'body schema'. With a parietal lobe lesion on one side of the brain, the representation of the other side of the body may be lost. The 'phantom limb' is something of the 'opposite' phenomenon. The limb is not actually there and yet the patient feels it present where it would normally be, and can feel the pain in it. The intriguing point is that 'something special' in the brain—the body schema—is needed for each of us to have even this most basic sense of our self, namely what limbs are currently part of our own body.

I consider the notion of the body schema in this sense as the first chapter of schema theory within the modern tradition of cognitive science. Then Frederic Bartlett, who was a student of Head's, published his book *Remembering* in 1932. He developed a constructive view of memory. There is a well-known party game where people sit around a table and one person writes down a short narrative and whispers it in the ear of her neighbor who whispers it to the next person, and so on. The last person writes it down as he hears it. Then he reads out both the original story and the final version—and everybody bursts into laughter because the stories are so different. The point is that remembering is not a passive process but a constructive one. Slightly different cognitive schemas inform each person's construction of the story. This notion of cognitive schema would, I think, be the next chapter in schema theory.

The next idea comes from a sequence of studies related to cybernetics, starting perhaps with Kenneth Craik's 1943 book on *The Nature of Explanation*, that suggest that the job of the brain is to model the world, so that when you act it is because you have been able to simulate the effects of your action before you do it. This idea was furthered in the 1960s by people like Donald MacKay, Richard Gregory, Marvin Minsky and others, who wrote about the model of the world in the mind or in the brain. The idea moved into artificial intelligence in the 1970s and the idea of schema became expressed in computer programs: Minsky used the word 'frames'; Schank used the word 'scripts'; others talked about 'semantic nets', and so forth.

SG: This concept is already getting complex. You have mentioned a body schema, a cognitive schema, and then more formal models that can be useful for artificial intelligence. You also mentioned Piaget (see e.g., 1976) but didn't he use the concept of schema in a slightly different way?

Arbib: Piaget belongs to another stream in schema theory, one that began with Kant rather than in neurology. Piaget offered a constructivist view of mental development that starts with sensorimotor skills. He suggested that the child at any time is building up a set of reproducible skills, or schemas, and that these make up what the child can do. These schemas change as the child moves through certain stages of development. The child, in a new situation, will try to make sense of it in terms of the schemas she already has. She tries to assimilate the situation to what she knows. From time to time she will find herself in a situation where these schemas are inadequate. She may then be forced to change the schemas, and Piaget calls this 'accommodation'; the schemas accommodate to the data they cannot assimilate.

I'm sympathetic with all of these ideas. When I talk about schema theory, however, I'm talking about my own brand, but building on all these contributions. For example, Piaget seems to talk as if the developmental stages are predetermined steps in maturation; in contrast, I understand the interaction of the schemas as being the determining aspect. From this interaction the schemas will develop a 'common style' and then we might be able to talk of a new stage. Accommodation continues and eventually a new style emerges, and this is another stage. Also, I think Piaget is more descriptive than explanatory; I try to develop a theory or computational model of how schemas change.

SG: I take it that on your conception when we think of a schema we should think of it as primarily something which functions in the brain. Doesn't schema theory become even more complex if one is attempting to provide an account of brain mechanisms for ongoing behavior?

Arbib: Even before we involve the brain, the very concept of schema has to change once we start worrying about the details of behavior. For Piaget a schema tends to be an overall skill manifested in a specific situation, whereas my theory requires a complex variety of schemas even in a single situation. For example, in a particular situation, a person has to recognize many things—the people sitting around the room, the furniture in the room, the location of a particular object the person is looking for—and this means that one has different schemas for recognizing the object, the furniture, and the people. Furthermore, such schemas may have to be combined in order to represent a totally novel situation. One thus calls upon the appropriate knowledge for making sense of that situation. I call this a schema assemblage. At any particular time there is a network of interacting schemas pulled together to represent the situation. And once we bring in motor schemas to integrate perception and action, we get what I call a coordinated control program. It's possible to provide a microanalysis of how schemas are integrated into abilities for recognizing objects and acting on them. This kind of integration gives you a wide ability to cope with novel situations in their complexity.

SG: And, just to be sure I understand this, your analysis is not just on a behavioral level, but also on a brain level? And you can think of this cognitively or as happening in the brain, for example, in terms of perception and motor control.

Arbib: In most of my work I am looking for brain mechanisms. I don't stop at saying, 'Here's a good description of a schema.' More importantly, I want to say, 'How could it occur in the brain?' There have to be mechanisms whereby perceptual schemas can be activated, pattern recognition routines, etc., whether 'bottom up' through analysis of sensory data or 'top down' on the basis of expectations generated by the currently active schema assemblage. One also has to specify how perceptual schemas can compete and cooperate with each other, and how they relate to output routines, motor schemas.

SG: You talk about a *neural schema theory*, and I have a quote here: you 'seek to understand how schemas and their interactions may indeed be played out over neural circuitry — a basic move from psychology and cognitive science as classically conceived (viewing the mind "from the outside") to cognitive neuroscience' (Arbib 1999). As you know Marc Jeannerod recently suggested that the notion of schema in this context is not adequate for explaining the brain mechanisms that must be involved for movement. I wonder if you want to respond to his criticism since he cites your work. For him the concept of schema describes the lowest and most elementary levels of motor representations.

Arbib: I would not restrict schemas to the lowest levels. The schema concept is hierarchical, bridging from the highest cognitive levels to networks of schemas localized in specific neural networks. Schema theory has long made contact with 'higher cognitive functions', including language (Arbib and Caplan 1979; Arbib and Hesse 1986 and Arbib, Conklin and Hill 1987). Elementary motor schemas are stored for 'automated actions', but they should be distinguished from *dynamic coordinated control programs* which can recursively define new schemas as a network of previously defined schemas which includes the ability to activate and deactivate these subschemas as the situation demands.

The point is that something like higher-order or intentional 'deliberation' may require explicit construction of a symbolic model (but that's still schemas!) to guide construction of the *executed* coordinated control program — which may then need to be restructured in the face of unexpected contingencies — and so we put stress on *dynamic planning*. The idea is that in general we *assemble* a stock of available schemas to handle a situation (cf. assimilation) though over time certain combinations may become stabilized and then tuned in a fashion that overrides their original schematic structure. Schemas contribute to the generation of an assemblage of schema instances and these in turn generate new tunable schemas. Marc and I agree that the new data from brain imaging require us to analyze psychological functions (vision, action, memory, planning, language and so on) in terms of the contributions made by specific brain regions and their interaction. However, Marc's description of a 'network of activation' that can be captured by brain imaging techniques is a restatement of schema theory as I see it, not a replacement for it.

Marc's description also seems to over-value the most activated regions seen for a task relative to others in an imaging study, ignoring the role of many less active regions in the current task. Synthetic PET was developed in part as a corrective to this (Arbib et al. 1994; 2000), using the detailed modeling of neural networks constrained by neurophysiological data on animals to make specific predictions about activity in homologous regions of the human brain. Let me add that it is rarely the case that a single neural network is assembled for a single task. Rather, it is a pattern of activation of networks that is controlled to mobilize the necessary resources. Schema theory clearly distinguishes the functional patterns (schemas) from the networks mobilized to implement them.

SG: So is it right to say that schemas are the functions of networks, that schemas are what networks do? That is, the concept of a schema is not simply an interpretation of or a way of speaking of the neural networks that brain imaging can capture. Could we say that the network is imaged only in its activation, and its activation is the temporary or the habitual schema of the network?

Arbib: Schema theory provides the vocabulary for the dialect between functions and the shifting alliances of structures which implement them. And brain imaging can capture such structures only in part. Just listing the most active areas does not provide a conceptual explanation. Schema theory can look for a causally complete explanation, augmenting known functions of the most active regions with schemas that 'fill in the gaps'. Moreover, an imaged brain region may be quite large, and we can use the language of schemas to suggest a variety of functions, then seek neurophysiological data to explore whether the schemas involve distinct brain regions or competitive cooperation across shared brain regions — at the next scale down. 'Whereof one cannot speak thereof one must be silent'. Schema theory lets one make scientific progress in analyzing a task in advance of — and thus preparing hypotheses for — experimental data. Schemas can express commonalities across varied tasks to which they contribute.

SG: Jeannerod suggests, however, that schemas are too static. This criticism has been reiterated in a recent article by Maxine Sheets-Johnstone (2003). She complains specifically that the notion of a body schema is not dynamic enough to capture real movement.

Arbib: Well, Head and Holmes (1911) said something about the body schema enabling a lady to feel the tip of the feather on her hat, which implies a certain dynamism. But I'm not trying to defend a century old view of schemas. Science is not static. For example, one of my most famous contributions to schema theory was inspired by experimental data of Jeannerod and Biguer (1982) which I had heard Marc present in 1979; my model (Arbib 1981) came out before the data were published! However, ten years later, data from Marc's group (Paulignan et al. 1990a,b) showed that the model was too simplistic to model the effect of perturbations. In response, Bruce Hoff and I (Arbib and Hoff 1994; Hoff and Arbib 1993) showed how to replace the schemas for arm and hand movement by control systems, and define a coordinating schema such that the revised assemblage matched the dynamical data from the Jeannerod lab. The dynamic nature of movement is represented in schema theory both by the 'bottom level' — basic schemas which may be dynamic systems, symbolic systems, or hybrids — and by the way in which these schemas are put together in coordinated control programs which show how copies of schemas may be activated or deactivated or interact with each other through processes of competition and cooperation. And of course — the neural networks of the brain are there functioning all the time, it is only their pattern of relative activation that is (partially) seen in neuroimaging. Much further research is still needed on the issue of learning how to deploy existing schemas. There may be a need to revive it and integrate it with progress in dynamic planning.

Philosophizing with a hammer

Let's return to Heidegger for a moment. His idea is that we are *in-the- world* in a pragmatic way before we start to think about the world in a conceptual way. His example is something like this. When an experienced carpenter is using a hammer to nail down a board, his relation to the hammer is not one in which he thinks about the hammer, or even one in which the hammer becomes a perceptual object. The hammer, Heidegger says, is 'ready-to-hand' in a way that is purely pragmatic. When I say that I have the know-how for hammering, it means that my hand knows what to do with the hammer. I don't have an explicit set of rules that I follow in order to hammer the nail; I simply pick the hammer up and start hammering. The hammer only becomes an object for consideration if something goes wrong (the hammer breaks) or something is not right (the hammer is too heavy). Then the hammer comes to center stage and I have to think about it.

When I start to think about the hammer, what is that like? The meaning of the hammer is tied to the particular context that defines my involvement with this or that project. We can think of this involvement context as a schema that plays an important role in the background when we think about the hammer. One could say that the relevant schema plays the same role in the act of thinking as the hammer did in the act of hammering. More generally, the relevant schema is ready-to-hand for the task of thinking about something. We might even push schemas further into the structural background if we translated this Heideggerian way of thinking about higher-order thought into terms that Merleau-Ponty would use. We could say that cognitive schemas work in thinking in the same way that body or motor schemas work when we pick up a hammer and start hammering. My hammering depends on that body-schematic system doing what it does to successfully use the hammer, and it does what it does in such a way that the hammer, while I am hammering, is something like an extension of my body schema, as Head, Merleau-Ponty, and many others have suggested.

Keeping this phenomenological view in mind, there are two ways that we can move from Arbib and Jeannerod's considerations of motor schemas to a discussion of higher-order cognition. The first is simply to pursue a continuation of schema theory and the development of the notion of cognitive schemas, as Arbib suggests. The second is to employ the Johnson-Lakoff concept of image-schemas (see below). Both of these paths will give us a way to talk about concept formation and conceptual content or meaning in higher-order thought. But another piece of this puzzle involves the logic, the rules and strategies that we use to manipulate these concepts on a conscious level—that is, when we think or try to solve problems conceptually. So one might say that there are thought contents (or meaning) and thought operations.

To conceive of thinking as involving thought contents and thought operations, however, is to conceive of it abstractly. If, for example, I am thinking through a problem in a way that is fully 'in my head', how I go about thinking of the problem, my cognitive strategy, is never divorced from the content that makes up that problem. In the same way that I use a hammer to drive a nail, I may be using the argument form *modus ponens* to formulate a conclusion, and although I may be doing this consciously (I'm consciously thinking of this particular problem that needs solving), I am not necessarily explicitly conscious of my use of *modus ponens*. I may be using *modus ponens* pre-reflectively, and I may (or may not) be able to report, if asked, how I went about thinking of the problem. But to produce a report I would likely have to introduce a metacognitive reflection, and that would be like looking at the hammer (taking the hammer as an object) rather than keeping my eye on the nail and using the hammer. The best way to describe thinking is not in terms of an abstract manipulation of rules or beliefs — the classical logic of propositional attitudes. It is rather a matter of doing things with the concepts and the rules, but in the same way that we do things with our hands when we hammer, or perhaps better, when we gesture.

Using a cognitive schema does not involve setting the vocabulary of the schema out in front of the user, or explicitly making adjustments to the schema. According to schema theory, one concept depends on a network of other concepts. When I think of a birthday party, concepts like gifts, cake, candles, the song, friends, family, and the various practices that go along with such events, support my thinking. Together they make up the birthday party schema. But unless I am metacognitively reflecting on what I do when I think of a birthday party, in my normal everyday thinking about a particular birthday party that I'm planning to attend, the schema vocabulary tends to stay in the background until needed. If I'm in charge of bringing the cake, then my thoughts may focus on what kind of cake, should I purchase it or bake it, do I have enough money to purchase it (the birthday party blends into an economic schema), how will I carry it, will it shift around in the car (the economic schema blends into a transportation schema), etc. etc. Much of our thinking and problem solving is pragmatic in this fashion. And it involves a process of constant semantic blending (see e.g., Brandt 2004; Fauconnier and Turner 2002), a point to which we shall shortly return.

The origin of these schemas are to be found in practices that are, first, bodily practices, movements, situated actions, intersubjective interactions, all of which become transformed by cultural practices and institutions. We can think of these processes as eventuating in what Johnson and

Lakoff call *image schemas*. An image schema is a repeatable cognitive structure or pattern that we employ in reasoning. According to Johnson (1987),
they originate in our bodily interactions, and take on metaphoric structure
through our linguistic practices; they 'emerge primarily as meaningful
structures for us chiefly at the level of our bodily movements through
space, our manipulation of objects, and our perceptual interactions' (Johnson 1987, 29). In cognitive linguistics image schemas are treated as
prelinguistic structures of embodied experiences that generate metaphor,
mapping basic body-environment structure into the conceptual realm.
Johnson's common example is the containment image schema, which naturally blends with other image schemas, like the OUT image schema. The
body itself is like a container; there is an inside to it. Bodily, I am often
located in, contained in, a space (a room or forest); or I am entering a space,
or leaving a space, etc. These basic bodily processes and movements are
reflected in a variety of statements (or thoughts) that are more and more
metaphorical by degree as they become more and more abstract.

> I am in the room.
> I am in the mood.
> He is in a deep depression.
> She is deeply in love.
> Mary walked out of the room.
> The team was sent out yesterday.
> We started out yesterday for Oregon.
> Don't leave any relevant details out of your argument.
> He eventually came out of his depression.
> I am out of the loop.

Here is Johnson's example of a typical morning routine where literal and
metaphorical meanings of containment are mixed like your breakfast por-
ridge: We wake up *out* of a deep sleep, drag ourselves *up out of* bed and *into*
the bathroom, where we look *into* the mirror and pull a comb *out from
inside* the cabinet. Later that same morning we wander *into* the kitchen, sit
in a chair and *open up* the newspaper and become lost *in* an article (1987,
30–32; see Rohrer 2005). The 'ins and outs' of image-schemas become metaphorical and abstract as they continue to shape our thinking. Abstract
reasoning is itself shaped by these kinds of spatial patterns that derive
from embodied practices. Johnson suggests, for example, that transitivity
and the law of the excluded middle in logic are based on the container
image-schema.

   If image-schemas really, and not just metaphorically, emerge from
sensory-motor schemas then there should be some evidence for this in the
part of the brain-body-environment that neuroscience is concerned with.
Tim Rohrer (2005) has reviewed evidence that suggests that the neural
basis of image-schemas are 'dynamic activation patterns that are shared

across the neural maps of the sensorimotor cortex'; that sensorimotor cortex is activated for the 'semantic comprehension of bodily action terms and sentences'; and that 'literal and metaphoric language stimuli activate areas of sensorimotor cortex consonant with the image schemata hypothesis' (ms. p 1). For example, fMRI studies of responses to action words involving different body parts (e.g., 'smile', 'punch' and 'kick') showed correspondingly differential responses in the somatomotor cortices (Hauk et al. 2004). Furthermore, when subjects were presented metaphorical sentences (e.g., 'he handed me the project', 'the ideas slipped through my fingers', 'I found the concept hard to grasp', and so on), activated areas of the sensory-motor cortexes overlapped with areas known to activate for hand activity, such as grasping, 'concentrated particularly in the hand premotor cortex and in hand sensorimotor regions along both sides of the central sulcus, as well as in a small region of the superior parietal cortex' (Rohrer 2001; 2005). The overlaps were more significant for literal than metaphoric sentences.

The evidence thus suggests, for example, that as you read the sentence — *'I'm going to hand you an idea that at first may seem hard to grasp, but if you turn it over and over again in your head until you finally get a firm handle on it, it will feel completely right to you'* — the areas that map hand and wrist in your primary motor and somatosensory cortices as well as premotor and secondary somatosensory areas are being activated (Rohrer 2005, 165). Accordingly, 'brain areas formerly thought to be purely sensorimotoric are turning out to have important roles in the so-called "higher" cognitive processes, e.g., language' (Ibid).

This suggests a direct connection between image schemas and the kinds of schemas that Arbib is talking about. It also suggests that language (both gestural and verbal) belongs to the same cortical fabric as action and cognition. Theories about schemas and image-schemas seem consistent with what McNeill and his colleagues have called the 'thought-language-hand' system (Cole et al. 1998; Cole et al. 2002; McNeill et al. 2005).. We can further suggest that what McNeill characterizes as the dialectical opposition between gestural and verbal language — that is, the idea that language functions by pulling together this opposition of simultaneity-succession, synthetic whole — compositional parts, functionally contextualized — functionally conventionalized elements into an unstable and spontaneously creative synthesis — is mirrored at the level of thought. What Arbib calls 'schema assemblage' is designed to pull together in a moment (as fast as our neurons can do it) a hierarchically organized schema that addresses the task at hand. In the realm of conceptual thought this kind of semantic engineering is referred to as 'semantic blending'. As Fauconnier and Turner (in press) point out, there is always built into a conceptual blend a mix of conventionality and novelty that derives from context.

Integration [blended] networks underlying thought and action are always a mix. On the one hand, cultures build networks over long periods of time that get transmitted over generations. Techniques for building particular networks are also transmitted. People are capable of innovating in any particular context. The result is integration networks consisting of conventional parts, conventionally-structured parts, and novel mappings and compressions (in press, ms, p. 2).

But this kind of assemblage or blending process needs to be kept dynamic. Schema assemblage/conceptual blending must always run along with a process that involves transitions to a new cause for assemblage, as we move from one task-step to the next, from one task to the next, from one context to the next, from one concept to the next. It's this running tension between the simultaneity of the schema, or the partially conventionalized syntax of blending, and the demands of the embodied context of action (where action may just be moving to the next logical task, or the next moment of narrative) that forms the unstable creativity of thought.

Chapter 11

Self and Self-consciousness

Throughout our discussions we have been suggesting that there is someone who is conscious, someone who moves, acts, interacts, gestures,
thinks, and so forth. *Who?* Recently cognitive scientists have answered this
question by invoking some version of 'the self', which is more appropriately an answer to the *What* question—'What is it that acts, interacts, gestures, thinks, and so forth?' The question then quickly transforms into the
How question: *how* does the brain generate a self, or a sense of self?
Depending on how neuroscientists answer that question, they may conclude that the self is nothing real, it's rather an illusion or fiction; or that it
is nothing other than the very real system itself, the brain. By this time,
however, it is not clear that we are anywhere near answering the original
question, Who? The *Who* question is the question of personal identity,
much discussed by philosophers. Do *I* (whatever *that* is) maintain identity
over time, and if so, *how?* This is a second *how* question. The two *how* questions—how does the brain generate a (sense of) self, and how do I maintain
identity over time—are not unconnected, and for this reason neither are
the *who* and *what* questions. Which makes it easy to get confused about
what question one is trying to answer. Answers to one question tend to
slip over into the answers to a different question. Answers that seem
appropriate on subpersonal levels tend to shift onto the personal level,
and vice versa.

Questions about the self are controversial ones that have relevance for a
number of different fields, including philosophy of mind, phenomenology, social theory, cultural studies, psychiatry, developmental psychology, and cognitive neuroscience. Perhaps not surprisingly, there is no
consensus in the scientific community concerning the scientific or philosophical legitimacy of the notion of self. Some, like Damasio (1999), claim
that the sense of self is an integral part of consciousness and that the ongoing search for the neural correlates of consciousness (NCC) must necessarily take this into account. Others, like Thomas Metzinger (2003), contend
that the self is not real, but simply a theoretical entity, which can be

explained in terms of brain processes, but which has no explanatory power itself. The controversy is often confused because when one defends or attacks the notion of self, it is not always clear what notion of self one is defending or attacking. And there are many notions. Here is the incomplete inventory given in Gallagher and Zahavi (2008).

1.   material self, social self, spiritual self (James 1890)
2.   ecological self, interpersonal self, extended self, private self, conceptual self (Neisser 1988)
3.   autobiographical self, cognitive self, contextualized self, core self, dialogical self, embodied self, empirical self, fictional self, minimal self, neural self (see, e.g., Damasio 1999; Gallagher and Shear 1999; Strawson 1999).

These different versions of the self are a product of the variety of methodological approaches taken within philosophy and in related interdisciplinary studies. The sense of the self that we end up talking about may depend on the particular mode of access or method that we pursue — through introspection, phenomenological analysis, linguistic analysis, the use of thought experiments, empirical research in cognitive and brain sciences, and studies of exceptional and pathological behavior. So one question is whether different methodological approaches target the same ontological subject matter, or lead to different models because on our chosen approaches we discover different conceptions of the self? This problem involves 'inter-theoretical coherency': do different characterizations of self signify diverse aspects of a unitary concept of selfhood, or do they pick out different and unrelated concepts. Let's explore some of these different ways of talking about the self.

How to split the brain and unify the self

Let's start by talking to one of the pioneers in the neuropsychology of split-brain research, Michael Gazzaniga. Split brains are of interest not only to neurosurgeons but also to philosophers and psychologists. A brain is split when, for medical reasons related to uncontrollable epilepsy, the corpus callosum, brain tissue that connects the two hemispheres, is severed. The result is relatively un-notable in regard to the patient's everyday existence, except, of course, that it controls his epileptic seizures. The patient seems normal in almost every way. But when you put the patient in a lab and start to do some well-designed experiments, some interesting things start to happen. It seem that each hemisphere has its own consciousness and the two consciousnesses can be isolated from each other at the behavioral level. Philosophers have used evidence from split- brain experiments to argue for the possibility that we each have more than one self, although for all practical purposes they are integrated as one self in non-split brains. What is clear is that the self is intricately connected to the brain. As Nagel puts it,

> I could lose everything but my functioning brain and still be me ... If my brain meets these conditions then the core of the self — what is essential to my existence — is my functioning brain ... I am not just my brain ... But the brain is the only part of me whose destruction I could not possibly survive. The brain, but not the rest of the animal, is essential to the self (1986, 40).

Gazzaniga, in his most recent book, *The Ethical Brain* (2006) argues that despite a modular brain, we maintain a unitary sense of self.

> Our brain is not a unified structure; instead it is composed of several modules that work out their computations separately, in what are called neural networks. These networks can carry out activities largely on their own. ... Yet even though our brain carries out all these functions in a modular system, we do not feel like a million little robots carrying out their disjointed activities. We feel like one, coherent self with intentions and reasons for what we feel are our unified actions. How can this be?

Gazzanaga suggests that there must be some part of the brain that monitors all of the other modular networks and attempts to interpret their activity in order to create a unifed self.

> Our best candidate for this brain area is the 'left-hemisphere inter-preter' ... [I]t includes a special region that interprets the inputs we receive every moment and weaves them into stories to form the ongoing narrative of our self-image and our beliefs. I have called this area of the left hemisphere the interpreter because it seeks explana-tions for internal and external events and expands on the actual facts we experience to make sense of, or interpret, the events of our life. (2005, 148).

> **Gazzaniga:** On the issue of one versus many selves, I would argue there is one self that can operate in many modes. I am a husband, father, scientist, skier, professor, etc. Each one of those modes calls upon different aspects of myself and each mode feels sort of differ-ent. There is no doubt that I am also capable of killing someone, if shot at. After all most soldiers are family men who are called upon to exercise an aspect of their self they would rather not see. All of this resides in the brain. Where else? In other words, the 'self' is the product of the workings of the brain. It may be somewhat misleading (or misguided) to discuss the 'self' as some unified, coherent entity except as the product of the operation of the brain.

SG: If we accept that the self is intricately related to the brain—possibly even reducible to the brain—it is also the case that a variety of theorists have conceived of this relation in different ways. Ramachandran and Hirstein (1997), for example, describe the self as a product of an executive mechanism, specifically a limbic executive rather than a frontal one. Nagel suggests that the whole brain is essential to the self. Damasio suggests that the emotional brain is central to what we call the self. How do you conceive of this relation between brain and self?

Gazzaniga: It's not simple. The split brain work allowed us to ask the question, does each separated hemisphere have its own self? At one level each can remember, emote, cognate and execute decisions. At some level of reasoning, each must have its own self. Over the years, however, it became clear that each hemisphere works at hugely different levels of understanding the world. The left hemisphere is completely self-aware, interprets its actions and feelings and those of the world. The right hemisphere doesn't do much of this and is an extremely poor problem-solver. In simple tests of self-awareness, such as showing pictures of the patient or of family members, each hemisphere seems to indicate recognition. But is each equally aware? It is hard to say as the recognition displayed by the right hemisphere might simply be an associative response. It is, of course, very difficult to interrogate the right hemisphere about its level of 'self-awareness' since it typically doesn't support spoken language.

But to answer Nagel's suggestion that the whole brain is necessary for the self more directly, it may be more reasonable to say that the self changes as a result of damage or disconnection and that less than the whole brain is capable of sustaining some sort of self. As you know, my proposal that the left hemisphere has an 'interpreter' that is constantly evaluating the state of the body and mind, plays a role here.

SG: Yes, perhaps you could say something more about the interpreter mechanism. If I understand it properly, it's a neuronal mechanism that monitors the subject's responses to the environment. But it monitors behavior on many different levels—cognitive as well as emotional, and as you say, it evaluates states of the body as well as mental states. Do you picture the interpreter as a complex neuronal location with inputs from all the relevant parts of the brain to track all of these dimensions, or is it a distributed process, albeit confined to the left hemisphere?

Gazzaniga: You said it all. It is the system that asks why and how and then tries to provide an answer. It is definitely in the left hemisphere but I can't be more specific.

Assuming that in some way what we call the self depends on the way the brain works, and considering the kinds of questions that philosophers ask about the continuity of the self over time, it may be important to consider whether changes in the brain necessarily entail changes in the self. Gazzaniga, however, presents a strong argument for genetic determinism, and rejects the notion that the brain has a large degree of plasticity, or that experience is essential for development.

SG: If that's the case, how do you explain the experimental data that indicate a large degree of brain plasticity, and that experience is necessary for proper development. I'm thinking of the famous work on critical periods in the visual system by Hubel and Wiesel (1963) and some of the more recent work by Carla Shatz (1992) and others which you discuss in your book, *The Mind's Past* (1998). You also cite the work by Merzenich (1984; 1987) on the owl monkey which showed that cortical representations of the body are subject to modification depending on the use of sensory pathways. Why doesn't this provide strong indication of the importance of experience for neuronal development?

Gazzaniga: There is no arguing there is some kind of plasticity mechanism in our brains. After all, we all learn things, like English, French, Japanese and our home telephone number. We can learn a new word in a flash, a new location in an instant. However, no one suggests that kind of learning is supported by the kinds of neural mechanisms you mention.

Shatz's beautiful work shows some activity-dependent development occurs way before the developing organism has any independent environmental experience. Surely that kind of dependency goes on, but I don't think there should be a wholesale importation of those concepts into how the brain gets built by psychological experience. There is a huge difference.

As for the extensive work by Merzenich and his colleagues, there can be little question that [neural] maps change as the result of experience. The question is, what does it mean? There are other results that show these changes may only occur when an alternative substrate is present for those changes to occur upon.

SG: Part of your evolutionary, genetic view depends on the concept of neural modules, or as you put it, 'neural devices that are built into our brains at the factory' (1998, xiii). One objection to this view comes from developmental psychology. For example, the idea that modular functions come 'on line' at certain critical moments in development has been questioned by Gopnik and Meltzoff (1997). Although they do not reject certain innate elements as important to development, they argue that at various times during development young children take up a completely inaccurate view of the world. In this case they wonder why evolution would have designed a sequence of incorrect modules rather than providing for the most direct and efficient course to maturity.

Gazzaniga: Does it really matter what we are like during transition from childhood to adulthood? Surely as brain development unfolds, the child is going through stages where interpretations of the world give rise to bizarre beliefs and perceptions. I don't see how that point argues against the idea many devices are built into our brains. Actually their bizarre beliefs serve up many of the endearments we all experience as parents.

SG: Would such childhood beliefs and misperceptions be the result of a developmental process related to the left-hemisphere interpreter? Or does the interpreter come pre-programmed, so to speak, and is it simply not getting the complete information it needs? I'm trying to understand where you might draw the line between a nativist account of brain development and one that would place the emphasis on perceptual experience.

Gazzaniga: I think the interpreter is doing its job in the child. During those years when it occasionally comes up with phantasmagorical stories about life, the child's knowledge system is not yet prepared to reject the idea served up by the interpreter. So the child plays with the idea, and the parents are amused. Pretty soon, however, the child realizes the Christmas canoe could not have fit down the chimney.

SG: You have embraced the latest version of the theory of the self as an illusion or a fiction. Perhaps Hume's account of the self as a product of an overworked imagination is the earliest of these theories. More recently narrative theory has suggested that selves are products of the stories we tell about ourselves. Dennett (1991) has worked out a theory of the self as a centre of narrative gravity, that is, as an abstract construct located at the intersection of the various tales we tell about ourselves. Metzinger (2004) has suggested that the self is nothing more than a model generated by brain processes. How does your theory differ from these?

Gazzaniga: Well I think Dennett borrows heavily from the idea of the interpreter to generate that idea, so I am in general agreement with his formulation.

SG: Even if the self is an illusion or fiction, would you agree that it plays an important practical role in our individual lives? I'm thinking of this question in relation to what you say about free will, that is, that the brain has already done the work before we become aware of it. How, in that case, are we able to talk about responsibility, or character, or ethics? A criminal might be tempted to argue that 'I didn't really do it, because, after all, I don't really exist (I'm nothing more than a fiction); and even if I did do it, I didn't freely choose to do it.'

Gazzaniga: The self is not a fiction. It is the centre of our personal narrative, as Dennett says. By trying to articulate how that develops, how the brain enables that sense of self, I do not mean to say the self is a fiction. It is that which the interpreter creates and gives narrative to. Now in my book *The Mind's Past* (2000) the lead chapter is called 'The Fictional Self' but that was to draw attention to the fact the interpreter calls upon all kinds of false information to build that narrative. So the construct that is derived comes from true facts of one's life as well as false facts that we believe to be true. The resulting spin that comes out as our personal narrative is, as a result, a bit fictional, like the idea we are in control of our behavior.

Having said that, I do not for a minute think this view relinquishes us from personal responsibility. I wrote about this at length in my book *The Social Brain* (1985). The late Donald M. MacKay made the argument over 30 years ago that even though we could view the brain as mechanical as clockwork, the idea of personal responsibility does not suffer (MacKay 1967). His long argument was based on the idea that in order for something to be true, it had to be true and public for all people. So, if you are sure that I am going to eat a Big Mac at noon, all I have to do to show you cannot predict my behavior is not eat it at noon. You respond, well what if I keep the prediction a secret? His argument was that the prediction might be true for you but that it wasn't true for the whole world. In order for that to occur, it had to be made public and the minute it was, I could negate it. It's a clever argument which I tend to agree with. Nonetheless, that argument aside, it also is obvious to me that people behave better when they believe they are in charge of their own behavior. That is good enough reason for me to support the concept.

SG: In *The Mind's Past* you suggest that 'autobiography is hopelessly inventive' and that false memories can be productive for a coherent life narrative. Now philosophers often worry about self-deception and how it's possible. But your claims about autobiographical inventiveness do not imply self-deception, that is, there is no level on which the individual knows that their false memories are false. Yet, philosophically, this conception of self-inventiveness should motivate in us some suspicion about who we are. Should we worry about this in any way?

Gazzaniga: We sure should. That is exactly the problem with false memories. In terms of our personal recollection, we can't tell the difference between true and false memories. When complex scalp recordings are made, the experimenter cannot detect that the brain responds differently to a true as opposed to a false memory. In short, both are part of the fabric of our personal narrative.

SG: I wonder if you would accept the name Platonic neuralism for your theoretical position. I have in mind your statement: 'Every newborn is armed with circuits that already compute information enabling the baby to function in the physical universe. The baby does not learn trigonometry, but knows it; does not learn how to distinguish figure from ground, but knows it; does not need to learn but knows, that when one object with mass hits another, it will move the object' (2000, 2). On this view, the child is much as Plato describes in his theory of recollection. Remember in Plato's dialogue, the *Meno*, when Socrates sits down with the slave boy and shows that the boy doesn't learn geometry, but already knows it. On some level, and with regard to some basics, we don't actually learn anything new, we simply recollect what we already know from prior lives (and here we could substitute the evolutionary explanation for the notions of reincarnation that Plato discussed). The knowledge is already in the brain.

Gazzaniga: I think the work of several of our leading developmental psychologists point to this conclusion. Elizabeth Spelke, Susan Carey and Rene Baillargeon all argue the point convincingly [see e.g. Baillargeon et al. 1985; Xu & Carey 1996]. For example, Mark Hauser and Susan Carey (2003) show that there seem to be some mental primitives that are shared by both the monkey and the young child. So yes, much of what we are is factory installed and may be from early in our evolutionary history.

Self-monitoring

If, as Gazzaniga suggests there is a part of the brain that monitors all other parts, what is the nature of this self-monitoring? One proposal is that we can learn more about it in cases where it fails? Our friend Chris Frith has studied this phenomenon in schizophrenics who experience delusions of control (when a patient thinks that someone else is making him move and act in certain ways) and thought insertion (when a patient thinks that someone else is inserting thoughts into her mind). Frith's original explanation (1992) was that in such cases, something goes wrong with our normal self-monitoring process that keeps track of our intentions and actions.

> **Frith:** The self-monitoring phenomenon relates to symptoms like delusions of control and thought insertion, and in fact the whole category of passivity disorders where the patient says that 'I am doing things, but it's not me that's doing them. They are being created by some external force'. And this includes inserted thoughts or inserted emotions, or making the arm move, and perhaps some kinds of auditory hallucinations, like the patient who says 'I hear my own thoughts spoken aloud'. So there's a whole class of symptoms like that, although in this respect there's a problem because a particular patient doesn't have all those symptoms, but maybe only one or two.

> **SG:** That makes schizophrenia a complicated thing to explain.

> **Frith:** Yes. You have the issue of why one patient has one symptom but not the other, and this seems totally mysterious. That idea has evolved quite a lot. The original story was that these symptoms were a step up from the negative symptoms.[1] Whereas the patient with negative symptoms doesn't have willed intentions, these patients with passivity experiences do have willed intentions, but they don't know about it. So their own actions appear out of the blue, as it were, and that makes it seem as if the actions are caused by some alien force. But I no longer believe that story. The most telling comparison for me now involves people with what we call the 'Anarchic Hand Sign'. These are the neurological patients in whom one arm, usually as the result of damage in the supplementary motor area, behaves all by itself without the patient intending — it grabs things, and so forth. What is so interesting about this syndrome, is that patients are fully aware that their hand is doing things they don't intend it to do, but they don't say that there's an alien force or agency controlling their hand. They usually say, 'something is wrong with my hand', and they try to stop it by holding it or even tying it down. In contrast, the patient with schizophrenia and delusions of control is exactly the opposite of this in all respects.

---

1   Schizophrenic symptoms are usually classified as either positive or negative. Positive symptoms include hallucinations, delusions of control, inserted thought, racing thoughts; negative symptoms include apathy, lack of emotion, and poor or nonexistant social functioning.

For example, Sean Spence did this nice experiment where he had schizophrenic patients in the scanner making random joystick movements. They experienced delusions of control while they did this (Spence et al. 1997). But, of course, they were doing what they intended to do — they were producing random movement as instructed. And they didn't try to stop it. And that is typically the case in schizophrenia. So it seems to me that if you analyze this thoroughly you would have to say that a patient with delusions of control has an intention to move his arm, and knows about it, and makes the movement which is consistent with his intention, as is shown by the fact that he doesn't try to stop himself, and yet still says that there is something about this experience that makes it seem that there's an alien force. The question is what does he mean, why does he interpret it in this way, why does he have this experience?

The new version, the new account, therefore, builds upon the old one. It's not that the patients are not aware of their intention to move. It's that they are not aware of the initiation of the movement.

SG: Self-monitoring breaks down at the point of initiation.

Frith: Yes. Normally, when we initiate an action, our awareness of the initiation is not based on the sensory feedback. It's based on predictions about what's going to happen. So the idea is that these predictions somehow do not enter awareness with these patients. So they get the sensory feedback without the experience of initiating the movement. That would certainly seem very odd. One could in principle do an experiment where you create that experience in normal people and see how they interpret it.

SG: It would seem like an involuntary movement, although in that case one would not have the intention.

Frith: Well here is my model, or my story about this. It would be like giving a lecture with a carousel projector where you press a button to make the slides move forward. But every time you're about to press a button, the slides move forward just before you press. I think the way you would interpret that, which would be reasonably correct, is that there is someone in the control box anticipating your needs and advancing the slide. So you are quite right, there is an agent. And it has to be an agent, because they are reading your intentions.

SG: Are there cases when in fact the intention is not there?

Frith: Well I think perhaps that patients with utilization behavior perform actions without intentions. These are people with large frontal damage who simply respond to objects in the environment in the canonical way in which one should respond to these objects, but not appropriate to the context. For example, whenever they see a tool, they will automatically pick it up and start using it. And there is this nice report by Lhermitte (1986) about taking this patient around his flat, and taking him into the bedroom. The patient sees the bed is turned down, and he undresses and gets into bed, including taking his wig off. Presumably these actions are driven by objects in the environment and they are no longer inhibited by the wider context or the appropriate intention. Interestingly, when you ask such patients 'Why did you do that'? they will say things like, 'I thought you wanted me to'. Which implies that they are not aware of any prior intention with which their action was incompatible. So I wonder if these are people who have no intentions. They are simply running off behavior automatically.

SG: No self-monitoring going on there either, but these patients are not schizophrenics. Even if they have no sense of self-agency, they don't try to attribute it to someone else, although they confabulate about why they did it.

Frith: Yes. We did an experiment on speaking a fairly long time ago, but we've never done it with hand movements. In principle you could do it with hand movements by measuring the EEG readiness potential that occurs just before you make a movement. You would use this potential to advance the carousel projector, for example. So the readiness potential would appear just before the subject pressed the button for the carousel projector and the slide would advance before the subject had pressed the button. The trouble is you can't do this in reality because the readiness potential can usually only be measured as an average of many trials. So what we did was to use the voice, because you can have a similar sort of explanation of auditory hallucinations (Cahill et al. 1996). We had patients and volunteers wear earphones and a throat microphone, so that they would hear their own voice very loudly through the earphones. We had to make it fairly loud to cover up feedback from bone conduction. And then we had a special effects box where you can distort what the subject hears. We didn't introduce distortions in time because if you hear your own voice delayed it interferes with speech production. Instead we altered the pitch. So you heard your voice in real time, with no delay, but at a different pitch. If I raise my voice by 2 semitones it sounds like a woman's voice. We had a very open ended situation where we varied the pitch distortion in various ways and got the subjects to talk to us. Then we asked them what they thought was going on. Normal volunteers, and even patients who were at that time reasonably well, said, not surprisingly, 'You're doing something to my voice with that box'. Whereas the acute patients with hallucinations and delusions at the time of testing would say things like 'Whenever I speak I hear someone else speaking'. More than one of them said 'It's the devil speaking'. Another one said, 'I keep hearing my brother saying the same things that I'm saying'. I'm pleased to say, by the way, that this is one of the rare experiments on the topic of schizophrenia that has actually been replicated by someone (Johns & McGuire 1999). What was particularly fascinating concerned the one who said 'I keep hearing my brother speaking whenever I speak'. Afterwards, obviously, we explained that it was all done with the special effects box, and showed how we turned the knob which changed the pitch. And the patient said, 'How does that box know what my brother sounds like'? What this experiment shows is that my model doesn't work.

SG: The original model (Frith 1992).

Frith: Right, the original model. Because what we predicted was if we produced this weird experience where the feedback is not what you expect, the normal subject should produce explanations similar to schizophrenic delusions. Obviously, the weird experience is not sufficient. To produce the delusional account you have to be schizophrenic as well.

SG: So on your original model the prediction would be that even normal subjects would suffer similar experiences as schizophrenics if the situation was rigged in the proper way. Specifically, as I recall, the model explained such delusions as caused by something going wrong with normal monitoring of motor or cognitive control mechanisms, removing a certain anticipatory sense of what was going to happen, and experimentally, this would be equivalent to the unanticipated altered pitch. Now, as you say, this can't be the entire story since under just such circumstances normal subjects don't experience delusions at all. So your original model could explain involuntary movement or the sort of unbidden thoughts we all experience, but not the schizophrenic's claim that someone else was the agent of these movements or thoughts. But currently you are still appealing to the idea of a 'forward model' of control — that is, a model that provides for the anticipatory sense of what you are going to do (see Frith, Blakemore and Wolpert 2000). How do you conceptualize this self-monitoring now? Is it something conscious, or something subpersonal?

Frith: Well, concerning basic motor control, there must be subpersonal or sub-conscious self-monitoring going on, otherwise we would all fall over. And presumably this aspect of the system is working reasonably well in schizophrenic patients since they do not fall over, bump into things, and so forth. So there must be a special high-level box in one's diagram of the self-monitoring system that says there is a conscious component, and that's where things go wrong. This is what I was talking about at the meeting we attended yesterday.[2] I asked, 'What's the purpose of this conscious component of the self-monitoring system that allows us to be aware of our actions?' My speculation is that it has very much to do with getting a sense of agency and being in control. One of the experiments we have done, which I always like to tell people about, is the tickling experiment.

SG: This is Sarah Blakemore's experiment?

Frith: Yes, Sarah's experiment (Blakemore et al. 2000; Blakemore, Wolpert and Frith 1998; 2000). The assumption was that, in schizophrenia, there is a problem with the awareness of the consequences of your action, perhaps because of a problem with predicting the consequences of your action. If this system is not working properly with these patients, then they should be able to tickle themselves. The reason we can't tickle ourselves is that we know in advance what it's going to feel like. So Sarah did this experiment on a group of schizophrenic patients, and indeed, those who were currently experiencing positive symptoms, like delusions of control, showed no difference between their ratings of self-tickling and her tickling them. So they were able to tickle themselves. We now have supporting data using force, which can be measured objectively, rather than tickliness, which is subjective. (Shergill et al. 2005).

SG: This is like the Frith and Done (1988) experiment. A loud sound will cause a large evoked potential in the EEG if it is sudden and unexpected. If a normal subject causes an auditory stimulus by pushing a button that creates a sound, they will have a greatly reduced evoked potential because they are not surprised by the outcome. But the schizophrenic is surprised — he fails to anticipate the outcome of his own action — and this generates a measurable response.

Frith: Yes. And these results were confirmed in experiments by Judy Ford at Stanford (Ford and Mathalon 2004). It's the same phenomenon. The big development in my thinking here has come from my meeting Daniel Wolpert who is a proper motor physiologist with engineering expertise who really knows about forward models. We're trying to get these ideas into a sensible framework in which the idea of a forward model provides a specific mechanism for under-

2   The original interview was conducted in Aarhus, Denmark, following the Conference on Brain and Cognition. Aarhus University Hospital, University of Aarhus, Denmark (February 2002). Frith presented a paper entitled, 'Attention to Action and Awareness of Other Minds'.

standing prediction in the motor system. And I find these developments quite exciting, because it leads on to the third area, which is
mentalizing or 'theory of mind' (see Wolpert, Doya and Kawato
2003).

Aspects of the minimal self

For Frith and his colleagues self-monitoring is much more distributed
than for Gazzaniga. That is, there is not necessarily one monitoring system
that keeps track of everything going on in the brain. Rather there are local
comparators that are responsible for keeping track of movement and
action. But in what sense is it possible to speak of self-awareness in these
subpersonal mechanisms? If we are aware of our movement in some way,
and of our action, we are in no way aware of the self-monitoring processes
themselves. There is no self in these processes. But is it possible for the self,
or some form of self-awareness to arise from such processes? If so, it is
what phenomenologists would call a pre-reflective self-awareness that
would help to constitute what Damasio (1999) calls the 'core' self, and
what some philosophers call the 'minimal' self (Gallagher 2000). Here is
one possible way to tell the story. Basically, it's a matter of code breaking.

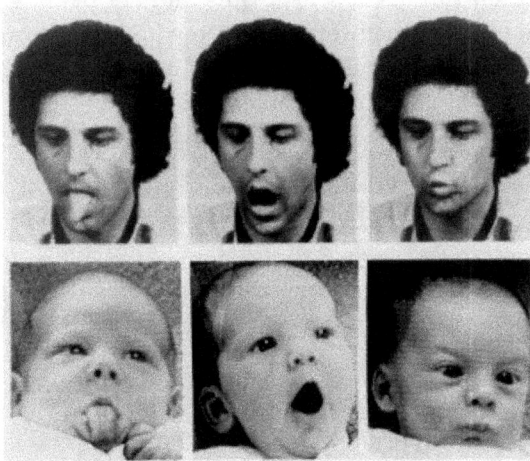

Figure 11.1 Neonate imitation. From Meltzoff and Moore (1977).

Infants are able to imitate facial gestures presented to them, starting just
after birth. Experiments by Meltzoff and Moore (1977; 1983; 1989) show
that infants can imitate tongue protrusion, mouth opening, and lip purs-
ing when less than an hour old. This is not a reflex movement because you
can delay their response and they will still imitate. Also, they improve

with practice. At first they may not perform the gesture accurately, but after a few tries they get it. This implies that infants already are able to discriminate self from non-self since they are able to see the difference between what they try to imitate, the other's facial gesture, and their own gesture (Gallagher and Meltzoff 1995). Part of what allows them to do this sort of imitation is the intermodal transformations that take place between vision (by which they see the other's face) and kinaesthesia or proprioception (by which they have some sense of what they are doing). Proprioception provides afferent feedback about the infant's own movements, and the infant is somehow able to match this up or compare it to what it sees. For this to happen proprioception and vision have to speak the same language, so to speak. They are articulated in the same code so there is no translation problem.

A comparator, of course, is instantiated as a subpersonal processing in the brain. For the simplest kind of sensory-motor comparator to work afferent feedback signals (proprioception, for example) have to be in the same code as efferent signals (motor command signals). The comparator compares afferent proprioceptive signals to a copy of the efferent signal sent to our motor cortex to initiate movement. If I turn my head with my eyes open, objects in my visual field shift in one direction; that's not because they moved, but because I moved. In order to explain why we can tell the difference between movement in our visual field because of movement in the world and movement in our visual field because of our own movement, von Holst & Mittelstaedt (1950) offered a simple model of a comparator which compared afferent input to efference copy. If there is a match between the afferent and the efferent the system registers the movement as our own; if they do not match, the system registers the movement as something happening in the environment. Our sensory-motor system is designed so that we have a built in way to register the difference between self and non-self.[3] But this is still all subpersonal. There is no conscious comparison going on between proprioception and vision. The brain 'knows' the difference between self and non-self even at the level where there is so self other than the organism itself. The supposition, however, is that when the actual information streams, i.e., afferent and efferent, are fed through the comparators in my brain, the neural activity generates some conscious sense that, for example, the action is mine, or not mine. Thus, Dorotheé Legrand (2006) has argued that when we move, the basic self/non-self distinction is generated by the comparator, such that a pre-reflective awareness of my bodily moving self is constituted. This would be a sense of self at the first-order level of consciousness.

---

3   Whether this difference is innate or not is a matter of debate. See Vosgerau & Newen (2007); Vosgerau (2007).

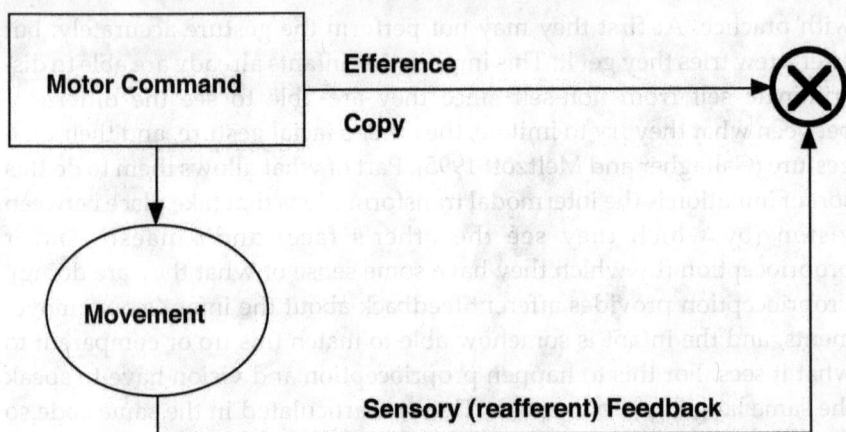

Figure 11.2 Simple sensory feedback comparator

As Legrand notes, the comparator model can be made more complex. In this regard, she stays with the simplest model while Frith goes to a more complex forward model.

> This model has been sophisticated enough to include intention and a [forward] internal model allowing for the prediction of the percep-tual consequences of the action (Wolpert, Ghahramani and Jordan 1995; Blakemore, Frith and Wolpert 1999). A comparator between intended, predicted and real reafferences is thus added to the com-parator between efference and afference. Although I do not deny the importance of such an internal model, my claim differs from Frith's since it implies the integration of efference with actual afferences, rather than with predicted afferences. (Legrand 2006, 111).

Legrand's position is based on 'action monitoring' rather than 'intention monitoring' in the forward model, so while Frith describes self-conscious-ness as relying on the latter, Legrand would rather describe self-con-sciousness as relying on the former.

One could, of course, prefer both the having and the eating of the cake. Certainly a full awareness of self, even in this minimal form, incorporates certain anticipations of its actions. Self-awareness, as phenomenologists like Legrand insist, is predicated on a basic temporality of experience which includes a sense of what my existence has just been, and what my existence is about to be.[4] So a system that can incorporate a sense of my potential or future movement on the basis of a forward model needs to be integrated with one that tells me what I have just done.

---

4   Here the phenomenologist would point to Husserl's analysis of time-consciousness which involves a retentional-protentional structure (see Husserl 1928; also Gallagher 1998; Gallagher and Zahavi 2008).

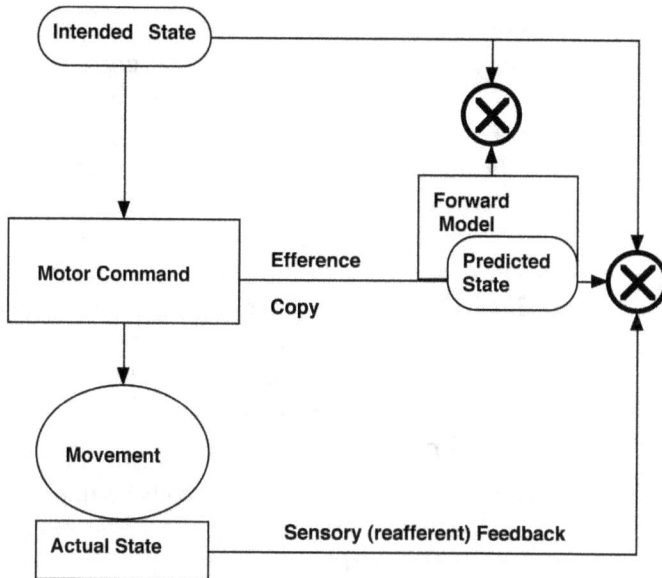

Figure 11.3 Comparator system with forward model

In terms of phenomenology, what these systems produce is first, a bodily *sense of ownership* — the experience of the moving body as *my* body, and thus of the movement as *my* movement; and second, a *sense of agency* — an experience that the movement has been initiated by me, that I am the cause of the action (Gallagher 2000).[5] Tsakiris and Haggard (2005) have provided evidence to the effect that the sense of ownership depends on sensory reafferent feedback while the sense of agency is tied primarily to efferent signals. This makes sense in regard to the difference between voluntary action (which involves both afference/sense of ownership and efference/sense of agency) and involuntary movement (which involves afference/sense of ownership — that is, I know that it is my body that is moving — but no efference/sense of agency — I am not the author of the action). This also seems to be a way to understand delusions of control in schizophrenia, which to the schizophrenic feels like involuntary action. As Frith suggests, something goes wrong in the comparator; efference copy goes astray or is mis-registered at the comparator, and the action feels alien.[6]

But the minimal sense of a bodily self is not just the result of all this activity in comparators. As we saw in earlier chapters, the body provides a

---

5   For studies of the neural correlates of the sense of agency, see Chaminade and Decety (2002); Farrer and Frith (2003); Farrer et al. (2003). For a critical discussion of these experiments, see Tsakris, Bosbach and Gallagher (2007) and Gallagher (2007c).

6   For more on this see Frith (1992). For why this doesn't work for thought insertion, see Gallagher (2004a). And for the additional explanation of why the schizophrenic attributes agency to someone else, see Gallagher (2007d).

perspective for perception and action, and that perspective comes with ecological (proprioceptive-kinesthetic) feedback that gives me a sense of my posture, location, and movement in the environment relative to the things around me. Furthermore, we have learned that the contribution of emotion is not insignificant. Jaak Panksepp's suggestion in this regard is that there is a primary sense of self that is based on the brain processes involved in emotion, which then gets reiterated at higher levels of cognition. Turning from schizophrenia to clinical depression, I suggested to Panksepp that this idea implies that when we medicate someone, for example for treatment of depression, and so when we start to change the balance of neurotransmitters in the system, we are not only addressing the depression, or introducing changes in consciousness, but we are also changing that person's feeling of self-identity.

Panksepp: That's certainly a reasonable hypothesis that could guide novel research initiatives. It is evident that evolutionary layers of control do exist in the brain, and the lower primary-processes permit higher secondary (learning) and tertiary (thought) processes to operate. I've taken the strong position that the slippery issue of self-representation does need to be neurologized, and the lower levels are essential for raw emotional feelings that higher cortical elaborations transform into more cognitive forms of self-identity, via self-referential information processing, as Georg Northoff puts it (see Northoff et al. 2006). The self is a very broad concept, with a lot of implications for the nature of mind. The self is surely a multi-layered process, but abundant evidence suggests the organization of lower levels more directly reflect the 'ancestral voices of the genes' while the higher levels are deeply epigenetic and experientially constructed. I think a solution to this puzzle will depend on clarity at the most foundational, primary-process level. Like everything else in living nature, things start from a seed that grows and elaborates. To make neuroscientific progress you have to identify where the initial neural 'seeds' are situated and then where in the brain self-referential growth ('mineness') and related information processing is concentrated.

SG: You've focused your search for these neural seeds in the midbrain for various reasons that are similar but also different from Damasio's reasons.

Panksepp: My focus is based upon the fact that there is more convergence of emotion-related neural systems within the Periaqueductal Grey (PAG), the most ancient regions of the midbrain, than anywhere else in the brain. It is here were ESB evokes the strongest emotional and affective responses with the lowest amount of electrical current. And this concentration, this massive interaction of emotional operating systems may have profound meaning. Certainly this deep and primitive midline system is massively connected to and functionally interrelated with higher medial brain regions all the way up to the medial frontal cortex, where insightful investigators, such as Georg Northoff, are demonstrating self-related cognitive-emotional information processing using human brain imaging approaches. So I think the concept of re-iteration simply has to be part of the whole package. For instance, the various neural chemistries that modify psychiatric disorders will have some effect on the neuronal tone of higher self-representation systems by initially having more primary interactions with the more ancient, genetically hard-wired aspects that permitted those systems to grow both evolutionarily and ontogenetically. We finally have a credible framework for studying such issues and progress will depend completely on the generation of testable (hence falsifiable) predictions. I think there is a whole new field of functional neuroscience to be cultivated here, especially for understanding primary-process affects.

The narrative self

The minimal self, as we have been using this term, is equivalent to a momentary or very short-term identity formed by a bodily and dynamic integration of sensory-motor, spatially perspectival, and emotional experience. It is the experiencing subject, plain and simple, although simple can still be complex insofar as one can discriminate a sense of ownership, sense of agency, embodied perspective, and specific feelings within this minimal ipseity. It has the same ontological status as the lived body, since it is nothing more than the individual's body in action, accompanied by what phenomenologists like Husserl, Merleau-Ponty, Zahavi, Legrand, and others call pre-reflective self-awareness. We should add to this the insight that an experiencing subject in action is most often in the company of other experiencing subjects in action, and gains in its sense of itself through its intersubjective interactions. We can see this from the very beginning in the infant's relations with others. Intersubjectivity presents a number of possibilities, which range from basic survival to being taken up into what Merleau-Ponty calls the 'whirlwind of language'. In this regard the minimal self operates as an anchor for the use of the first-person pronoun, and for further development of more sophisticated experiences of self-consciousness that are fully situated in the give and take of intersubjective communicative situations (see Stawarska 2008 for some of the fine details of how this works in terms of pronouns). If the infant comes to recognize herself in the mirror, it's because there is already a self to recognize. If, in effect, she thinks 'That's me', the 'me' has already been there in the form of the minimal self; and has already been reflected in the perspectives of others. The child starts to see herself as others see her, and this is something more than minimal self-awareness.

Use of the first-person pronoun, of course, arrives on the scene relatively early, with minimal linguistic ability. What do we do with language – or what does language do with us? Communicating with others, expressing what we want; these language events suddenly find themselves entering a transformative loop because others are asking us what and why and so forth. More than that, people start telling us stories, and they begin to elicit our story. Developmentally, our self-narratives are initiated and shaped by others and by those kinds of narratives that are common and possible in the culture surrounding the child. Because we develop in social contexts and normally acquire the capacity for narrative in those contexts, the development of self-narrative necessarily involves others. Katherine Nelson (2003) points out that a certain limited ability for narrative emerges in 2-year olds, 'with respect to the child's own experience, which is forecast and rehearsed with him or her by parents'. As we noted before, self-narrative requires building on our experiences of others and their narratives, so 'children of 2–4 years often "appropriate" someone else's story as their own' (Nelson 2003, 31). Furthermore, to occupy a position within a self-narrative requires more than a minimal, non-conceptual self-awareness – it requires a conceptual, objective, narrative self that is aware of itself as having a point of view that is different from others.

The importance of narrative in the development of a more nuanced and sophisticated self-identity has been emphasized by Jerome Bruner (2004). In a recent lecture in Oxford he recommends that we take narrative as a serious enterprise.

> Why are we so intellectually dismissive towards narrative? Why are we inclined to treat it as rather a trashy, if entertaining, way of thinking about and talking about what we do with our minds? Storytelling performs the dual cultural functions of making the strange familiar and ourselves private and distinctive. (March 2007, cited in Crace 2007).

The kind of discourse that narrative is contributes to its ability to shape the self. As Bruner puts it, 'self is in part a product of discourse – a function of the discourses in which you chose to enter' (Shore 1997, 23) – but also in part a function of the discourses you find yourself in, over above any choice you make. Narratives, to speak metaphorically, have a life of their own that carry individuals along with them. They carry us further into our intersubjective relations and our cultural milieu.

The narrative self can be conceived in several ways. Dennett (1988; 1991) offers an account consistent with recent developments in our understanding of distributed neuronal processing. In that account, there is no real neurological center of experience. No Cartesian pineal gland that would operate as the theater of consciousness. But insofar as humans have language they can create a relatively stable center of life at the intersection of the stories they tell about themselves. Indeed, for Dennett, we cannot prevent ourselves from 'inventing' our selves. We are hardwired to become language users, and once we are caught up in the web of language and begin spinning our own stories (*or they spinning us* – Dennett and Merleau-Ponty are on the same page in this respect), we are not totally in control of the product. An important product of this spinning is the narrative self. The narrative self, however, is nothing substantially real. Rather, according to Dennett, it is an empty abstraction. Specifically, Dennett (1991) defines a self as an abstract 'center of narrative gravity'. He compares it to the theoretical fiction of the center of gravity of any physical object. On this view an individual self consists of the abstract and movable point where one's various autobiographical stories meet up. In a televised interview with Wim Kayzer, Dennett explains this idea.

Dennett: What a person is, is, in effect, information.

Kayzer: An abstraction?

Dennett: It's an abstraction, yes. What you are is an abstraction. I talk about what I call the self as a center of narrative gravity. And just the way that the center of gravity is an object, it is not an atom, it's not a pearl, it's not a bit of stuff; it's a very important abstraction, but it is an abstraction. So, what you are, what a self is, is an abstract object which is definable in terms of a certain set of information. (Kayzer 1993).

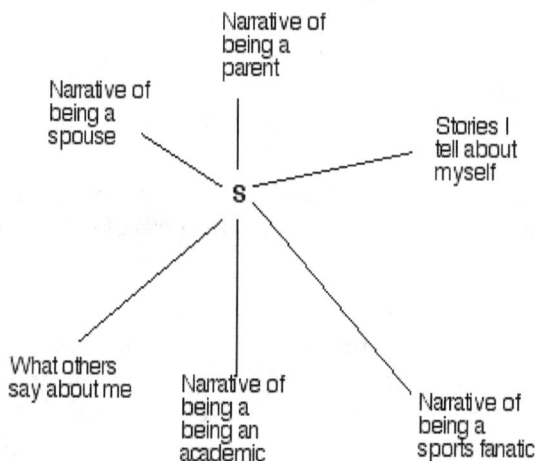

Figure 11.4 Self as center of narrative gravity

This center can shift around as various narratives take on more importance throughout life or as the information quality or quantity increases or
diminishes.

Dennett's view, as Gazzaniga noted, is consistent with the notion of the
left-hemisphere 'interpreter'. In Gazzaniga's model, the interpreter
weaves together autobiographical fact and inventive fiction to produce a
personal narrative that enables the sense of a continuous self. Gazzaniga,
however, contends that the self, in this regard, is not a fiction because the
normal functioning of the interpreter tries to make sense of what actually
happens to the person. At most, in the nonpathological case, it may be only
'a bit fictional'. It seems likely that we do enhance our personal narratives
with elements that smooth over discontinuities and discrepancies in our
self-constitution.

Other theorists, like Paul Ricoeur (1984; 1992) and Alistair MacIntyre
(1981), have explored these issues in different ways and have reached con-
clusions that are not inconsistent with the views of Bruner, Dennett,
Gazzaniga, and others. In contrast to Dennett, however, Ricoeur conceives
of the narrative self, not as an abstract point at the intersection of various
narratives, but as something richer, more complicated. Ricoeur shows that
one's own self-narrative is always entangled in the narratives of others.
On this view we might say that the self is the sum total of its narratives,
and includes within itself all of the equivocations, contradictions, strug-
gles and 'inconclusions' that find expression in personal life. In contrast to
Dennett's center of narrative gravity, this extended self is dynamically
intersubjective, decentered, distributed and multiplex. At a psychological
level, this view allows for conflict, moral indecision and self-deception, in
a way that the metaphor of an abstract point would be hard pressed to
capture.

The narrative self is much more contextualized than the minimal self;
the minimal self by itself is something of an abstraction that gets fleshed
out in the narrative accounts of *what* I am doing and *why* or *for whom*. At the
same time, the minimal self is as real as the embodied agent, and without it
self-narrative would be unanchored and adrift—it wouldn't be *self*-narra-
tive at all.

In self-narrative, our identity—*who* we are—is framed and reinforced.
As Francisco Varela indicated, however, this kind of identity is difficult to
pin down.

> **Varela:** What's involved in identity are one's cognitive and moral
> decisions, one's temperament, but also actions, behaviors and mem-
> ories as they characterize an individual life. None of this is isolated
> from our associations with others. Neuroscience tells us that all of
> this originates in a set of dynamic interactions in the brain that mirror
> the dynamic interactions—the perceptions which are necessarily tied

to actions — in the coupling between organism and world. This kind of identity, however, is of a totally peculiar nature. On the one hand one can say that it definitely exists, and we can see this in our everyday interactions with others who we treat as individuals and who treat us as individuals. On the other hand, this process is like all emergent processes, unlocalizable. I cannot point to it and say 'Here, this is my self'. This is because we have a purely relational identity. And so that's why it becomes impossible to find anything like the neural correlates of self-identity. It's not possible because it's a relational identity that exists only in the dynamic process as an emerging and changing pattern.

Chapter 12

Free Will and Moral Responsibility

At the beginning of the 18th century, the German philosopher Leibniz wrote that our conscious thoughts are influenced by sensory stimuli of which we are not aware:

> ... at every moment there is in us an infinity of perceptions, unaccompanied by awareness or reflection. ... That is why we are never indifferent, even when we appear to be most so. ... The choice that we make arises from these insensible stimuli, which ... make us find one direction of movement more comfortable than the other. (1981, 53).

Everything depends on how strongly one interprets the word 'arises'. Do these sub-conscious processes influence or motivate our choices, or do they cause them? It seems that if there is something that we call a self, part of what we have in mind by that term is not only some kind of entity capable of self-conscious action, but an entity that takes responsibility for that action—in effect, someone with the status of moral agency. Where in previous ages this was a huge controversy in theological contexts (see, for example, St. Augustine, and Leibniz himself: if God knows what I'm going to do before I do, am I not already predetermined and without free will?), today this is still a huge controversy, but now in contexts informed by neuroscience (if the brain knows what I am going to do before I do, am I not already determined and without free will?). The brain has taken the place of God, at least in this corner of the discussion.

The sense of effort and free will

Remember the conversation between Princess Elisabeth and Descartes about how the mind is able to move the body (Chapter 2). Elisabeth was quite puzzled about how this was possible given Descartes's definition of the mind as an unextended, thinking thing. Descartes himself seemed not to be troubled. He offers the following explanation.

> Now the action of the soul consists entirely in this, that simply by willing it makes the small [pineal] gland to which it is closely united move in the way requisite for producing the effect aimed at in the volition ... when we will to walk or to move the body in any manner, this volition causes the gland to impel the spirits toward the muscles which bring about this effect (Descartes 1649, §§ xli, xliii).

Concerning the will he also writes:

> Our volitions, in turn, are also of two kinds. Some actions of the soul terminate in the soul itself, as when we will to love God, or in general apply our thought to some non-material object. Our other actions terminate in our body, as when from our merely willing to walk, it follows that our legs are moved and that we walk (1649, § xviii).

Descartes's answer to this question still frames the discussion today. So, for example, two neuropsychologists who have done some important experiments on the question of free will, Patrick Haggard and Benjamin Libet frame the question in exactly the same way, referring to it as the traditional concept: 'how can a mental state (my conscious intention) initiate the neural events in the motor areas of the brain that lead to my body movement?' (Haggard and Libet 2001,47). If we substitute 'the pineal gland' for 'neural events in the motor areas', this is precisely Descartes' question. Neuroscientists, of course, are interested in identifying the precise area of the brain responsible for the movement in question. The kind of responsibility they are interested in is *causal* responsibility. For philosophers who are interested in the question of *moral* responsibility two questions come immediately to mind. First, does causal responsibility stretch back to include the mental state that seemingly gets the relevant neural mechanisms going (with some arguing that the mental state is nothing other than another set of neural mechanisms, or something caused by another set of neural mechanisms). Second, to what degree is moral responsibility dependent on causal responsibility?

In Lyon I asked Marc Jeannerod about some of the details and basic concepts of volitional action, will and effort.

> **SG:** In your book (Jeannerod 1997) you talk about 'the effort of the will' as related to a sense of heaviness of the limb.
>
> **Jeannerod:** I am referring to a particular situation where the experiment involves modified conditions of the limb, such as partial paralysis or fatigue (e.g., McCloskey, Ebeling and Goodwin 1974). Imagine that you have one arm partially paralyzed or fatigued, and you are asked to raise a weight with that arm (the reference weight).

Then, by using the other, normal arm, you are asked to select a weight that matches the reference weight: the weight selected by the normal arm will be heavier than the reference weight. This means that, in selecting a weight, you refer not to the real reference weight, but to the effort that you have to put into lifting it. Because your arm is partially paralyzed or fatigued, you have to send an increased motor command to lift the reference weight, and you will read this as an increased weight. You need more motor commands to recruit more muscle units, because they have less force.

SG: So the state of the muscles determines the phenomenology — how heavy the weight seems. In this regard I was puzzled because I thought that the sensation of the heaviness involved was due to peripheral feedback, whereas, if it is dependent on a quantity of motor commands, it is not really peripheral feedback, is it?

Jeannerod: Right. When you lift something in the case of fatigue or partial paralysis, the illusion of an increased weight is due to increased motor commands.

SG: So you would be using more muscle commands to accomplish the same thing that you could accomplish with less muscle when not fatigued or partially paralyzed.

Jeannerod: In normal life, you calibrate the muscle command based on visual cues or cognitive cues — you know that this particular object is heavy.

SG: The idea of a sense of effort and corresponding discharges in the motor system reminds me of Libet's experiments and how they tie into the question of free will. I think you cite his experiments.

Jeannerod: Yes, I like them very much. If one looks in great detail, as Libet has done, at the timing of execution of a voluntary movement, the movement preparation begins 300 or 400 milleseconds prior to the consciousness that you have of it. This duration fits quite well with what we found in our experiment with Castiello (Castiello and Jeannerod 1991; Castiello, Paulignan and Jeannerod 1991) where subjects had to simultaneously reach for an object which suddenly changed its position, and to tell us when they noticed the change. The conscious awareness of the change lagged behind the motor correction to the change by about 350 milliseconds. This means that one can initiate an action non-consciously and become aware later, as we illustrated earlier with your snake anecdote [see p. 62 above]. Of course, what remains unsolved in these experiments is the theoretical issue: how can it be that the brain decides before me?

SG: Right. People say this has to do with free will. But consciousness comes back into it and qualifies what happens unconsciously.

Jeannerod: And in fact this is what Libet tends to say.

We better review the Libet experiments to make sure we understand them (see Libet et al. 1983). One experiment goes like this. Libet places an array of surface electrodes on your scalp to monitor brain activity. He asks you to rest one of your hands on a table top and to flick your wrist whenever you want to. Just before the flick, there is 50 milleseconds of activity in the motor nerves descending from motor cortex to your wrist. But this is preceded by several hundred (500-800) milleseconds of brain activity known as the readiness potential (RP). Libet allows you to view a large clock with a rotating red ball designed to register fractions of a second. He asks you where the red ball is when you decide to move your wrist, or when you were first aware of the urge to do so. The results are that on average, 350 ms before you are conscious of deciding to move, or of having an urge to move, your brain is already working on the motor processes that will result in the movement (Figure 12.1). The readiness potential is already underway before you know that you are going to move.

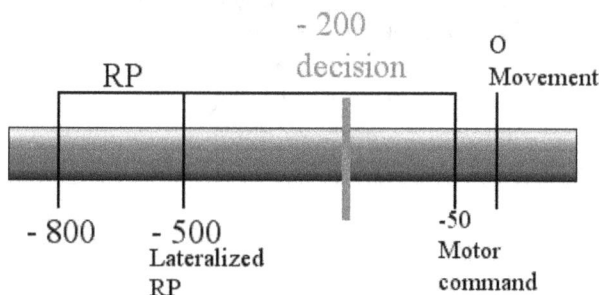

Figure 12.1 Timeline for Libet experiment

Thus, Libet concludes, voluntary acts are 'initiated by unconscious cerebral processes before conscious intention appears' (Libet 1985). Libet continues to the main question: 'The initiation of the freely voluntary act appears to begin in the brain unconsciously, well before the person consciously knows he wants to act. Is there, then, any role for conscious will in the performance of a voluntary act?' Now although some (e.g., Wegner 2002) have used this evidence to argue that free will is an illusion, Libet himself contends that we can still save free will — because there is still approximately 150 ms of brain activity left after we are conscious of our decision, and before we move. We have time to consciously veto the movement — a kind of Libetarian freedom.

SG: Let's go back to something we were talking about earlier, the idea that consciousness is slower than some forms of bodily movement; that some movement is so fast that our consciousness has to play catch up. The experiments with Castiello, for example, show that a subject's motor system will have already made proper adjustments to a target that unexpectedly moves, and these motor adjustments occur prior to the subject's awareness of the movement. In summarizing the results of these experiments you make the following statement (Jeannerod 1997, 86–7). 'The fact that the delay of a visual stimulus remained invariant, whereas the time to the motor response was modulated as a function of the type of task (correcting for a spatial displacement or for a change in object size), reveals that awareness does not depend on a given particular neural system to appear. Instead it is an attribute related to particular behavioral strategies.'

Jeannerod: I was comparing two experiments. In one, the target is displaced at the time where you start moving to it. Your motor system makes a fast adjustment and you correctly grasp the target before being aware of the change. In the second experiment, the size, not the position, of the target is changed at movement onset (we had a system where an object could be suddenly made to appear larger). In this case, the shape of the finger grip has to be changed in time for making a correct grasp. Instead of seeing very fast corrections as we saw for the changes in object position, we found late corrections in grip size, the timing of which came close to the time of consciousness. This is because the timing of corrections for the grasp is much slower than for the reach. The important point is that, although the time to corrections may change according to the type of perturbation, the time to consciousness is invariant.

SG: So there is a delay for the subjective awareness of the change in visual stimulus, and that delay remains invariant across the two situations.

Jeannerod: It remains invariant. Whether it is a change in position or a change in size, it will always take more or less the same time to become aware of that.

SG: Whereas the time to the motor response ...

Jeannerod: ... which is either the time to the adjustment of the reach or to the change in grip size, will be different. The motor system will have to execute very different types of movements in the two situations

SG: The time to that is modulated as a function of the task. That's fine. This reveals that 'awareness does not depend on a given particular neural system to appear'?

Jeannerod: Now I understand your puzzle.

SG: I think I read the emphasis to be on a *particular* neural system in order to appear, and you mean that it is consistent across both of those experimental cases. But then you conclude, 'Instead it is an attribute of a particular behavioral strategy.' This last part is where I am puzzled.

Jeannerod: This is only partly true. Awareness can be shown to depend on the behavioral strategy when you are trying to isolate automatic actions from other aspects of your behavior, mostly in experimental situations. In everyday life, you have a constant flow of consciousness because automatic and controlled strategies, perception and action, etc, always go together.

Willed intentions

Certainly, in our ordinary, everyday tasks we tend to proactively formulate intentions — for example, I may decide to go shopping — and then we carry them out. So we normally think that we are in control of our actions and not just vetoing an action that had been decided by the brain or some force beyond our control. But neuroscientists seem rather insistent on rethinking this. Chris Frith suggests that one function of intentions is precisely to eliminate all the other competing possibilities.

> **Frith:** Every one remembers Libet's demonstration that the brain activity associated with the intention to act precedes the awareness of the intention to act (Libet et al. 1983). But most of us had forgotten (until Patrick Haggard reminded us, Haggard et al. 1999) that Libet also showed that the physical initiation of the act occurs *after* the awareness of the initiation. It seems that the awareness of the initiation and the awareness of the intention are really pulled very close together in this self-monitoring system, giving you a stronger sense that you are controlling your actions. You decide to do something and then, after a very short interval, you do it. There is a series of clever experiments by Dan Wegner (2002) showing that you can mess this system up. The relation between the intention to act and the initiation of the action is simply one of contingency, but we perceive the intention as causing the action. Wegner does experiments where the intention doesn't cause the action, but the subject still experiences causation. One example relates to the controversial technique of

facilitative communication. This has been used with autistic children. You have a helper who puts her hand on top of the child's hand to help him type onto a keyboard, and then you get very unusual things happening. Sometimes a child who has never spoken seemingly starts writing paragraphs or poems. The facilitator is absolutely convinced that it is the child doing this, but there are experiments that show it is in fact the facilitator who is producing the actions. So in this case the facilitator has attached his or her motor initiations to his or her strong beliefs about the child's intentions. Wegner would say that free will is an illusion, because you believe there is this causal relationship between the intention and the action, but it is only a correlation and you can fool people into making mistakes about the causation. I guess that this is the system where something very peculiar is going wrong in patients with schizophrenia.

SG: Can you tell me about some of the experiments that you have been doing in this regard?

Frith: Most of the things I do still derive from my interest in schizophrenia. Schizophrenia is very complex and patients with schizophrenia have many different problems. I think I still believe in the idea that there are three particular problems they have, which relate to different clusters of signs and symptoms. The first of these involve problems with 'willed action'. They have no difficulty responding to external cues but they have great difficulty doing things spontaneously. When I started to do [brain] imaging, one of the first experiments we did was on willed action (Frith et al. 1991). The experiment involved volunteers simply lifting one or other of their fingers. They had to decide which finger they were going to lift each time, in contrast to lifting a predetermined finger. It is a bit like the Libet task, except that the variation in his case was that subjects lifted one finger at whatever time they felt like (Libet et al. 1983). In our experiment the subject chooses between two fingers and the time was set. This is a minimum possible example of choice. And we found activity in the dorsolateral prefrontal cortex (DLPFC). Libet commented on this, that it was not the same as his task, because the volunteers were not allowed to choose the time of their response. But my colleague Marjan Jahanshahi actually did the experiment again so that the subjects were allowed to lift one finger whenever they felt like it, rather than making a choice between fingers, and she also saw activity in DLPFC (Jahanshahi et al. 1995). I remember discussing these experiments with Dick Passingham because one of the problems is that you could say that all we are looking at is working memory rather than choice. In order to be 'spontaneous', you have to remember what you've done before and try to be different. We've been doing various experiments to try to follow up, and I think we've shown that the DLPFC activity relates to choice, not memory. We did an experiment where you have to complete a sentence with the last word missing — you have to provide the missing word (Nathaniel-James and Frith 2002). The trick there is that we have access to this marvelous database of sentences from Bloom and Fischler (1980), in which the constraint for the last word is varied. So you have a sentence like, 'He posted the letter without a _____'. And 99% of American psychology students who express an opinion say 'stamp'. And then you have other sentences like, 'The police have never seen a man so _____'. And I think the commonest response there is 'drunk'. But that is only 9% of the answers. So there are twenty or thirty alternatives. And what you find with this task is that the more alternatives there are available for ending a particular sentence the more activity you see in the DLPFC. In such cases, you don't have to remember what you did last time at all.

SG: The more choices that are intrinsically available, the more activity you get?

Frith: Yes, and actually, the subjects are a bit slower. So that's slightly problematic in its own way. Luckily, as seems often to be the case with me, someone in California had done an experiment just before (Desmond et al. 1998). Instead of using sentences they used word stems. So you saw three letters like 'MOR', and then you had to make a word of that. And you could do exactly the same trick. For something like 'MOV' there is essentially only one possibility, which is 'move' or related words, whereas for 'MOR' there are lots and lots of possibilities, such as 'moral' and 'morbid', and 'more' and so on. The ones with the few alternatives are the difficult ones, and they slow the responses. But in terms of brain activity, you get exactly the same effect. So the more alternatives there are the more activity you see in the DLPFC.

SG: So it's not the degree of difficulty for the task, but the fact that one must make a choice that generates the activity in the prefrontal cortex.

Frith: Yes. I also did an experiment with Marjan, which was an explicit random number generation task (Jahanshahi et al. 2000). So subjects, paced by a metronome, were asked to give a number between 1 and 9. On every tick they had to give a number. Again you find activity in the DLPFC. And what we found here I think is very interesting. If you increase the rate at which you have to do the task, when you get to one number a second, or even two numbers a second, it becomes very difficult, and the randomness, which you can measure, basically by looking at whether they say 1,2 or 7, 8, i.e., numbers in sequential order signifying less randomness, decreases. What I think was very interesting in terms of brain activity was that when it became too difficult and the randomness decreased, so did the activity in the DLPFC. Whereas I had expected, naively, that it would increase because at high rates you would have to work very hard to cope with the problem. What I think is happening is that this is in fact a dual task situation. You have two requirements: to give a response when the signal comes, and to give an appropriately random response. And sometimes you don't have time to come up with the appropriately random response, so you just give the first one that comes into your head, without thinking any further. That suggests that in order to give this inappropriate response, activity in the DLPFC has to be suppressed.

SG: So the activity is inhibited in some way so as to allow for a more automatic, less willed response.

Frith: Yes. So my fantasy is that what this region is doing is specifying an arbitrary collection of suitable responses and suppressing those that are not suitable. The problem with all of this is the homunculus. What is it in there that is making the choice in the end? I think that this formulation is saying that it is not the DLPFC, because all that this region is doing is specifying what is a proper response.

SG: And then something else is actually making the choice.

Frith: Yes, and what I'm wondering about is, does the choice matter at this stage? I mean once you've restricted everything to a subset of possible responses, anyone of these will do. So one could be chosen randomly, being triggered by some external event, or whatever.

SG: So once the possible responses are set, things can go back to automatic again? But if you think of it that way, aren't you saying that it is not really a matter of the will, it's simply a matter of sorting things properly? It's all cognition, and once you're done the cognitive task, things happen automatically and there is no extra thing called the will.

Frith: Yes, that's the way I'm thinking of it. And that would apply even to moral instances, so that there are certain things that I was brought up to know that I should not do.

SG: So when you make a choice, it's simply a matter of eliminating and eliminating until you get it down to the one thing, or a few things, and that's it. But then you have to act on it, you have to put it into effect in some way.

Frith: You mean you have to do the elimination?

SG: I mean, once you have eliminated certain possibilities and discovered just the thing to do, you have to go further and carry through on the action. I'm thinking about moral contexts. So, for example, you might narrow it down and say 'Yes, but I don't really want to do *that*. But I guess I should do it'. So the will pushes you along to the right action.

Frith: Well, my own personal trick in situations like that—I think I discovered that I do this after coming up with some of these formulations—is that if there is something that I think I ought to do but I don't wish to do, which is usually telephoning someone, because I don't like complaining to people especially on the phone, then I say to myself, right, I'm going to do this exactly at 2 o'clock, and then when the clock goes, that's the signal, and I do it automatically. So I try to have an external cue to take over for me.

SG: So you eliminate your free will altogether if you can.

Frith: Right. Or at least you push it back into the past. Going back to the experiments, the pathological groups that have problems with these tasks are those with Parkinson's disease. The crude formulation would be that they know what they want to do, but they have great difficulty in initiating an action in the absence of an external stimulus. Yet they have no, or much less difficulty in responding to a stimulus, so they catch something if it falls off the table. I have no idea what the explanation is, but I guess that in the sort of terminology I'm thinking in, you always have this balance between the elimination of the things you don't want and the activation of the things you do want. I think that in this case, the balance is such that everything gets eliminated, or there's not enough left over to motivate the appropriate action, unless there is an external cue. Parkinson's patients do tricks to provide themselves with external cues. One person, for example, was unable to go across a threshold, but he could if there was a line there to walk over. So he had two walking sticks that he held upside down so the crooks created a line, and he could walk over them. Now in contrast, the patients with late stages of schizophrenia, who have so-called negative features and don't do anything, are different from Parkinson patients. It's not that they know what to do but they can't do it. It's as if they don't actually wish to do anything.

SG: Yes, so on your model, the Parkinson's patients can do the cognitive activity, and figure out what they ought to do, what the choice is, but they just can't put it into effect.

Frith: Yes, and the schizophrenic patients can't work out what it is they are supposed to do. You find a similar thing in frontal patients. In the Wisconsin Card Sorting Test (WCST) you have to switch from one cue to another, so you either sort by color or form. You learn how to sort by color and then the experimenter unbeknown to you switches the rule, so you have to stop using color and use another dimension. Frontal patients perseverate on the old rule. If you ask them about this, however, as Brenda Milner (1963) once reported, they will say, 'Yes, I know that it is not color', but they continue to sort by color. There's an anecdote about a patient with problems of this sort, who was living in the States, I presume, in a house with vicious air conditioning. His wife instructed him to always put on his pullover whenever he comes into the house. He would frequently come into the house and not put on his pullover, and she would say, 'What are you supposed to do when you come into the house'? And he would say, 'Put on my pullover'. Well I think that this kind of schizophrenic patient is similar to that.

SG: So they seem to know what should be done, but they still don't do it, because they can't work out how to go about doing it.

Frith: I think this is also like what Damasio reports about a patient with social difficulties. If you ask him what should you do, whether you should avoid taking up with dubious people, and so on, he will tell you exactly what you should do, but he doesn't actually do it himself. Well they're all a bit like that.

SG: So they have the cognitive part of it, but they are still missing something. But that goes back to the previous question. If you say that all there is is the cognitive part, and once you work out the choice then things go to automatic, there nonetheless seems to be something else that you need to put it into action.

Frith: I think there must be two stages. First you have to use your knowledge to suppress inappropriate responses. This stage seems to fail in some patients with frontal lesions. They know they should suppress the responses, but they don't actually suppress them. Then you have to initiate one of the appropriate responses. I guess that what I would predict is that you need some sort of cue, and in the extreme cases, only external cues will work. The question is whether we manage this by creating virtual cues.

SG: But even cues would not work for the schizophrenic, or for the frontal patient who comes into the house but does not put on his pullover.

Frith: Yes, that's true.

SG: But perhaps he simply does not take that as a cue.

Frith: Yes. In regard to this particular question of willed action, that's where I'm stuck.

SG: In any case, the whole story isn't located in the dorsal lateral prefrontal cortex. There is something else that has to be said.

Frith: Certainly, if I'm right, and it's all about creating this appropriate selection of responses, then we haven't identified the key element of will, if there is such a thing.

SG: So that's where you are in regard to willed action.

Frith: Yes. But let me note that in the last few years the study of decision-making has been revolutionized by new work on reward systems in the brain and by bringing in ideas from economics: Neuroeconomics (see, e.g., Schultz 2006; Fehr and Camerer 2007).

Freedom, responsibility, and the ability to thwart the brain

The positions of Libet and Frith are very similar. In both cases one is put in a position (by one's brain) to either allow the action to proceed or to veto it. And you don't have much time to do it in. Frith also points out that there are various ways things can go wrong if something is not just right with your brain. Whether the brain is properly functioning or not, however, since it is the brain that is doing most of the work, seemingly delivering a short menu of things you can allow happen or prevent, it's not clear how extensive we can conceive moral responsibility to be.

Libet's experiments have made a great impact on the field of neuroscience and how contemporary researchers are thinking about free will. Thomas Ramsøy, in his interview with Christof Koch asks about the fact that some of what we consider to be the decision making processes in the brain work below the level of consciousness. Doesn't this contradict our everyday experience of agency?

> **Koch:** Well, yes, but we knew that at least since Benjamin Libet's seminal experiments on the readiness potential that can appear many hundreds of milliseconds before the subject became aware of wanting to initiate the action on the surface of her brain (and can be picked up by EEG electrodes). Something in her brain made the decision to lift the arm or whatever else the voluntary action consisted of and this decision was only later communicated to the stages of the brain accessible to conscious perception of agency or authorship.
>
> Immanuel Kant had argued two centuries earlier against the possibility of a physical event occurring without a prior, physical cause,

that is, against the idea of a truly free will. Every scientist knows perfectly well that whenever something happens somewhere at sometime, this event has to be caused by something else (or a combination of other factors; the universe is causally closed as the philosophers like to say).

Yet, of course, I perfectly well feel that I am in charge, that it is me, Christof, that decided to type this text on my laptop. That is, from a psychological point of view, my actions are not predetermined (in general, and excluding things like rage, intoxication etc). The question is what are the neuronal correlates of this conscious feeling of agency, of being in charge? What are the computational algorithms that are underlying its outputs and what are the sources of information this module uses (prior intentions, sensory-motor feedback, efference copy signals and so on)? All of these are experimentally accessible questions.

The successful conclusion of my quest, identifying and understanding the neuronal correlates of all aspects of consciousness, is bound to have significant consequences for ethics. They may give rise to a new conception of what it is to be human, a view that might radically contradict the traditional images that men and women have made of themselves throughout the ages.

Ramsøy: This also points to the function of consciousness. In the free will discussion, one could ask why we should have a sense of agency at all, if it is really an after-the-fact phenomenon. Actions, if they are indeed selected and executed without our awareness, would function just the same. What function do you think the sense of agency plays? And would you say that the sense of agency is thus an illusion of free will?

Koch: It is important to point out that this tension between the causal closedness of the universe—nothing from outside the universe can cause anything within it to happen—and the perceived freedom of action is a major, unresolved empirical and theoretical problem. One solution is to argue that all agency is illusory. While under laboratory conditions, it can be shown that some free acts are influenced—in an unconscious manner—by previous ones, the assumed illusory nature of free will simply does not accord with our everyday experience in which I choose one course of action over another. As John Searle has remarked somewhere, I don't go to a restaurant, look at the menu, and then tell the waiter 'I'm a determinist, I'll just wait and see what I order.'

For those who believe that free will does not exist, the perception of agency must carry some evolutionary function. Dan Wegner has suggested that it gives the system a sense of purpose, that it will act in the world on the belief that its action can influence events. Think of the difference between an optimist, who thinks that by acting he can make a difference in the world, and a pessimist, who thinks that all is lost and nothing really makes a difference. Who will shape the future more? Surely the optimist, because he tries, even if half of the time the outcome is negative. And so it may be with the sense of freedom of action.

Michael Gazzaniga defends the concept of free will on similar pragmatic grounds. Going back to the idea that our personal narrative is generated by a left-hemisphere interpreter, there is still a question of whether we control it. From the neuroscientific perspective Gazzaniga takes a determinist viewpoint. You will recall, however, that Gazzaniga takes a pragmatic view on personal responsibility—that people behave better when they believe they are in charge of their own behavior, and in this regard he cites an argument made by MacKay. MacKay's argument is that if I have complete knowledge of the present state of your brain, and of all the laws that your brain follows, and of all the inputs between now and some time in the future, x, I should be able to predict your action at x. But if you know the prediction, you can simply do something different at x. So in some sense you are not determined by your brain.

SG: Let's look again at MacKay's argument. The only way I could predict with certainty that you were going to eat a Big Mac at noon is if I knew your current brain state and all of the inputs to the system that will come along between now and noon. Since right now I can't know all of the precise inputs that will occur between now and noon, I can't really predict anything about your action with a large degree of certainty. But even assuming perfect knowledge, my prediction itself, if it is known to you, is another input that I would have to consider in my prediction. At that point we have an obvious paradox involving public predictions. Perhaps we could we get around that difficulty by placing the prediction in a sealed envelope in a public place. If we did that, there are still two possible outcomes. (1) My prediction might be right, and this might count as evidence for your lack of free will. (2) My prediction might be wrong, because I still might not know all of the social and environmental inputs—you might get in an accident on the way to MacDonalds. The fact that my prediction is wrong does not show that you have free will, it shows that I don't have enough information.

Gazzaniga: MacKay's point is that in order for your prediction to be true for everyone it has to made available to me as well. There is no such thing as a private set of Kepler's laws. They are true because they hold for one and all. That means you can have no secret predictions. And in MacKay's hands he jumps ahead of the current problem of knowing all the inputs, etc. He assumes someday brain scientists will know this sort of thing. So, at this point I really can't find a problem with his analysis. His classic paper, 'Freedom of Action in a Mechanistic Universe' (1967), spells out the issue in detail. And as a result, I still stand with the idea of the great importance of taking moral responsibility for one's actions.

Actually the paradox involved in public predictions may even support MacKay's conclusion. Let's assume there are two people, A and B, and that they have perfect knowledge about the brain and happen to know what all of the inputs into their own and the other person's brain will be over the next hour. That means that A can predict that in five minutes B is going to predict what A is going to be doing at the end of the hour. Let's leave aside the problem of infinite regress that we get into right here—A predicts that B is going to predict; and of course B knows that A has predicted his prediction; and A also must know that B knows, etc. That aside, it would follow from MacKay's argument that successful predictions would never be possible in this situation, since if A knows what B is predicting, A can thwart the prediction by doing something different. Since B knows that A can thwart the prediction, but also has perfect knowledge about A's brain, etc., he should also know whether A will thwart his prediction or not. If he knows that A is going to thwart his prediction, he has to change his prediction. But A will also know that and can thwart his new prediction by fulfilling the original one. This suggests that B can never successfully predict what A is going to do (or that there can never be true predictions in this regard), which supports MacKay's conclusion anyway.

Of course we should keep three things in mind. First, we don't have perfect knowledge (and let's make the more realistic assumption that we never will given that we are finite humans). Second, that's part of the problem. The problem is not about someone making predictions; it's about us not knowing enough about the brain or the current and future states of the system to thwart what the brain is deciding for us. The real issue is not between A and B, but between A and his brain. A can only thwart B's predictions because he has perfect knowledge about brains; but he can neither thwart B's predictions or his own brain if he does not have perfect knowledge about brains. The upshot of this would be that until we gain perfect knowledge about our brains, we don't have the wherewithall to thwart its 'decisions'—we don't have free will. Third, and most importantly, all of this is based on the premise that the brain does in fact decide what we are going to do before we know it. That's what motivates MacKay's argument in the first place. But is this premise justified?

In defense of free will

We are still faced with the problem of making free will consistent with the idea that the brain does its work before we become aware of it. Faced with the Libet experiments, and many other facts of behavior (see Wegner 2002), is it a problem for ethical accounts of moral responsibility to say that the brain not only decides and enacts in a preconscious fashion, but also inventively tricks consciousness into thinking that we consciously decide matters and that our actions are personal events? Is free will nothing more than the illusion of free will, as Wegner proposes?

I've argued elsewhere that the mistake is to think of free will in terms of the very short time frame of milliseconds involved in the brain processes Libet was measuring (see Gallagher 2005; 2006). Once we understand that deliberation and decision are processes that are spread out over longer time periods, even if, in some cases, relatively short amounts of time, then there is plenty of room for conscious components that are more than accessories after the fact. To the extent that consciousness enters into the ongoing production of action, and contributes to the production of further action, *even if significant aspects of this production takes place nonconsciously*, our actions are intentional and to some extent under our free control. As Gazzaniga's work shows, some kind of self-interpretation comes into the process and introduces a temporally extended 'looping effect' (Hacking 1995). That is, conscious deliberation by the agent, which involves memory and knowledge about the world, has real effects on behavior, and it does so by changing the brain states of the agent, among other things. Our lives are not composed of a series of automatic reactions, like the super-fast amygdala reaction to a snake in the grass. Even if we experience such a reaction after the brain causes it, we do *experience* it, and we consciously realize what just happened and why. This consciousness, however, goes on to shape what we do about it. I could, for example, decide to catch the snake for my snake collection, and no one could say that this is merely an action that is caused by neurons firing, since it already depends on my becoming conscious of the snake and consciously deciding something in reference to my snake collection, and since the snake and the snake collection that motivate me are part of the world and not reducible to firing neurons, and my ability to reach and to grasp are dependent on something other than just my brain.

What we call free will cannot be conceived as something instantaneous, a knife-edge moment located between being undecided and being decided. If that were the case it would indeed completely dissipate in the three hundred and fifty milliseconds between a brain event and our conscious awareness. Free will involves temporally extended feedback or looping effects that are transformed and enhanced by the introduction of interpretational consciousness, and the kind of situated reflection that can engage. This means that the conscious sense of free will, even if it did start out as an illusion or accessory generated by the brain, is itself a real force that counts as further input in the formation of our future action, makes that action free, and bestows responsibility on the agent. To paraphrase Jean-Paul Sartre, no more is needed in the way of a philosophical foundation for an ethics (see Sartre 1957, 106). In contrast to Sartre, however, this doesn't give us anything close to an absolute freedom or an absolute responsibility since, as Leibniz suggested, the subject is not absolute consciousness but subject to an infinity of perceptions and continuous brainstorms.

References

Abell, F., Krams, M., Ashburner, J., Passingham, R., Friston, K., Frackowiak, R., Happé, F., Frith, C.D. and Frith, U. (1999), 'The neuroanatomy of autism: A voxel-based whole brain analysis of structural scans', *NeuroReport*, 10, pp. 1647–51.

Aglioti, S., DeSouza, J.F.X. and Goodale, M.A. (1995), 'Size contrast illusions deceive the eye but not the hand', *Current Biology*, 5 (6), pp. 679–85.

Arbib, M.A. (1964/1987), *Brains, Machines, and Mathematics* (New York: Springer).

Arbib, M.A. (1972), *The Metaphorical Brain: An Introduction to Cybernetics as Artificial Intelligence and Brain Theory* (New York: Wiley-Interscience).

Arbib, M.A. (1981), 'Perceptual structures and distributed motor control', in *Handbook of Physiology, Section 2: The Nervous System, Vol. II, Motor Control, Part 1*, ed. V.B. Brooks (American Physiological Society).

Arbib, M.A. (1982), 'Rana Computatrix: An evolving model of visuo-motor coordination in frog and toad', in *Machine Intelligence* 10, ed. J.E. Hayes, D.Michie and Y.H. Pao (Chichester: Ellis Horwood Publishers).

Arbib, M.A. (1985a), *In Search of the Person: Philosophical Explorations in Cognitive Science* (Amherst, MA: University of Massachusetts Press).

Arbib, M.A. (1985b), 'Schemas for the temporal organization of behaviour', *Human Neurobiology*, 4, pp. 63–72.

Arbib, M.A. (1999), 'Crusoe's brain: Of solitude and society', in *Neuroscience and the Person: Scientific Perspectives on Divine Action*, ed. Russell, R.J., Murphy, N., Meyering, T.C., and Arbib, M.A. (Vatican City State: Vatican Observatory Publications/Berkeley, CA: Center for Theology and the Natural Sciences).

Arbib, M.A. (2002), 'The mirror system, imitation, and the evolution of language', in *Imitation in Animals and Artifacts*, ed. C. Nehaniv and K. Dautenhahn (Cambridge, MA: The MIT Press).

Arbib, M.A. (2003), 'Rana computatrix to human language: Towards a computational neuroethology of language evolution', *Phil. Trans. R. Soc. Lond. A*, 361, pp. 2345–79.

Arbib, M. A. (2005), 'From monkey-like action recognition to human language: An evolutionary framework for neurolinguistics, *Behavioral and Brain Sciences* 28, pp. 105–167.

Arbib, M. A. (2008), 'From grasp to language: Embodied concepts and the challenge of abstraction. *Journal of Physiology* (Paris).

Arbib, M.A., Billard, A., Iacoboni,M. and Oztop, E. (2000), 'Synthetic brain imaging: Grasping, mirror neurons and imitation', *Neural Networks*, 13, pp. 975–97.

Arbib, M.A., Bischoff, A., Fagg, A.H. and Grafton, S.T. (1994), 'Synthetic PET: Analyzing large-scale properties of neural networks', *Human Brain Mapping*, 2, pp. 225–33.

Arbib, M.A. and Caplan, D. (1979), 'Neurolinguistics must be computational', *Behavioral and Brain Sciences*, 2, pp. 449–83.

Arbib, M.A., Conklin, E.J. and Hill, J.C. (1987), From Schema Theory to Language (Oxford: OUP).

Arbib, M.A., Fagg, A.H. and Grafton, S.T. (2003), 'Synthetic PET imaging for grasping: From primate neurophysiology to human behavior', in *Exploratory Analysis and Data Modeling in Functional Neuroimaging*, ed. F.T. Sommer and A. Wichert (Cambridge, MA: The MIT Press), pp. 231–250.

Arbib, M. A. and Fellous, J. M. (2004), 'Emotions: from brain to robot', *Trends in Cognitive Sciences*, 8(12), pp. 554–561.

Arbib, M.A. and Hesse, M.B. (1986), *The Construction of Reality* (Cambridge: Cambridge University Press).

Arbib, M.A. and Hoff B (1994), 'Trends in neural modeling for reach to grasp', in *From Insights Into Reach To Grasp Movement*, ed. K.M.B. Bennett and U. Castiello (Elsevier Science B.V.).

Arbib, M.A., Iberall, T. and Lyons, D.M. (1985), *Coordinated Control Programs for Movements of the Hand Exp. Brain Res.* #10 (Berlin: Springer-Verlag).

Arbib, M.A., Iberall, T. and Lyons, D.M. (1987), 'Schemas that integrate vision and touch for hand control', in *Vision, Brain and Cooperative Computation*, ed. Arbib, M.A., Hanson, A.R. (Cambridge, MA: MIT Press).

Arbib, M.A. and Manes, E.G. (1974), 'Foundations of system theory: decomposable systems', *Automatica*, 10, pp. 285–302 .

Armstrong, D. (1968), *A Materialist Theory of the Mind* (London: Routledge).

Auvray, M., C. Lenay, et al. (2006), 'The attribution of intentionality in a simulated environment: the case of minimalist devices', Paper presented, Tenth Meeting of the Association for the Scientific Study of Consciousness, Oxford, UK.

Baars, B.J. (1997), *In the Theater of Consciousness: The workspace of the mind* (New York: Oxford University Press).

Baillargeon, R., Spelke, E.S. and Wasserman, S. (1985), 'Object permanence in five-month-old infants', *Cognition*, 20, pp. 191–208.

Baron-Cohen, S. (1995), *Mindblindness* (Cambridge: MIT Press).

Bartlett, F.C. (1932), *Remembering* (Cambridge: Cambridge University Press).

Beck, D.M., Rees, G., Frith, C.D. and Lavie, N. (2001), 'Neural correlates of change detection and change blindness', *Nature Neuroscience*, 4, pp. 645–50.

Beer, R.D. (1990), *Intelligence As Adaptive Behavior: An Experiment In Computational Neuroethology* (San Diego, CA: Academic Press).

Benvenuto, S. (2001), La coscienza nelle neuroscienze: Interviste, Francisco Varela. Enciclopedia Multimediale delle Scienze Filosofiche 7 (http://www.emsf.rai.it/interviste/interviste.asp?d=452); translated by T. Bruce (2002), Consciousness in the neurosciences: A conversation with Francisco Varela. *Journal of European Psychoanalysis* 14 (http://www.psychomedia.it/jep/number14/varela.htm). .

Billard, A., Robins, B., Dautenhahn, K. and Nadel, J. (2006), 'Building Robota, a mini-humanoid robot for the rehabilitation of children with autism', *RESNA Assistive Technology Journal*. 19 (1).

Blakemore, S.-J. and Decety, J. (2001), 'From the perception of action to the understanding of intention', *Nature Reviews: Neuroscience* 2, pp. 561–7.

Blakemore, S.J., Smith, J., Steel, R., Johnstone, E.C. and Frith, C.D. (2000), 'The perception of self-produced sensory stimuli in patients with auditory hallucinations and passivity experiences: evidence for a breakdown in self-monitoring', *Psychological Medicine*, 30, pp. 1131–9.

Blakemore, S.J., Wolpert, D.M. and Frith, C.D. (1998), 'Central cancellation of self-produced tickle sensation', *Nature Neuroscience*, 1, pp. 635–40.

Blakemore, S.-J., Wolpert, D. & Frith, C.D. (2000), 'Why can't you tickle yourself?', *NeuroReport*, 11, R11–R16 .

Blakeslee, S. (2006), 'Cells that read minds', *New York Times*, January 10, 2006. http://www.nytimes.com/2006/01/10/science/10mirr.html. Accessed January 2006; May 2007.

Block. N. (1995), 'On a Confusion about a Function of Consciousness', *Behavioral and Brain Sciences*, 18 (2), pp. 227–287.

Bloom, P.A., Fischler, I. (1980), 'Completion norms for 329 sentences', *Memory and Cognition* 8, pp. 631–42.

Bonaiuto, J., Rosta, E. & Arbib, M. (2007), 'Extending the mirror neuron system model, I: Audible actions and invisible grasps', *Biol Cybern* 96, pp. 9–38.

Bosbach, S., Cole, J.D., Prinz, W. and Knoblich, G. (2005), Inferring another's expectation from action: the role of peripheral sensation. *Nature Neuroscience*, 8, 1295-1297.

Boulton, D. (2007), 'Language, writing, mind, and consciousness: An interview with John Searle', *Children of the Code*,
(http://www.childrenofthecode.org/interviews/searle.htm).

Braitenberg, V. (1965), 'Taxis, kinesis and decussation', *Progress in Brain Research*, 17, pp. 210–22.

Braitenberg, V. (1984), *Vehicles: Experiments in Synthetic Psychology* (Cambridge, MA: MIT Press).

Braitenberg, V. and Onesto, N. (1960), 'The cerebellar cortex as a timing organ', *Congress Inst Medicina Cibernetica, First Naples Atti.*, pp. 239–55.

Brandt, P. A. (2004), *Spaces, Domains, And Meaning: Essays In Cognitive Semiotics*, European Semiotics, Vol. 4. (Peter Lang Publishing).

Brentano, F. (1973), *Psychology from an Empirical Standpoint*, trans. A. C. Rancurello, D. B. Terrell & L.L. McAlister (London: Routledge & Kegan Paul).

Brooks, R. A. (1988), 'Intelligence without Representation', in J. Haugeland (ed.), *Mind Design* (Cambridge, MA: The MIT Press), pp. 395–420.

Brockman, J. (1995), *The Third Culture: Beyond the Scientific Revolution*. New York: Simon & Schuster.

Brockman, J. (1997), 'Parallel memories: Putting emotions back into the brain: A talk with Joseph LeDoux', *Edge* (http://www.edge.org/3rd_culture/ledoux/ledoux_p1.html).

Brockman, J. (2001), 'The computational perspective: A talk with Daniel C. Dennett', *Edge* (http://www.edge.org/video/dsl/dennett.html).

Browning, R. (1895). 'How They Brought the Good News from Ghent to Aix' in C. W. Eliot (ed.), *English Poetry III: From Tennyson to Whitman*. Harvard Classics, Vol. 42 (New York: P.F. Collier & Son, 1909–14; Bartleby.com, 2001).

Bruner, J. (2004), Life as narrative, *Social Research* 71, 691–710.

Cahill, C., Silbersweig, D. and Frith, C.D. (1996), 'Psychotic experiences induced in deluded patients using distorted auditory feedback', *Cognitive Neuropsychiatry* 1, pp. 201–11.

Calder, A., Keane, J., Cole, J.D., Campbell, R. and Young, A. (2000), 'Facial identity and expression recognition in Moebius Syndrome', *Cognitive Neuropsychology* 17, (1/2/3), 73–87.

Calvin, W. H. and Ojemann, G. A. (1980), *Inside the Brain: Mapping the Cortex, Exploring the Neuron* (New York: New American Library).

Carruthers, P. (1996), *Language, Thoughts and Consciousness. An essay in philosophical psychology* (Cambridge: Cambridge University Press).

Castiello, U. and Jeannerod, M. (1991), 'Measuring time to awareness', *Neuroreport*, 2, pp. 797-800.

Castiello, U., Paulignan, Y. and Jeannerod, M. (1991), 'Temporal dissociation of motor responses and subjective awareness: A study of normal subjects', *Brain*, 114, pp. 2639-55.

Chalmers, D. (1995), 'Facing up to the problem of consciousness', *Journal of Consciousness Studies*, 2, pp. 200-19.

Chalmers, D. (1996), *The Conscious Mind. In Search of a Fundamental Theory* (New York: Oxford University Press).

Chaminade, T. and Decety, J. (2002), 'Leader or follower? Involvement of the inferior parietal lobule in agency', *Neuroreport* 13 (1528), pp. 1975-78.

Clark, A. (1997), *Being There: Putting Brain, Body, and World Together Again* (Cambridge, MA: MIT Press).

Clark, A. and Grush, R. (1999), 'Towards a cognitive robotics', *Adaptive Behavior*, 7 (1), pp. 5-16.

Clements, W.A. and Perner, J. (1994), 'Implicit Understanding of Belief', *Cognitive Development*, 9 (4), pp. 377-95.

Cliff, D. (1992), 'Neural networks for visual tracking in an artificial fly', in *Towards a Practice for Autonomous Systems: Proceedings of the First European Conference on Artificial Life* (ECAL91), ed F. Varela and P. Bourgine (Cambridge, MA: MIT Press).

Coetzee, J.M. (2003), *Elizabeth Costello* (New York: Viking).

Cole, J.D. (1995), *Pride and a Daily Marathon* (Cambridge, MA: MIT Press) .

Cole, J. (1998), *About Face* (Cambridge, MA: The MIT Press).

Cole, J. (2004), *Still Lives: Narratives of Spinal Cord Injury* (Cambridge, MA: The MIT Press).

Cole, J.D. Gallagher, S. and McNeill, D. (2002). 'Gesture following deafferentation: A phenomenologically informed experimental study', *Phenomenology and the Cognitive Sciences*, 1 (1), pp. 49–67.

Cole, J., Gallagher, S., McNeill, D., Duncan S., Furuyama, N. and McCullough, K-E. (1998), 'Gestures after total deafferentation of the bodily and spatial senses', in S. Santi et al. (ed.), *Oralité et gestualité: Communication multi-modale, interaction* (Paris: L'Harmattan), pp. 65–69.

Cole, J.D. and Sedgwick, E.M. (1992), 'The perceptions of force and of movement in a man without largemyelinated sensory afferents below the neck', *Journal of Physiology*, 449, pp. 503–15.

Cole, J.D., Merton, L.W., Barrett, G., Treede, R.-D., Katifi, H. (1995), 'Evoked potentials in a deafferented subject', *Canadian Journal of Physiology and Pharmacology*, 73, pp. 234–45.

Corcoran, R., Mercer, G. and Frith, C.D. (1995), 'Schizophrenia, symptomatology and social inference: Investigating "theory of mind" in people with schizophrenia', *Schizophrenia Research*, 17, pp. 5–13.

Cotterill, R.M.J. (1998), *Enchanted Looms: Conscious Networks in Brains and Computers* (Cambridge: Cambridge University Press).

Crace, J. (2007), Jerome Bruner: The lesson of the story, *The Guardian* (27 March 2007). http://education.guardian.co.uk/higher/profile/story/0,,2043337,00.html.

Craik, K. (1943), *The Nature of Explanation* (Cambridge: Cambridge University Press).

Crick, F. & Koch, C. (1995), 'Are we aware of neural activity in primary visual cortex?' *Nature*, 375, pp. 121–123.

Crick, F. & Koch, C. (2000), 'The unconscious homunculus', in *The Neuronal Correlates of Consciousness*, T. Metzinger (ed.), pp. 103–110 (Cambridge: MIT Press).

Csibra, G. (2005), 'Mirror neurons and action observation. Is simulation involved?' *ESF Interdisciplines*. http://www.interdisciplines.org/mirror/papers/.

Churchland, P. S. (1986), *Neurophilosophy* (Cambridge, MA: MIT Press).

Damasio, A.R. (1994), *Descartes' Error: Emotion, Reason, and the Human Brain* (New York: Putnam Publishing).

Damasio, A. (1997), 'Thinking and feeling: Review of LeDoux's The Emotional Brain', *Scientific American* June 1997. (http://world.std.com/%7Eawolpert/gtr400.html).

Damasio, A.R. (1999), *The Feeling of What Happens: Body and Emotion in the Making of Consciousness* (New York: Harcourt Brace & Company).

Davidson, D. (2001), *Essays on Actions and Events* (Oxford: Clarendon Press).

Dautenhahn, K. (2006), 'Interview', BBC News, 27 January 2006, http://news.bbc.co.uk/1/hi/magazine/4654332.stm.

Davis, E. (1994), 'Mind Waves: An Interview with Francisco Varela', originally appeared in *Shamballah Sun*, 1994 (http://purifymind.com/MindWaves.htm).

Decety, J. (2002), 'Naturaliser l'empathie', *L'Encéphale*, 28, pp. 9–20.

Decety, J. (2003), 'L'empathie ou l'émotion partagée', *Pour La Science*, 309, pp. 46–51.

Decety, J. (2004), 'Empathie et mentalisation a la lumiere des neurosciences sociales', *Neuropsychiatrie: Tendances et Debats*, 23, pp. 25–35.

Decety, J. (2005), 'Perspective taking as the royal avenue to empathy', in: Malle, B.F., Hodges, S.D. (Eds.), *Other Minds: How Humans Bridge the Divide between Self and Other* (New York: Guilford Publications), pp. 135–149.

Decety, J. and Grèzes, J. (2006), 'The power of simulation: Imagining one's own and other's behavior', *Brain Research*, 1079(1), pp. 4–14.

Decety, J., Grèzes, J., Costes, N., Perani, D., Jeannerod, M., Procyk, E., Grassi, F. and Fazio, F. (1997), 'Brain activity during observation of actions: Influence of action content and subject's strategy', *Brain*, 120, pp. 1763–77.

Decety, J. and Jackson, P. L. (2004), 'The functional architecture of human empathy. *Behavioral and Cognitive Neuroscience Reviews* 3 (2), pp. 71–100.

Decety, J. and Jeannerod, M. (1996), 'Fitts' law in mentally simulated movements', *Behavioral Brain Research*, 72, pp. 127–36.

Decety, J. Perani, D., Jeannerod, M., Bettinardi, V., Tadary, B.,Woods, R., Mazziotta, J.C. and Fazio, F. (1994), 'Mapping motor representations with PET', *Nature*, 371, pp. 600–2.

Dehaene, S. & Naccache, L. (2001), 'Towards a cognitive neuroscience of consciousness: basic evidence and a workspace framework', *Cognition*, 79, pp. 1–37.

Dennett, D. C. (1969), *Content and Consciousness* (London: Routledge and Kegan Paul). .

Dennett, D. C. (1971) 'Intentional systems', *The Journal of Philosophy* 68 (4), pp. 87–106.

Dennett, D. (1988), 'Why everyone is a novelist', *Times Literary Supplement* Sept.16-22, pp. 1016, 1028–1029.

Dennett, D.C. (1991), *Consciousness Explained* (Boston, MA: Little, Brown & Co.).

Dennett, D.C. (1994), 'Tiptoeing past the covered wagons: A response to Carr', in 'Dennett and Carr Further Explained: an exchange', Emory Cognition Project, Report #28, Department of Psychology, Emory University, Apr. 1994; and at http://cogprints.org/278/0/tiptoe.htm.

Dennett, D. (2003), 'Who's on first? Heterophenomenology explained' *Journal of Consciousness Studies* 10 (9–10), pp. 19–30.

Descartes, R. (1641), Meditationes de prima philosophia: In *qua Dei existentia, et animæ humanæ à corpore distinctio, demonstratur.* (http://www.wright.edu/cola/descartes/medl.html).

Descartes, R. (1643), 'Letter to Elizabeth on May 21, 1643', in M. Atherton (ed.), *Women Philosophers of the Early Modern Period* (Indianapolis: Hackett, 1994), pp. 12–15.

Descartes, R. (1649), The Passions of the Soul (I, XXXI). In E.S. Haldane and G.R.T. Ross (ed.), *The Philosophical Works of Descartes* v. 1 (Cambridge: Cambridge University Press, 1969).

Descartes, R. (1958), *Philosophical Writings*, ed. and trans. N. K. Smith (New York: Modern Library).

Desmond, J.E., Gabrieli, J.D.E. and Glover, G.H. (1998), 'Dissociation of frontal and cerebellar activity in a cognitive task: Evidence for a distinction between selection and search', *Neuroimage* 7, pp. 368–76.

De Jaegher, H. 2006, 'Social interaction rhythm and participatory sense-making: An embodied, interactional approach to social understanding, with some implications for autism. Ph.D. Thesis, Sussex University. .

de Waal, F. and Thompson, E. (2005). 'Primates, monks and the mind: The case of empathy', interview by J. Proctor, *Journal of Consciousness Studies*, 12 (7), pp. 38–54. .

Dewey, J. (1928), 'Body and mind', *Bulletin of the New York Academy of Medicine*, 4, pp. 3–19.

DeYoe, E.A., Felleman, D.J., Van Essen, D.C. & McClendon, E. (1994), 'Multiple processing streams in occipitotemporal visual cortex', *Nature* 371, pp. 151–154.

Didday, R.L. (1970), 'The simulation and modeling of distributed information processing in the frog visual system', PhD Thesis, Stanford University.

Di Paolo, E. A. (2000), 'Behavioural coordination, structural congruence and entrainment in a simulation of acoustically coupled agents', *Adaptive Behaviour* 8(1), pp. 27–48. .

Di Paolo, E. A., Rohde, M. and Iizuka, H. (2008). Sensitivity to social contingency or stability of interaction? Modelling the dynamics of perceptual crossing, *New Ideas in Psychology*, doi:10.1016/j.newideapsych.2007.07.006 (http://www.informatics.sussex.ac.uk/users/ezequiel/newideas.pdf).

Di Pellegrino, G. Fadiga, L., Fogassi, L., Gallese, V. and Rizzolatti, G. (1992), 'Understanding motor events: a neurophysiological study', *Exp. Brain Res.* 91, pp. 176–180.

Dreyfus, H. and Dennett, D. (1997), 'Big Blue Wins', *The News Hour*, 12 May 1997 – ghttp://www.pbs.org/newshour/bb/entertainment/janjune97/ big_blue_5-12.html.

Dreyfus, H. (2002), 'Intelligence without representation Merleau-Ponty's critique of mental representation: The relevance of phenomenology to scientific explanation', *Phenomenology and the Cognitive Sciences* 1, pp. 367–383.

Dreyfus, H. (2007), 'Why Heideggerian AI failed and how fixing it would require making it more Heideggerian', *Artificial Intelligence* 171 (18), pp. 1137–1160.

Eccles, J.C., Ito, M. and Szentágothai, J. (1967), *The Cerebellum as a Neuronal Machine* (New York: Springer Verlag).

Edelman, G. (1993), *Bright Air, Brilliant Fire* (New York: Basic Books). .

Fadiga, L., Fogassi, L. Pavesi, G. and Rizzolatti, G. (1995), 'Motor facilitation during action observation: a magnetic stimulation study', *Journal of Neurophysiology*, 73, pp. 2608–2611.

Faillenot, I. Decety, J. & Jeannerod, M. (1999), 'Human brain activity related to the perception of spatial features of objects', *Neuroimage*, 10, pp. 114–24.

Farrer, C., Franck, N. Georgieff, N. Frith, C.D. Decety, J. and Jeannerod, M. (2003), 'Modulating the experience of agency: a positron emission tomography study', *Neuroimage* 18, pp. 324–333.

Farrer, C. and Frith, C.D. (2001), 'Experiencing oneself vs. another person as being the cause of an action: the neural correlates of the experience of agency', *NeuroImage* 15, pp. 596–603.

Fauconnier, G. and Turner, M. (2002), *The Way We Think: Conceptual Blending and the Mind's Hidden Complexities* (New York: Basic Books).

Fauconnier, G. and Turner, M. (in press), 'Rethinking metaphor', In Ray Gibbs, ed. *Cambridge Handbook of Metaphor and Thought* (Cambridge: Cambridge University Press).

Fehr, E., and Camerer, C. F. (2007), 'Social neuroeconomics: the neural circuitry of social preferences', *Trends Cogn Sci* 11, pp. 419–427.

Felleman, D.J. & Van Essen, D.C. (1991), 'Distributed hierarchical processing in the primate cerebral cortex'. *Cereb. Cortex*, 1, pp. 1–47.

Fellous, J.-M. & LeDoux, J. E. (2005), Toward Basic Principles for Emotional Processing: What the Fearful Brain Tells the Robot. In J.-M. Fellous & J. E. LeDoux (eds.), *Who Needs Emotion* (Oxford: Oxford University Press), pp. 79–116.

Feser, E. and Postrel, S. 2000, 'Reality principles: An Interview with John R. Searle', *Reasononline 2000*, http://www.reason.com/news/show/27599.html.

Flanagan, O. (1993), *Consciousness Reconsidered* (Cambridge, MA: MIT Press).

Flor, H., Denke, C., Schaefer,M., Grusser, S. (2001), 'Effect of sensory discrimination training on cortical reorganisation and phantom limb pain', *Lancet*, 357 (9270), pp. 1763–4.

Fodor, Jerry A. (1981), *RePresentations* (Cambridge, MA: MIT Press).

Fogassi, L., Ferrari, P.F., Gesierich, B., Rozzi, S., Chersi, F. and Rizzolatti, G. (2005), 'Parietal lobe: from action organization to intention understanding', *Science* 308, pp. 662–667.

Fogel, A. (1993), 'Two principles of communication: co-regulation and framing', in J. Nadel and L. Camaioni (eds.), *New Perspectives in Early Communicative Development* (London, Routledge).

Ford, J. M., and Mathalon, D. H. (2004), 'Electrophysiological evidence of corollary discharge dysfunction in schizophrenia during talking and thinking', *Journal of Psychiatric Research*, 38, pp. 37–46.

Fourneret, P. and Jeannerod, M. (1998), 'Limited conscious monitoring of motor performance in normal subjects', *Neuropsychologia*, 36 (11), pp. 1133–40.

Fourneret, P., Paillard, J., Lamarre, Y., Cole, J., Jeannerod, M. (2002), 'Lack of conscious knowledge about one's own actions in a haptically deafferented patient', *Neuroreport*, 13 (4), pp. 541–7.

Frak, V.G., Paulignan, Y. and Jeannerod, M. (2001), 'Orientation of the opposition axis in mentally simulated grasping', *Experimental Brain Research*, 136, pp. 120–27.

Freedberg D. and Gallese V. (2007), 'Motion, emotion and empathy in esthetic experience', *Trends in Cognitive Sciences*, 11, pp. 197–203.

Freud, S. (1960), *Jokes and their relation to the unconscious*, trans. J. Strachey. (New York: Norton).

Frith, C.D. (1992), *The Cognitive Neuropsychology of Schizophrenia* (Hillsdale, NJ: Lawrence Erlbaum Associates).

Frith, C. D. (2007), *Making up the Mind: How the Brain Creates our Mental World* (Oxford: Blackwell).

Frith, C.D., Blakemore, S.J. and Wolpert, D. (2000), 'Explaining the symptoms of schizophrenia: Abnormalities in the awareness of action', *Brain Research Reviews*, 31, pp. 357-63 .

Frith, C.D. and Done, D.J. (1988), 'Towards a neuropsychology of schizophrenia', *British Journal of Psychiatry*, 153, pp. 437-43.

Frith, C.D., Friston, K.J., Liddle, P.F. and Frackowiak, R.S.J. (1991), 'Willed action and the prefrontal cortex in man: A study with PET', *Proceedings of the Royal Society of London, Series B*, 244, pp. 241-6.

Frith, C.D. and Frith, U. (1999), Interacting minds — A biological basis. *Science*, 286: 1692-95.

Gallagher, S. (1986), 'Lived body and environment', *Research in Phenomenology*, 16, pp. 139-70.

Gallagher, S. (1998), *The Inordinance of Time* (Evanston: Northwestern University Press).

Gallagher, S. (2000), 'Philosophical conceptions of the self: implications for cognitive science', *Trends in Cognitive Sciences* 4 (1), pp. 14-21.

Gallagher, S. (2001), 'The practice of mind: Theory, simulation, or interaction?', *Journal of Consciousness Studies*, 8 (5-7), pp. 83-107.

Gallagher, S. (2004a). 'Neurocognitive models of schizophrenia: A neurophenomenological critique', *Psychopathology* 37, pp. 8-19.

Gallagher, S. (2004b), 'Understanding interpersonal problems in autism: Interaction theory as an alternative to theory of mind', *Philosophy, Psychiatry, and Psychology*, 11 (3), pp. 199-217. .

Gallagher, S. (2005), *How the Body Shapes the Mind* (Oxford: Oxford University Press).

Gallagher, S. (2006), 'Where's the action? Epiphenomenalism and the problem of free will', in W. Banks, S. Pockett, and S. Gallagher (eds.), *Does Consciousness Cause Behavior? An Investigation of the Nature of Volition* (Cambridge, MA: MIT Press), pp. 109-124.

Gallagher, S. (2007a), 'Simulation trouble', *Social Neuroscience*, 2 (3-4), pp. 353-65.

Gallagher, S. (2007b), 'Logical and phenomenological arguments against simulation theory', in D. Hutto and M. Ratcliffe (eds.), *Folk Psychology Re-assessed* (Dordrecht: Springer Publishers), pp. 63-78.

Gallagher, S. (2007c), 'The natural philosophy of agency', *Philosophy Compass* 2 (j.1747-9991.2006.00067.x).

Gallagher, S. (2007d), 'Sense of agency and higher-order cognition: Levels of explanation for schizophrenia', *Cognitive Semiotics* 0, pp. 32-48.

Gallagher, S. (2008), 'Are minimal representations still representations?' *International Journal of Philosophical Studies* 16 (3) – in press.

Gallagher, S. and Cole, J. (1995), 'Body schema and body image in a deafferented subject', *Journal of Mind and Behavior*, 16, pp. 369-90.

Gallagher, S. and Hutto, D. (2008), 'Understanding others through primary interaction and narrative practice', in J. Zlatev, T. Racine, C. Sinha and E. Itkonen (eds). *The Shared Mind: Perspectives on Intersubjectivity* (Amsterdam: John Benjamins), pp. 17-38.

Gallagher, S. and Marcel, A. J. (1999) 'The self in contextualized action', *Journal of Consciousness Studies*, 6 (4), pp. 4-30.

Gallagher, S. and Meltzoff, A. (1996), 'The earliest sense of self and others: Merleau-Ponty and recent developmental studies,' *Philosophical Psychology*, 9, pp. 213-36.

Gallagher, S. and Shear, J. eds. (1999), *Models of the Self* (Exeter: Imprint Academic).

Gallagher, S. and Varela, F. (2003), 'Redrawing the map and resetting the time: Phenomenology and the cognitive sciences', *Canadian Journal of Philosophy*, (Supplementary) 29, pp. 93-132.

Gallagher, S. and Zahavi, D. 2008. *The Phenomenological Mind* (London: Routledge).

Gallese, V. (2001), 'The "shared manifold" hypothesis: from mirror neurons to empathy', *Journal of Consciousness Studies*, 8 (5-7), pp. 33-50.

Gallese, V. (2003), 'The manifold nature of interpersonal relations: the quest for a common Mechanism', *Philosophical Transactions of The Royal Society London*, B 358, pp. 517-528.

Gallese, V., Fadiga, L., Fogassi, L. and Rizzolatti, G. (1996), 'Action recognition in premotor cortex, *Brain*, 119, pp. 593-609.

Gallese, V. L. and Goldman, A. (1998), 'Mirror neurons and the simulation theory of mind-reading', *Trends in Cognitive Sciences*, 2, pp. 493–501.

Gallese, V. L. and Lakoff, G. (2005), 'The brain's concepts: The role of the sensory-motor system in conceptual knowledge', *Cognitive Neuropsychology* 22, pp. 455–479.

Garnham,W.A. and Ruffman, T. (2001), 'Doesn't see, doesn't know: Is anticipatory looking really related to understanding of belief?', *Developmental Science*, 4 (1), pp. 94–100.

Garnham, Wendy A. and Perner, Josef (2001), 'Actions really do speak louder than words—But only implicitly: Young children's understanding of false belief in action', *British Journal of Developmental Psychology*, 19 (3), pp. 413–32.

Gazzaniga, M.S. (1985), *The Social Brain* (New York: Basic Books).

Gazzaniga, M.S. (1998), *The Mind's Past* (Berkeley: University of California Press).

Gazzaniga, M. 2005. The Ethical Brain (Washington: Dana Press).

Georgieff, N. and Jeannerod, M. (1998), 'Beyond consciousness of external events: A Who system for consciousness of action and self-consciousness', *Consciousness and Cognition*, 7, pp. 465–77.

Glenberg, A. M. and Kaschak, M. P. (2002), 'Grounding language in action', *Psychonomic Bulletin and Review*, 9, pp. 558–65.

Goldin-Meadow, S. (1999), 'The role of gesture in communication and thinking', *Trends in Cognitive Sciences*, 3, pp. 419–429.

Goldman, A. I. (2002), 'Simulation theory and mental concepts', in J. Dokic and J. Proust (eds.), *Simulation and Knowledge of Action* (Amsterdam: John Benjamins), pp. 1–19.

Goldman, A. (2005a), 'Mirror systems, social understanding and social cognition', *Interdisciplines*. (http://www.interdisciplines.org/mirror/papers/3).

Goldman, A. (2005b), 'Imitation, mind reading, and simulation', in S. Hurley and Chater (eds.) *Perspectives on Imitation* II (Cambridge, MA: MIT Press), pp. 79–94.

Goldman, A. (2006), *Simulating Minds: The philosophy, psychology and neuroscience of mindreading* (Oxford: Oxford University Press).

Goldman, A. I. Sripada, C. S. (2005), 'Simulationist models of face-based emotion recognition', *Cognition*, 94, pp. 193–213.

Goodale, M.A. and Milner, A.D. (1992), 'Separate visual pathways for perception and action', *Trends in Neuroscience*, 15, pp. 20–25.

Gopnik, A. and Meltzoff, A. (1997), *Words, Thoughts, and Theories* (Cambridge, MA: MIT Press).

Grezes, J. and Decety, J. (2001), 'Functional anatomy of execution, mental simulation, observation, and verb generation of actions: A meta-analysis', *Human Brain Mapping*, 12, pp. 1–19.

Grusser, S.M., Winter, C., Muhlnickel, W., Denke, C., Karl, A., Villringer, K., Flor, H. (2001), 'The relationship of perceptual phenomena and cortical reorganization in upper extremity amputees', *Neuroscience*, 102 (2), pp. 263–72.

Hacking, I. (1995), 'The looping effects of human kinds', in *Causal Cognition: A Multidisciplinary Debate*, ed. D. Sperber, D. Premack and A. J. Premack (New York: Oxford University Press).

Haggard, P., and Libet, B. (2000), 'Conscious intention and brain activity', *Journal of Consciousness Studies* 8 (11), pp. 47–63.

Haggard, P., Newman, C. and Magno, E. (1999), 'On the perceived time of voluntary actions', *Br J. Psychol.*, 90, pp. 291–303.

Harcourt. (2000), 'Interview with Antonio Damasio', (http://www.harcourtbooks.com/authorinterviews/bookinterview_damasio.asp). .

Hauk, O., Johnsrude, I. and Pulvermüller, F. (2004), 'Somatotopic representation of action words in human motor and premotor cortex', *Neuron*, 41, pp. 301–7.

Hauptli, B. W. (2005), *Descartes and Princess Elizabeth Correspondence*. (http://www.fiu.edu/~hauptli/DescartesandPrincessElizabethCorrespondenceLecture Supplement.htm).

Hauser, M. D. and Carey, S. (2003), 'Spontaneous representations of small numbers of objects by rhesus macaques: Examinations of content and format', *Cognitive Psychology*, 47, pp. 367–401.

Haywood, J. and Varela, F. (1992), *Gentle Bridges: Conversations with the Dalai Lama on the Sciences of Mind* (Boston: Shambala).

Head, H. (1920), *Studies in Neurology*, Volume 2 (Oxford: The Clarendon Press).

Head, H. and Holmes, G.M. (1911), 'Sensory disturbances from cerebral lesions', *Brain*, 34, pp. 102–254.

Heidegger, M. (1996), *Being and Time*, trans. J. Stambaugh (Albany: SUNY Press).

Hoff, B. and Arbib, M.A. (1993), 'Simulation of interaction of hand transport and preshape during visually guided reaching to perturbed targets', *Journal of Motor Behavior* 25, pp. 175–92.

Holland, J. H. (1975), *Adaptation in Natural and Artificial Systems* (Ann Arbor: U. of Michigan Press; reprinted, MIT Press, 1992).

Howe, M. L. (2000), *The Fate of Early Memories: Developmental science and the retention of childhood experiences* (Cambridge, MA: MIT Press).

Hubel, D.H., and Wiesel, T.N. (1963), 'Receptive fields of cells in striate cortex of very young, visually inexperienced kittens', *Journal of Neurophysiology*, 26, pp. 994–1002.

Husserl, E. (1928), 'Vorlesungen zur Phänomenologie des inneren Zeitbewussteins', Herausgegeben von Martin Heidegger. Jahrbuch für Philosophie und phänomenologische Forschung, 9, pp. 367–498.

Husserl, E. (2001), *Logical Investigations*, 3 vols., trans. J.N. Findlay, (London: Routledge).

Hutto, D. (2008), *Folk Psychological Narratives* (Cambridge, MA: MIT Press).

Iacoboni, M. and Dapretto, M. (2006), 'The mirror neuron system and the consequences of its dysfunction', *Nature Reviews Neuroscience* 7, pp. 942–951.

Jacob, P. (2008), 'What do mirror neurons contribute to human social cognition?' *Mind & Language* 23 (2), pp. 190–223.

Jacob, P. and Jeannerod, M. (2003), *Ways of Seeing: The Scope and Limits of Visual Cognition* (Oxford: Oxford University Press).

Jahanshahi, M., Dirnberger, G., Fuller, R. & Frith, C.D. (2000), 'The role of the dorsolateral prefrontal cortex in random number generation', *Neuroimage* 12, pp. 713–25.

Jahanshahi, M., Jenkins, H., Brown, R.G., Marsden, C.D., Passingham, R.E. and Brooks, D.J (1995), 'Self-initiated versus externally triggered movements. 1. An investigation using measurement of regional cerebral blood-flow with pet and movement-related potentials in normal and Parkinsons-Disease subjects', *Brain*, 118, pp. 913–33.

James, W. (1890), *The Principles of Psychology* I-II. London: Macmillan and Co. (New York: Dover, 1950).

Jeannerod, M. (2001a), 'Neural simulation of action: A unifying mechanism for motor cognition', *Neuroimage* 14, pp. S103–S109.

Jeannerod, M. (2001b), 'Simulation of action as a unifying concept for motor cognition', in *Cognitive Neuroscience. Perspectives on the Problem of Intention and Action*, ed. S.H. Johnson. (Cambridge, MA: MIT Press).

Jeannerod, M. (1997), *The Cognitive Neuroscience of Action*. (Oxford: Blackwell).

Jeannerod, M. (1994), 'The representing brain: Neural correlates of motor intention and imagery', *Behavioral and Brain Sciences*, 17, pp. 187–245.

Jeannerod, M. and Biguer, B. (1982), 'Visuomotor mechanisms in reaching within extrapersonal space', in *Analysis of Visual Behavior*, ed. Ingle, D.J., Goodale, M.A.and Mansfield, R.J.W. (Cambridge, MA: MIT Press).

Jeannerod, M. and Frak, V.G. (1999), 'Mental simulation of action in human subjects', *Current Opinion in Neurobiology*, 9, pp. 735–9.

Jeannerod, M. and Gallagher, S. (2002), 'From action to interaction: An interview with Marc Jeannerod', *Journal of Consciousness Studies*, 9 (1), pp. 3–26.

Jeannerod, M. and Pacherie, E. (2004), 'Agency, simulation, and self-identification', *Mind and Language*, 19(2), pp. 113–46.

Johns, L.C. and McGuire, P.K. (1999), 'Verbal self-monitoring and auditory hallucinations in schizophrenia', *The Lancet*, 353 (9151), pp. 469–470. .

Johnson, M. (1987), *The Body in the Mind: The Bodily Basis of Meaning, Imagination, and Reason* (Chicago: University of Chicago Press).

Kampe K.K., Jones R.A., and Auer D.P. (2000), 'Frequency dependence of the functional MRI response after electrical median nerve stimulation', *Human Brain Mapping*, 9, pp. 2106–114.

Kayzer, W. (1993), 'Interview with Dennett', A Glorious Accident: Understanding Our Place in the Cosmic Puzzle. (Televised interview) VPRO Television, Netherlands.

Kenny, A. (tr. & ed.) (1970), *Descartes: Philosophical Letters*. (Oxford: Clarendon Press).

Kilmer, W.L., McCulloch, W.S. and Blum, J. (1969), 'A model of the vertebrate central command system', *Int. J. Man-Machine Studies*, 1, pp. 279–309.

Koch, C. (2004), *The Quest for Consciousness. A Neurobiological Approach* (Englewood, CO: Roberts and Company Publishers).

Kohler E., Keysers C., Umiltà M.A., Fogassi L, Gallese V. and Rizzolatti G. (2002), 'Hearing sounds, understanding actions: Action representation in mirror neurons', *Science*, 297, pp. 846–8.

Lakoff, G. and Johnson. M. (1980), *Metaphors We Live By* (Chicago: University of Chicago Press).

Lakoff, G. & Núñez, R. (2000), *Where Mathematics Comes From: How the Embodied Mind brings Mathematics into Being.* (New York: Basic Books).

Lambie, J.A. & Marcel, A.J. (2002), 'Consciousness and emotion experience: A theoretical framework', *Psychological Review*, 109, pp. 219–59.

LeDoux, J. (1998). *The Emotional Brain: The Mysterious Underpinnings of Emotional Life* (New York: Simon and Schuster).

Lee, S-H., Blake, R., and Heeger, D.J. (2007). 'Hierarchy of cortical responses underlying binocular rivalry'. *Nature Neuroscience* 10, pp. 1048–1054.

Legrand, D. (2006), 'The bodily self: The sensori-motor roots of pre-reflexive self-consciousness', *Phenomenology and the Cognitive Sciences* 5(1), 89–118.

Leibniz, G.W. 1981. 'Preface', *New Essays on Human Understanding*, tr. & ed. P. Remnant & J. Bennett, (Cambridge: Cambridge University Press).

Lettvin J.Y., Maturana, H.R., McCulloch W.S. and Pitts, W.H. (1959), 'What the frog's eye tells the frog's brain', *Proceedings of the IRE* 47 (1959) 1940–1951.

Levine, J. (1983), 'Materialism and qualia: The explanatory gap', *Pacific Philosophical Quarterly*, 64, pp. 354–61.

Lhermitte, F. (1986), 'Human autonomy and the frontal lobes. Part II: Patient behavior in complex and social situations: The "environmental dependency syndrome"', *Ann. Neurol.*, 19, pp. 335–43.

Libet, B. (1985), 'Unconscious cerebral initiative and the role of conscious will in voluntary action', *Behavioral and Brain Sciences* 8, pp. 529–66.

Libet, B., Gleason, C.A.,Wright, E.W. & Pearl, D.K. (1983), 'Time of conscious intention to act in relation to onset of cerebral activity (readiness potential): The unconscious initiation of a freely voluntary act', *Brain*, 106, pp. 623–42.

Lipps, T. (1903), 'Einfulung, innere nachahmung und organenempfindung', *Archiv. F. die Ges. Psycologie*, I, part 2 (Leipzig: W. Engelmann).

Locke, J. (1690), *An Essay Concerning Human Understanding*, 2nd edn. 1694, A. C. Fraser (ed.), (New York: Dover, 1959).

Lotze, M., Grodd, W., Birbaumer, N., Erb, M., Huse, E., Flor, H. (1999), 'Does use of a myoelectric prosthesis prevent cortical reorganisation and phantom limb pain?', *Nature Neuroscience*, 2 (6), pp. 501–2.

Lutz, A., Lachaux, J.-P., Martinerie, J., and Varela, F. J. (2002), 'Guiding the study of brain dynamics using first-person data: Synchrony patterns correlate with on-going conscious states during a simple visual task'. *Proceedings of the National Academy of Science USA*, 99, pp. 1586–1591.

Lycan, W.G. (1997), 'Consciousness as Internal Monitoring', in N. Block, O. Flanagan & G. Güzeldere (eds.), *The Nature of Consciousness* (Cambridge, MA: MIT Press), pp. 754–771.

McIntyre, A. (1981), *After Virtue: A Study in Moral Theory* (Notre Dame: University of Notre Dame Press).

MacKay, Donald M. (1967), Freedom of Action in a Mechanistic Universe, The Eddington Lecture (Cambridge: Cambridge University Press).

MacLean, P.D. (1990), *The Triune Brain In Evolution* (New York: Plenum).

Macmillan, M. (2000), The Phineas Gage Information Page, website at http://www.deakin.edu.au/hmnbs/psychology/gagepage/.

Manuela, L. (2005), 'Feeling our emotions: Interview with Antonio Damazio', *Scientific American Mind*, 16 (1), pp.14–15.

Marcel, A.J. (1992), 'The personal level in cognitive rehabilitation', in *Neuropsychological Rehabilitation*, ed. VonSteinbuchel, N., Poppel, E. and von Cramon, D. (Berlin: Springer), pp. pp. 155–168.

Marcel, A. J. (1998), 'Blindsight and shape perception: deficit of visual consciousness or of visual function?', *Brain* 121(8), pp. 1565–88.

Maturana, H. R. and Varela, F. G. (1987), *The Tree of Knowledge: The Biological Roots of Human Understanding* (Boston: Shambhala).

McCloskey, D.I., Ebeling, P., and Goodwin, G.M. (1974), 'Estimation of weights and tensions and apparent involvement of a "sense of effort",' *Experimental Neurology*, 42, pp. 220–32.

McGinn, C. (1989), *Wittgenstein on Meaning* (Oxford: Basil Blackwell).

McGuire, P.K., Silbersweig, D.A., Murray, R.M., David, A.S., Frackowiak, R.S.J. and Frith, C.D (1996), 'Functional anatomy of inner speech and auditory verbal imagery', *Psychological Medicine*, 26, pp. 29–38.

McNeill, D. (1992), *Hand and Mind: What Gestures Reveal about Thought* (Chicago: University of Chicago Press).

McNeill, D. Duncan, S. Cole, J. Gallagher, S. & Bertenthal, B. (2008) 'Neither or both: Growth points from the very beginning', *Interaction Studies*, 9 (1), pp.117–132.

McNeill, D., Bertenthal, B., Cole, J. and Gallagher, S. (2005), 'Gesture-first, but no gestures? Commentary on Michael A. Arbib', *Behavioral and Brain Sciences*, 28, pp. 138–39.

Mead, G.H. (1974), *Mind, Self, and Society From the Standpoint of a Social Behaviorist*, C.W. Morris ed. and introduction, (Chicago: University of Chicago Press).

Meltzoff, A. and Moore, M. K. (1977), 'Imitation of facial and manual gestures by human neonates', *Science*, 198, pp. 75–78.

Meltzoff, A. and Moore, M. K. (1983), 'Newborn infants imitate adult facial gestures', *Child Development*, 54, pp. 702–709.

Meltzoff, A. and Moore, M. K. (1989), 'Imitation in newborn infants: Exploring the range of gestures imitated and the underlying mechanisms', *Developmental Psychology*, 25, pp. 954–62. .

Merzenich, M.M. et al. (1984), 'Somatosensory cortical map changes following digital amputation in adult monkey', *Journal of Comparative Neurology*, 224, pp. 591–605.

Merzenich, M.M., et al. (1987), 'Variability in hand surface representations in areas 3b and 1 in adult owl and squirrel monkeys', *Journal of Comparative Neurology*, 258, pp. 281–96.

Merleau-Ponty, M. (1945), *Phénoménologie de la perception* (Paris, Éditions Gallimard).

Merleau-Ponty, M. (1962), *Phenomenology of Perception*, trans. C. Smith (London: Routledge and Kegan Paul).

Merleau-Ponty, M. (1964), *The Primacy of Perception* (Chicago: Northwestern University Press).

Merleau-Ponty, M. (1996), *Texts and Dialogues: On Philosophy, Politics, and Culture*, ed. and trans. H. Silverman and J. Barry (Amherst, NY: Prometheus Press).

Metzinger, T. (2004). *Being No One* (Cambridge, MA: MIT Press).

Miall, R. & Cole, J. (2007), 'Evidence for stronger visuo-motor than visuo-proprioceptive conflict during mirror drawing performed by a deafferented subject and control subjects', *Experimental Brain Research*, 176 (3), pp. 432–439.

Milner, A.D. and Goodale, M.A. (1995), *The Visual Brain in Action* (Oxford: Oxford University Press).

Milner, B. (1963), 'Effects of different brain lesions on card sorting', *Archives of Neurology*, 9, pp. 90–100.

Mulder, A. (2000), The Deep Now, in J. Brouwer (ed.), *Machine Times* (Rotterdam: NAI Publishers).

Murray, L. and Trevarthen, C. (1985), 'Emotional regulations of interactions between two-month-olds and their mothers', in T. M. Field and N. A. Fox (eds.) *Social Perception in Infants* (Norwood, NJ: Ablex), pp. 177–197.

Nadel, J., I. Carchon, et al. (1999), 'Expectancies for social contingency in 2-month-olds', *Developmental Science*, 2(2), pp. 164–173. .

Nagel, T. (1986), *The View from Nowhere* (Oxford: Oxford University Press).

Nathaniel-James, D. A., and Frith, C. D. (2002), 'The role of the dorsolateral prefrontal cortex: evidence from the effects of contextual constraint in a sentence completion task', *Neuroimage* 16, pp. 1094–1102.

Neisser, U. (1988), 'Five kinds of self-knowledge', *Philosophical Psychology*, 1, pp. 35–59.

Nelson K. (2003), 'Narrative and the emergence of a consciousness of Self', in *Narrative and Consciousness*, G. D. Fireman, T. E. J. McVay and O. Flanagan (eds.). Oxford: Oxford University Press.

Newman-Norlund, RD. Noordzij, ML. Meulenbroek, RGJ, Bekkering, H. (2007), 'Exploring the brain basis of joint attention: Co-ordination of actions, goals and intentions', *Social Neuroscience*, 2 (1), pp. 48–65.

Nielsen, T.I. (1963), 'Volition: A new experimental approach', *Scandinavian Journal of Psychology*, 4, pp. 225–3.

Nobe, Shuichi. (2000), 'Where do most spontaneous representational gestures actually occur with respect to speech?' In D. McNeill (ed.), *Language and Gesture* (Cambridge: Cambridge University Press), pp. 186–198.

Noë, A. (2004), *Action in Perception* (Cambridge, MA: MIT Press).

Norman, D.A. and Shallice, T. (1986), 'Attention to action:Willed and automatic control of behaviour', in *Consciousness and Self Regulation: Advances in Research*, Vol. IV, ed. Davidson, R.J., Schwartz, G.E. and Shapiro, D. (New York: Plenum).

Northoff, G., Heinzel, A., de Greck, M., Bermpohl, F. and Panksepp, J. (2006), 'Our brain and its self: The central role of cortical midline structures', *Neuroimage*, 15, pp. 440–457.

Nougier, V., Bard, C., Fleury,M., Teasdale, N., Cole, J., Forget, Y. et al. (1996), 'Control of single joint movements in deafferented subjects: evidence for amplitude coding rather than position control', *Experimental Brain Research*, 109, pp. 473–82.

Oberman, L. M. and Ramachandran, V. S. (2007), 'The simulating social mind: The role of the mirror neuron system and simulation in the social and communicative deficits of autism spectrum disorders. *Psychological Bulletin* 133 (2): 310–327.

Oberman, L. M., McCleery, J. P., Ramachandran, V. S. and Pineda, J. A. (2007), 'EEG evidence for mirror neuron activity during the observation of human and robot actions: Toward an analysis of the human qualities of interactive robots', *Neurocomputing*, 70, pp. 2194–2203.

Onishi, K.H., and Baillargeon, R. (2005), 'Do 15-month-old infants understand false beliefs?' *Science*, 308 (5719), pp. 255–8.

O'Regan, J. K. and Noe, A. (2001), 'A sensorimotor account of vision and visual consciousness', *Behavioral and Brain Sciences*, 24(5), pp. 939–73.

Oztop, E. and Arbib, M.A. (2002), 'Schema design and implementation of the grasp-related mirror neuron system', *Biological Cybernetics*, 87, pp. 116–40.

Oztop, E., Bradley, N., and Arbib, M.A. (2004), 'Infant grasp learning: A computational model', *Experimental Brain Research*, 158 (4), pp. 480–503.

Paillard, J. (1960), 'The patterning of skilled movements', *Handbook of Physiology-Section I: Neurophysiology*, (American Physiological Soc. Washington, DC) 3, pp. 1679–1708.

Panksepp, J. (2006), 'Emotional endophenotypes in evolutionary psychiatry', *Progress in Neuro-Psychopharmacology & Biological Psychiatry*, 30, pp. 774–84.

Panksepp, J. (1998), *Affective Neuroscience: The foundations of human and animal emotions* (New York: Oxford University Press).

Parsons, L.M. (1994), 'Temporal and kinematic properties of motor behavior reflected in mentally simulated action', *Journal of Experimental Psychology: Human Perception and Performance*, 20, pp. 709–30.

Paulignan, Y., Frak, V.G., Toni, I. and Jeannerod, M. (1997), 'Influence of object position and size on human prehension movements', *Experimental Brain Research*, 114, pp. 226–34.

Paulignan, Y., Jeannerod, M., MacKenzie, C. and Marteniuk, R. (1991a), 'Selective perturbation of visual input during prehension movements: 2. The effects of changing object size', *Experimental Brain Research*, 87, pp. 407–20.

Paulignan, Y., MacKenzie, C., Marteniuk, R. and Jeannerod, M. (1991b), 'Selective perturbation of visual input during prehension movements: 1. The effects of changing object position', *Experimental Brain Research*, 83, pp. 502–12.

Phillips, C.G. (1985), *Movements of the Hand* (Liverpool: Liverpool University Press).

Piaget J. (1976), *The Grasp of Consciousness: Action and concept in the young child*, trans. S. Wedgwood (Cambridge, MA: Harvard University Press).

Pickup, G.J. and Frith, C.D. (2001), 'Schizotypy, theory of mind and weak central coherence', *Schizophrenia Research*, 49 (1–2 Supplement), p. 118.

Ramachandran, V.S. and Hirstein, W. (1997), 'Three laws of qualia: What neurology tells us about the biological functions of consciousness', *Journal of Consciousness Studies*, 4 (5–6), pp. 429–57.

Ramachandran, V. S., Rogers-Ramachandran D. C. & Cobb, S. (1995), 'Touching the phantom', *Nature*, 377, pp. 489–490.

Ramsøy, T. Z. (2004), 'Interview with Christof Koch', *Science and Consciousness Review*, November 5, 2004; http://sci-con.org/2004/11/interview-with-christof-koch/.

Ramsøy, T. Z. (2006), 'How the body shapes the mind: An interview with Shaun Gallagher'. *Science and Consciousness Review*, January 19, 2006; http://sci-con.org/2006/01/how-the-body-shapes-the-mind-an-interview-with-shaun-gallagher/.

Ratcliffe, M. (2006), *Rethinking Commonsense Psychology: A Critique of Folk Psychology, Theory of Mind and Simulation* (Basingstoke: Palgrave Macmillan).

Ricoeur, P. (1984), *Time and Narrative*, 3 Vols. (Chicago: University of Chicago Press).

Ricoeur, P. (1992), *Oneself As Another* (Chicago: University of Chicago Press).

Rizzolatti, G. and Arbib, M.A. (1998), 'Language within our grasp', *Trends in Neurosciences*, 21, pp. 188–94.

Rizzolatti, G., Fadiga, L., Gallese V. and Fogassi, L. (1996), 'Premotor cortex and the recognition of motor actions', *Cognitive Brain Research*, 3, pp. 131–41.

Robinson, J. (2003), 'Management wisdom from a neuroscientist: Q&A with Joseph LeDoux', *Gallup Management Journal*, December 11, 2003. http://gmj.gallup.com/content/9844/1/Management-Wisdom-From-a-Neuroscientist.aspx.

Rohrer, T. (2005), 'Image schemata in the brain', in *From Perception to Meaning: Image Schemas in Cognitive Linguistics*, B. Hampe and J. Grady, eds. (Berlin: Mouton de Gruyter), pp. 165–196.

Rohrer, T. (2001), 'Understanding through the body: fMRI and of ERP studies of metaphoric and literal language', Paper presented at the 7th International Cognitive Linguistics Association conference, July 2001.

Rolls, E.T. (1999), *The Brain and Emotion* (Oxford: Oxford University Press).

Rolls, E.T. (2005), *Emotion Explained* (Oxford: Oxford University Press).

Rosenthal, D.M. (1986), 'Two concepts of consciousness', *Philosophical Studies*, 94(3), pp. 329–359.

Rosenthal, D.M. (1997), 'A Theory of Consciousness', in N. Block, O. Flanagan & G. Güzeldere (Eds.), *The Nature of Consciousness* (Cambridge, MA: MIT Press), pp. 729–753.

Ross, G. M. (1975–1999), *Sections of Descartes' Replies* (http://www.philosophy.leeds.ac.uk/GMR/hmp/texts/modern/descartes/dcindex.html).

Rowlands, M. (2006), *Body Language* (Cambridge, MA: MIT Press).

Roy, J-M. (2007), 'Heterophenomenology and phenomenological skepticism', *Phenomenology and the Cognitive Sciences* 6 (1–2), pp. 1–20.

Ruby, P. and Decety, J. (2001). 'Effect of subjective perspective taking during simulation of action: a PET investigation of agency', *Nature Neuroscience*, 4(5), pp. 546–50.

Rudebeck, P. H., Buckley, M. J., Walton, M. E., and Rushworth, M. F. (2006), 'A role for the macaque anterior cingulate gyrus in social valuation'. *Science*, 313, pp. 1310–1312.

Ryle, G. (1949), *The Concept of Mind* (New York: Barnes and Noble).

Samson, D., Apperly, I. A., Chiavarino, C., and Humphreys, G. W. (2004), 'Left temporoparietal junction is necessary for representing someone else's belief'. *Nat Neurosci*, 7, pp. 499–500.

Sartre, J-P. (1956), *Being and Nothingness* (New York: Philosophical Library).

Sartre, J.-P. (1957), *The Transcendence of the Ego*, trans. F. Williams & R. Kirkpatrick (New York: The Noonday Press).

Shallice, T. (1988), *From Neuropsychology to Mental Structure* (Cambridge: Cambridge University Press).

Scharmer, C. O. (2000), 'The three gestures of becoming aware: Conversation with Francisco Varela', *Dialog on Leadership*. (http://www.dialogonleadership.org/varela-2000.html).

Schultz, J., Friston, K. J., O'Doherty, J., Wolpert, D. M., and Frith, C. D. (2005), 'Activation in posterior superior temporal sulcus parallels parameter inducing the percept of animacy', *Neuron*, 45, pp. 625–635.

Schultz W. (2006), 'Behavioral theories and the neurophysiology of reward', *Annu Rev Psychology* 57, pp. 87–115.

Searle, J. (1983), *Intentionality: An Essay in the Philosophy of Mind* (Cambridge: Cambridge University Press).

Shatz, C.J. (1992), 'The developing brain', *Scientific American (U.K.)*, 267 (3), pp. 35–41.

Sheets-Johnstone,M. (2003), 'Kinesthetic memory', *Theoria et Historia Scientiarum*, 7 (1), pp. 69–92.

Shergill, S. S., Samson, G., Bays, P. M., Frith, C. D., and Wolpert, D. M. (2005), 'Evidence for sensory prediction deficits in schizophrenia', *American Journal of Psychiatry*, 162, pp. 2384–86.

Shewmon, D.A., Holmes, G.L.and Byrne, P.A. (1999), 'Consciousness in congenitally decorticate children: developmental vegetative state as self-fulfilling prophecy', *Developmental Medicine and Child Neurology*, 41, pp. 364–74.

Shoemaker, S. (1999), 'Self, body, and coincidence', *Proceedings of the Aristotelian Society*, Supplementary Volume 73, pp. 287–306.

Shore, B. (1997), 'Keeping the conversation going: An interview with Jerome Bruner', *Ethos*, 25 (1), pp. 7–62.

Slachewsky, A., Pillon, B., Fourneret, P., Pradat-Diehl, Jeannerod, M. and Dubois, B. (2001) 'Preserved adjustment but impaired awareness in a sensorimotor conflict following prefrontal lesions', *Journal of Cognitive Neuroscience*, 13, pp. 332–40.

Smith, N. K. (ed.), (1952). *Descartes' Philosohical Writings* (London: Macmillan).

Sørensen, J.B. (2005), 'The alien hand experiment', *Phenomenology and the Cognitive Sciences*, 4, 73–90.

Spence, S.A., Brooks, D.J., Hirsch, S.R., Liddle, P.F., Meehan, J. and Grasby, P.M. (1997), 'A PET study of voluntary movement in schizophrenic patients experiencing passivity phenomena (delusions of alien control)', *Brain*, 120, pp. 1997–2011.

Sprong. M., Schothorst, P., Vos, E., Hox, J., van Engeland, H. (2007), 'Theory of mind in schizophrenia: meta-analysis, *Br J Psychiatry*, 191, pp. 5–13.

Stanfield, A.C., McIntosh, A.M., Spencer, P.R., Gaur, S., Lawrie, S.M. (2007), 'Towards a neuroanatomy of autism: A systematic review and meta-analysis of structural magnetic resonance imaging studies', *European Psychiatry*. [Epub ahead of print; PMID: 17765485].

Star, A. (2000), 'Questions for Dr. Antonio Damasio: What feelings feel like', *New York Times Magazine* (May 1, 2000), p. 31.

Stawarska, B. (2008), 'You and I, here and now: Spatial and social situatedness in deixis. *International Journal of Philosophical Studies* 16 (3), pp. XXX.

Steenstrup, M., Arbib, M.A. and Manes E.G. (1983), 'Port automata and the algebra of concurrent processes', *J. Comput. Syst. Sci.*, 27 (1), pp. 29–50.

Stern, D. (2002), *The First Relationship: Infant and Mother* (Cambridge, MA: Harvard University Press). .

Steuber, K. (2006), *Rediscovering Empathy: Agency, Folk Psychology, and the Human Sciences* (MIT Press 2006).

Stokoe,W.C. (2001), *Language in Hand: Why Sign Came Before Speech* (Washington, DC:GallaudetUP).

Strawson, G. (1999), 'The self and the SESMET', in S. Gallagher and J. Shear (eds.), *Models of the Self* (Exeter: Imprint Academic), pp. 483–518.

Stuss, D. T., Gallup, G. G., Jr., and Alexander, M. P. (2001). 'The frontal lobes are necessary for "theory of mind"'. *Brain*, 124, pp. 279–286.

Surian, L., Caldi, S., and Sperber, D. (2007), 'Attribution of beliefs by 13-month-old infants', *Psychol Sci*, 18, pp. 580–586.

Tai, Y. F. Scherfler, C. Brooks, D. J. Sawamoto N. and Castiello, U. (2004, 'The human premotor cortex is mirror only for biological actions', *Current Biology*, 14, pp. 117–120.

Teitelbaum, P., Teitelbaum, O., Nye, J., Fryman, J. and Maurer, R.G. (1998), 'Movement analysis in infancy may be useful for early diagnosis of autism', *PNAS*, 95, pp. 13982–7.

Thelen, E. & Smith, L. (1994), *A Dynamic Systems Approach to the Development of Cognition and Action* (Cambridge, MA: MIT Press).

Thompson, E. 2001a. Empathy and consciousness, *Journal of Consciousness Studies* 8(5–7) (2001): 1–32.

Thompson, E. 2001b. *Between Ourselves: Second Person Issues in the Study of Consciousness*. Imprint Academic, 2001.

Tierney, J. 2007. 'A world of eloquence in an upturned palm', *New York Times*, Science section (28 August 2007). http://www.nytimes.com/2007/08/28/science/28tier.html.

Tononi, G. & Edelman, G.M. (1998), 'Consciousness and complexity'. *Science*, 282, pp. 1846–51.

Toombs, K. (1993), *The Meaning of Illness* (Dordrecht: Kluwer).

Trevarthen, C. (2000), 'Intrinsic motives for companionship in understanding: Their origin, development, and significance for infant mental health', *Infant Mental Health Journal*, 22, pp. 95–131.

Trevarthen, C. (1998), 'The concept and foundations of infant intersubjectivity', in S. Bråten (ed.), *Intersubjective Communication and Emotion in Early Ontogeny* (Cambridge, Cambridge University Press), pp. 15–46.

Trevarthen, C. B. (1986), 'Neuroembryology and the development of perceptual mechanisms', in F. Falkner and J. M. Tanner (eds.), *Human Growth: A Comprehensive Treatise*, 2nd edn (New York: Plenum Press), pp. 301–383. .

Trevarthen, C. B. (1979), Communication and cooperation in early infancy: A description of primary intersubjectivity', in M. Bullowa (ed.), *Before Speech*. (Cambridge: Cambridge University Press), pp. 321–347.

Trevarthen, C. (1970), 'Two mechanisms of vision in primates', *Psychologische Forschung*, 31, pp. 299–337.

Trevarthen, C. and Hubley, P. 1978. Secondary intersubjectivity: Confidence, confiding and acts of meaning in the first year. In A. Lock (ed.), *Action, Gesture and Symbol: The Emergence of Language* (London: Academic Press), pp. 183–229.

Tsakiris, M. Bosbach S. and Gallagher, S. (2007), 'On agency and body-ownership: Phenomenological and neuroscientific reflections', *Consciousness and Cognition* 16 (3), pp. 645–60.

Tsakiris, M. and Haggard, P. (2005), 'Experimenting with the acting self', *Cognitive Neuropsychology* 22 (3/4), pp. 387–407.

Van Essen, D.C., Anderson, C.H. & Felleman, D.J. (1992), 'Information processing in the primate visual system: an integrated systems perspective'. *Science*, 255, pp. 419–423.

Van Gelder, T. (1995), 'What might cognition be, if not computation?' *The Journal of Philosophy*, 92(7), pp. 345–381.

Varela, F. J. (1996), 'Neurophenomenology: A methodological remedy for the hard problem'. *Journal of Consciousness Studies*, 3 (4), pp. 330–49.

Varela, F. J., Thompson, E. and Rosch, E. (1991), *The Embodied Mind: Cognitive Science and Human Experience* (Cambridge: MIT Press).

von Holst, E. & Mittelstaedt, H. (1950), 'Das Reafferenzprinzip', *Die Naturwissenschaften*, 20, pp. 464–476.

Vosgerau, G. & Newen, A. (2007), 'Thoughts, motor actions, and the self', *Mind & Language* 22(1), pp. 22–43.

Vosgerau, G. 2007. Mental Representation and Self-Consciousness in Humans. Ph.D. Dissertation, Bochum Universität.

Walker, C. (2000), 'Interview with Francisco Varela', *Wild Duck Review*, 4(1), pp. 1–6.

Walter, G. (1953/1961), *The Living Brain* (New York: W.W. Norton).

Watt, D. (2007), 'Towards a neuroscience of empathy: Integrating cognitive and affective perspectives', *Neuropsychoanalysis*, 9(2), pp. 119–140.

Wegner, D. (2002), *The Illusion of Conscious Will* (Cambridge, MA: MIT Press).

Weiskrantz, L. (1986), *Blindsight: A Case Study and Implications*, (Oxford: Oxford University Press).

Weiskrantz, L., Warrington, E.K., Sanders, M.D., and Marshall, J. (1974), 'Visual capacity in the hemianopic field following a restricted occipital ablation', *Brain*, 97, pp. 709–728.

Wheeler, M. (2005), *Reconstructing the Cognitive World: The next step* (Cambridge, MA: MIT Press).

Wheeler, M. (1996), 'From robots to Rothko', in Boden, M. (ed), *The Philosophy of Artificial Life* (Oxford: Oxford University Press), pp. 209–36.

Wimmer, H. & Perner, J. (1983), 'Beliefs about beliefs: Representation and constraining function of wrong beliefs in young children's understanding of deception', *Cognition*, 13, pp. 41–68.

Witelson, S.F., Kigar, D.L., and Harvey, T. (1999), The exceptional brain of Albert Einstein', *The Lancet* 353, pp. 2149–53; http://www.bioquant.com/gallery/einstein.html.

Wittgenstein, L. (1980). *Remarks on the Philosophy of Psychology*. 2 vols. (Oxford: Basil Blackwell).

Wolpert, D. M., Doya, K., and Kawato, M. (2003), 'A unifying computational framework for motor control and social interaction', *Philosophical Transactions of the Royal Sociery of London: Series B Biological Sciences*, 358, pp. 593–602.

Wolpert, D.M., Grahramani, Z. and Flanagan, J.R. (2001), 'Perspectives and problems in motor learning', *Trends in Cognitive Sciences*, 5, pp. 487–94.

Wolpert, D. M., Ghahramani, Z. and Jordan, M.I. (1995), 'An internal model for sensorimotor integration', *Science*, 269 (5232), pp. 1880–1882.

Xu, F. And Carey, S. (1996), 'Infants' metaphysics: The case of numerical identity', *Cognitive Psychology*, 30 (2), pp. 111–53.

Yuille, A., and Kersten, D. (2006), 'Vision as Bayesian inference: analysis by synthesis?' *Trends Cogn Sci*, 10, pp. 301–308.

Zahavi, D. (2001), 'Beyond empathy: Phenomenological approaches to intersubjectivity', *Journal of Consciousness Studies* 8 (5–7), pp. 151–167.

Zahavi, D. (2005), *Subjectivity and Selfhood: Investigating the first-person perspective* (Cambridge, MA: The MIT Press).

Index